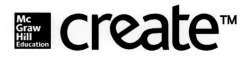

Annual Editions: Aging, 30/e

Elaina F. Osterbur

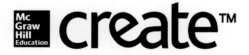

http://create.mheducation.com

ISBN-10: 1260488349   ISBN-13: 9781260488340

Contents

Detailed Table of Contents

Unit 3: Societal Attitudes Toward Old Age

Social and Health Disparities in Aging: Gender Inequities in Long-term Care, Nancy R. Hooyman, *Generations*, 2015
This article suggests that the bulk of family caregiving is performed by women. Family caregiving, in general, is undervalued even though the economic value is estimated to be $450 billion. The low status of caregiving encourages gender-based social and health disparities in aging.

The Public Policies We Need to Redress Ageism, Robert B. Blancato and Meredith Ponder, *Generations*, 2015
The authors suggest in this article that ageism exists in some federal programs. The failure exists in the current caregiving challenges not addressed in federal programs, benefit disparity based on gender in Social Security, age-based discrimination in the workplace, access to benefit programs, and others. Society needs to take action to address these issues.

Health Disparities among Lesbian, Gay, and Bisexual Older Adults: Results from a Population-Based Study, Karen I. Fredriksen-Goldsen, et al., *American Journal of Public Health*, 2013
The author points out the need for tailored interventions to address health disparities among lesbian, gay, and bisexual older adults. Furthermore, there is also a need for ongoing research across the life course to better understand health disparities by sexual orientation and age.

Attitudes about Aging: A Global Perspective, *Pew Research Center*, 2014
The Pew Research Center study suggests that most global populations are concerned about their standard of living as they age. They are concerned about the shrinking of the working age population group who will be tasked to support social insurance systems.

Sexual Orientation, Socioeconomic Status and Healthy Aging, Bridget K. Gorman and Zelma Oyarvide, *Generations*, 2018
The authors suggest that socioeconomic status is important to healthy aging. Disparities exist in socioeconomic status across groups, especially for older adults. This study suggests that across age groups, bisexual elders have the lowest rates of completed schooling, and live in lower-income households than to heterosexual, gay or lesbian older adults.

Unit 4: Problems and Potentials of Aging

Physician Supply and Demand Through 2025: Key Findings, *Association of American Medical Colleges*, 2016
This article is a summary of the study performed by IHS Inc. "*The Complexities of Physician Supply and Demand: Projections from 2014 to 2025*" on behalf of the Association of American Medical Colleges. The key findings include growth of demand for physicians, shortages by specialty, and brief suggested solutions.

Sexuality in Later Life, *National Institute on Aging*, 2017
This article suggests the problems experienced in sexuality in later life. Normal changes versus abnormal changes are discussed. The article further distinguishes the physical differences between men and women that occur as we age.

The Edinburgh Social Cognition Test (ESCoT), R. Asaad Baksh, et al., *PLoS ONE*, 2018
The authors suggest inconsistent findings in the effects of healthy aging on social cognition measures. The study examined the effects of age, measures of intelligence and the Broader Autism Phenotype (BAP) on the ESCoT and established tests of social cognition.

Gastric Balance: Heartburn Not Always Caused by Excess Acid, James English, *NutritionReview.org*, 2018
This article discusses the changes that take place in the ability to absorb minerals, vitamins and other nutrients with advancing age. These changes can affect digestive function over time. The authors define the symptoms and diseases that may accompany poor digestive function.

Preface

The global population of older adults is rising due in part to improved public health and economic conditions. The number of older persons (age 60 years and over) is expected to more than double by 2050. According to the United Nations, the average life expectancy is 83.7 years in Japan for both males and females and is one of the highest in the world. Along with the observed increased life expectancy, the world total fertility rate is declining. The increase in longevity and the decrease in fertility rates have created this demographic shift whereby people 65 and over now account for a larger proportion of the world population.

What does this mean to an aging population? Historically societies were plagued by infectious diseases that caused much of the morbidity and mortality of the times. Since then aging societies have transitioned morbidity and mortality rates from infectious disease to non-communicable chronic disease as the cause of disability and death. Living longer means greater planning on the part of both the older adult and his/her family. Thus older adults and families have reacted with the demand for increased medical technologies that will not only allow for longer life, but also to allow older people to live at home longer with greater degree of independence. Increased longevity also means that planning finances from younger years may not spread far enough during the retirement years and thereby are requesting increased opportunities for work from employers. Greater options in health insurance coverage are demanded along with a variety of options for long-term care insurance. These advances in technologies are creating a peripheral legal marketplace that has reacted in ways that require advance directives, living wills, long-term care insurance options and other lifespan planning devices. The culmination of opportunities, needs and expectations of older adults brought forth through longevity have the popular press, researchers and the media scrambling to provide pertinent information to the masses.

This volume represents the field of gerontology in that it is interdisciplinary in its approach, including articles from the biological sciences, medicine, nursing, psychology, sociology, and social work. The articles are taken from the popular press, government publications and scientific journals. They represent a wide cross-section of author's perspectives, and issues related to the aging process. They were chosen because they address the most relevant and current problems in the field of aging and present divergent views on the appropriate solutions to these problems. The topics covered include demographic trends; the aging process; the quality of later life; social attitudes toward old age; problems and potentials of aging; retirement; death; living environments in later life; and social policies, programs and services for older Americans.

The articles are organized into an anthology that issued for both the student and the teacher. *Learning Outcomes* outline the key concepts that students should focus on as they read the material. *Critical Thinking* questions allow students to test their understanding of the key concepts, and a list of recommended *Internet References* guides them to the best sources of additional information on a topic. The goal of Annual Editions: Aging is to choose articles that are pertinent, well-written, and helpful to those concerned with the field of gerontology. Comments, suggestions, and constructive criticism are welcome to help improve future editions of this book.

Editor

Dr. Elaina F. Osterbur is an associate professor at Saint Louis University in St. Louis, Missouri. After receiving a Master's Degree in Gerontology, Elaina received her PhD in Epidemiology at the University of Illinois Urbana-Champaign. Her research interests include gynecological cancer screening in older women and family caregiving.

Academic Advisory Board

Members of the Academic Advisory Board are instrumental in the final selection of articles for the *Annual Editions* series. Their review of the articles for content, level, and appropriateness provides critical direction to the editor(s) and staff. We think that you will find their careful consideration reflected in this book.

Gloria Aguilar, Florida
A&M University

Padmini Banerjee, Delaware
State University

James Blackburn
Hunter College

Karen Dorman
St. Johns University

Ric Ferraro
University of North Dakota

Deloris Fields-Jones
Daemen College

Gregory Green
Fort Valley State University

Lisa Hardy
Bethel College

Lisa Hollis-Sawyer
Northeastern Illinois University

Curtis Hosier
Indiana University/Purdue University

Ft. Wayne Robert C. Intrieri
Western Illinois University

Barry Johnson
Davidson County Community College

Charles Kaiser
College of Charleston

Rona Karasik
Saint Cloud State University

Nancy Karlin
University of Northern Colorado

Rosalind Kopfstein
Western Connecticut State University

Denise C. Lewis
University of Georgia

Karen Lynch
National Louis University Chicago

Shannon Mathews
Winston-Salem State University

Willis McAleese
Idaho State University

Glen McNeil
Fort Hays State University

P. James Nielsen
Western Illinois University

Natasha Otto
Morgan State University

Sarah Pender
Folsom Lake College

Sharon Marie Rice
South Texas College

Terry Salem
Lake Land College

Susan Schlicht
St. Cloud Technical & Community College

Laurence Segall
Housatonic Community College

Kim Shifren
Towson University

Shirley R. Simon
Loyola University

Luceal Simon
Wayne State University

Joyce Sween
DePaul University

Mieke Thomeer McBride
University of Alabama at Birmingham

Stephanie Travers
Luther College

Dean D. VonDras
University Wisconsin-Green Bay

Fedder Williams
nvSouth Piedmont Community College

Unit 1

UNIT

Prepared by: Elaina Osterbur, *Saint Louis University*

The Phenomenon of Aging

The phenomenon of aging includes biological, psychological, sociological, and behavioral changes. Biologically, the body gradually loses the ability to renew itself. Various body functions begin to slow, and the vital senses become less acute. Psychologically, aging persons experience changing sensory processes; perception, motor skills, problem-solving ability, and drives and emotions are frequently altered. Sociologically, this group must cope with the changing roles and definitions of self that society imposes on individuals. For instance, the role expectations and the status of grandparents differ from those of parents, and the roles of retirees are quite different from those of employed persons. Behavioral changes are common across the life span. However, as we age, these changes may be based on retirement, physical health changes, mobility, and loss of a loved one.

Those studying the process of aging often use developmental theories of the lifecycle—a sequence of predictable phases that begins with birth and ends with death to explain individuals' behavior at various stages of their lives. An individual's age, therefore, is important because it provides clues about his or her behavior at a particular phase of the lifecycle—be it childhood, adolescence, adulthood, middle age, or older age. There is, however, the greatest variation in terms of health and human development among older people than among any other age group. We find that by age 65, some people are in good health, employed, and performing important work tasks. Others of this cohort are retired but in good health or are retired and in poor health. Still others have died prior to the age of 65.

Another important phenomenon includes demographic changes in an aging world. Every day, 10–1000 people all over the world turn 65. This trend will continue for the next 20 years. In the United States alone, waves of the 78 million baby boomers have begun to turn 65 years. This generation will have great expectations regarding health care, long-term care, housing, finances, technology, work, and even the return to college. The articles in this section attempt to explain the phenomenon of aging both nationally and globally, as well as the resulting choices in lifestyle and cultural implications of an older population.

Article   Prepared by: Elaina Osterbur, *Saint Louis University*

Demography Is Not Destiny: The Challenges and Opportunities of Global Population Aging

The world's population is aging: eventually there will be more older people than younger. Population patterns in three countries offer a projected, diverse view of the possibilities that await.

PETER UHLENBERG

Learning Outcomes

After reading this article, you will be able to:

- Identify the challenges of an aging population.

- Identify the reasons for an aging world.

- Discuss the social changes necessary to appreciate an aging population.

The world is undergoing a major demographic restructuring of its population: in nearly every country around the globe, the proportion of children is declining and the proportion of old people is increasing.

Population aging began in Sweden and France in the nineteenth century as a consequence of their declining fertility rates, and was pervasive across all developed countries by 1950. Nevertheless, as recently as 1950, only 5 percent of the world's population was older than age 65, and 34 percent were children under age 15. (Unless otherwise noted, all population statistics are taken from the United Nations Department of Economic and Social Affairs, 2011).

Population projections suggest that by 2060, the proportion of people older than age 65 will almost equal the proportion younger than age 15 (18 percent versus 20 percent). And in the more developed regions of the world in 2060, there will be 156 people older than age 65 for every 100 children younger than age 15.

Demographers thoroughly understand the reasons for global population aging and the patterns of population aging across countries. The more interesting and complex questions concern the social, political, and economic implications of this phenomenon. This article offers a brief explanation of why populations around the world are growing older, compares patterns of population aging in three countries to illustrate the diversity that exists, and provides a foundation for thinking about a future where older people are more numerous than children.

Why Populations Age

The age composition of a population is determined by its past patterns of fertility, mortality, and international migration. Of these three variables, fertility decline is by far the most important factor leading to population aging. As women have fewer children, the proportion of children in the population declines and the proportion of older people increases. The reason developed countries have older populations than do developing countries is because fertility decline occurred far earlier in developed countries than it did in developing countries. In

Western Europe, where low fertility rates persisted over most of the twentieth century, 20 percent of the population will be older than age 65 in 2015. In Eastern Africa, where fertility rates remained high until recently, only 3 percent of the population will be older than age 65 in 2015. Looking ahead, fertility rates are falling in Eastern Africa, and projections indicate that by 2060, the proportion of older adults in the population will increase to 7 percent. But because very low fertility is expected to persist in Western Europe, that region of the world is expected to have more than 27 percent elders by 2060. In Japan, where there is extremely low fertility, 35 percent of the population is projected to be older than age 65 in 2060.

The effect of declining mortality on population aging is more complex than declining fertility. Declining mortality among infants and children actually works to make populations younger. On the other hand, decreasing death rates at older ages increases the proportion of older adults in a population. Historically, declining mortality among the young caused gains in life expectancy as countries moved from high to moderate levels of mortality. But as most people survive to old age, declining death rates in later life become the primary reason for increased levels of life expectancy; future improvements in life expectancy in low-mortality countries will contribute to further aging of their populations. But the impact of declining mortality on population age composition is small compared with that of fertility change.

The effect of declining mortality on population aging is more complex than declining fertility.

Contrary to some popular thinking, international migration has only a small effect on population aging. Net positive immigration of young adults has an immediate effect of making a population younger, but in the long run, these immigrants age. A steady flow of in-migrants will lead to a slightly younger population over time, but demographers agree that immigration at any reasonable level will not significantly affect population aging in countries with low fertility (Keely, 2009). The relatively small effect of even large-scale immigration on population aging can be illustrated by comparing two projections of what percent of the U.S. populace will be older than age 65 in 2050. Assuming a steady stream of 820,000 immigrants annually produces a projection of 20 percent of the populace being older than age 65; assuming zero immigration yields a projection of 22 percent (United States Census Bureau, 1996). Without immigration, the population would be older, but only slightly.

Variability of Global Population Aging

In discussing global population aging, it is important to recognize the large demographic and social variability across regions and countries. The demographic contrast between Western Europe and Eastern Africa was mentioned above. Equally important are the large differences that exist across societies regarding the role of the state versus the family in caring for dependent elders. Because of this, population aging may have different implications for different societies. A comparison of population aging in three countries (Sweden, China, and the United States) illustrates the importance of examining aging within a social and historical context.

Sweden

Sweden was one of the first countries to experience population aging—8 percent of its population was older than age 65 in 1900. Across the twentieth century, the percentage of elders in Sweden more than doubled (to 17 percent in 2000), and this trend will continue in the coming decades, reaching a level of 26 percent of the populace older than age 65 in 2060. Although Sweden no longer has the oldest population (Japan tops the list), what is occurring there is of interest because of Sweden's long history of population aging, combined with its generous welfare state. One goal of the Swedish welfare state has been to allow elders to maintain a high standard of living and to keep their independence in old age by providing them with state pensions, healthcare, housing, and access to social services. Providing these benefits requires a high tax rate on the working population. How viable this welfare-state model is—as the older population expands significantly relative to the working population-is a major question being asked in more developed countries at this time.

Population aging may have different implications for different societies.

While future adjustments to the welfare state in Sweden are uncertain, the choices made thus far suggest that changes can be made without abandoning popular welfare policies. The pension system was redesigned in the late 1990s to provide strong incentives for delaying retirement age and continuing to work past age 60, and average age at exit from the labor force increased by two years between 2001 and 2010. Greater restrictions on public financing of homecare and institutional care have increased the importance of family care for older people needing assistance. Survey evidence shows that only 5 percent of older Swedes in need of assistance with activities of daily living depend exclusively on in-home help if they are married and have a child, while 80 percent depend exclusively on family help (Sundstrom, 2009).

The tax base supporting the welfare state is being expanded by policies that increase the percentage of the population in the workforce and increase the hours worked by those who are employed. Sweden provides an example of a country that, in the face of aging, has made adjustments to welfare polices while continuing to provide a high level of support for its older population (and its younger populations).

Critics of a generous welfare state model have argued that as the state assumes more responsibility for the welfare of its population, the role of the family in providing care is undermined. However, a growing body of evidence suggests this has not been the case in Sweden. Not only does the family continue to be responsive to its older members, but elders continue to be involved in caring for their grandchildren. Given the high level of welfare support for children and working parents in Sweden, few Swedish grandparents co-reside with their grandchildren or provide regular childcare. But most Swedish grandparents care for grandchildren on an occasional basis, and they overwhelmingly agree that grandparents should help their grandchildren when needed (Albertini, Kohli, and Vogel, 2007). All evidence suggests that intergenerational bonds remain strong in Sweden.

China

Population aging in China stands out—and merits special attention—because of its magnitude, the speed with which it will occur, and the timing of its occurrence relative to China's economic development. One-fifth of the older people in the world now live in China, and by 2060, the older population of China will exceed the total older population living in developed countries (357 million versus 343 million). While most discussions of population aging focus on aging in wealthy countries such as Japan and those in Europe and North America, a global perspective calls attention to the fact that two-thirds of all older people live in developing countries. That fraction will increase to four-fifths by 2060.

The proportion of China's population that is older than age 65 doubled (or soon will) between 1950 and 2015 (from 5 percent to 10 percent), but between 2015 and 2060, that proportion will triple again, to 30 percent. The rapidity of this aging is unprecedented in world history—to go from a 10 percent elderly population up to 28 percent is taking 100 years in Western Europe (from 1950 to 2050), but this phenomenon will occur in merely forty years in China (from 2015 to 2055). This accelerated pace is because of the dramatic decline in fertility that occurred after institutionalization of the one-child policy in 1979. Some authors have warned of the devastating economic and social

consequences that China will face as it encounters this so-called old age tsunami, but alarmist prophecies about the future consequences of demographic change tend to miss the mark because they fail to appreciate how social institutions adapt to changing conditions.

There is no question that rapid population aging will present challenges to China over the next several decades. China will become old before becoming rich. In contrast to most developed countries, China's state pension system does not cover most of the workforce, and it is largely unfunded. The availability of working-age people to support the older population is now favorable in China, but that will change dramatically. In 2015, there will be 7.7 people of ages 15 to 64 for every person older than age 65; by 2060, there will be only 1.9. Traditionally older people in China have depended upon their children for support, but in the future, older adults will have relatively few children (Chen and Liu, 2009).

Another factor to consider is China's unbalanced sex ratio from selective abortion under the one-child policy; this means that daughters to provide care to elderly parents and other family members will be in short supply. Healthcare for the aging population also presents challenges because the cost of providing healthcare for the old greatly exceeds that of caring for the young. Despite these challenges, demography is not destiny. The failure of economists to foresee the economic growth that occurred in China in recent decades should be a caution for those who think that the challenges of population aging cannot be overcome.

The United States

Between 1900 and 2010 there was a gradual aging of the U.S. population as the percentage of those older than age 65 increased from 4 percent to 13 percent. However, a much more rapid aging of the population will occur between 2010 and 2030 as the baby boomer cohort enters old age. By 2030, 20 percent of the population will be older than age 65. After 2030, population aging will again be gradual, with those older than 65 reaching 22 percent by 2060. The aging of baby boomers in the United States has stimulated a great deal of discussion about the challenges of population aging. Most attention has been directed at issues facing Social Security, Medicare, and Medicaid—although both experts and average citizens disagree about what changes should be made to these programs. Equally important, but less discussed, is a question about how population aging might impact the supply of informal care for older people by spouses, children, and siblings. Data from the 2004 National Long-Term Care Survey shows that 79 percent of the care received by older people with disabilities who lived in the community was provided by family members (Houser, Gibson, and Redfoot, 2010). But the declining fertility that leads to population aging also leads to a decrease in the number of adult children and siblings available to provide informal care. How serious are these concerns? The following four observations provide some perspective.

Compared to other developed countries, the United States is exceptional in having a low level of population aging. Projections show 26 percent of the population in the more developed regions of the world, and 33 percent in Spain, will be older than age 65 in 2050, compared to only 21 percent in the United States. Why? Because fertility in the United States remains relatively high.

Other countries already have populations as old as the United States' population will be in 2030, after the baby boomer cohort passes age 65. But reaching this level of population aging has not inevitably resulted in significant social and economic upheaval. For example, Sweden now has an age composition similar to that expected in the United States in 2030. While no one knows how the United States will respond to population aging over the next several decades, other countries can provide insight into what is possible.

Alarmist writing on implications of population aging tends to exclude considerations of elders as resources. If reaching age 65 meant dependency and an end to productive activity, one might have cause for deep concern. But viewing old age as a long stage of life marked by dependency and unproductivity is a negative stereotype unsupported by empirical evidence. Along with growing labor force participation among those older than age 65, findings show high levels of volunteer work and engagement in family caregiving. Furthermore, aging is malleable and there is potential for greatly increasing the productivity of older people through greater opportunities and incentives, such as reducing age discrimination toward older workers, increasing recruitment of older volunteers, and providing them with more support and training and recognition.

Concerns have also been raised about the effects of population aging on the well-being of children (Uhlenberg, 2009). As the proportion of the populace that is older than age 65 increases from 15 percent to 21 percent between 2015 and 2050, the proportion that is younger than age 15 declines only from 20 percent to 19 percent. In other words, the demands on the working population to support children will not decrease as the demands of supporting the older population increase. The potential tension between supporting the old and supporting the young, sometimes referred to as the intergenerational equity issue, could be further complicated by the changing racial-ethnic composition of age groups. In 2050, it is expected that a majority of elders (66 percent) will be non-Hispanic whites, but only 43 percent of children will be in this category (United States Census Bureau, 1996). While conflict across generational lines has not yet been revealed in survey data on attitudes toward old-age entitlements, attention should be given to possible growing competition for scarce resources.

Thinking Clearly about Population Aging

In response to population aging, all societies face a number of common issues. The following points may provide a starting place for future discussions of global population aging.

There is no viable demographic way to avoid population aging. Countries with very low fertility might try to slow aging by encouraging women to have more babies, but efforts to implement pronatalist policies have not succeeded. No country is likely to adopt a policy of increasing death rates for the older population. And the level of immigration required to make a significant difference is politically infeasible. In a world with low fertility, low mortality, and restricted immigration, countries must deal with the reality of having 20 percent or 30 percent of their populations older than age 65.

As a country experiences the transition from high to low birth rates, shifts in its age composition are dynamic. In the early phase, which lasts at least three or four decades, the proportion of children in the population drops, while the proportion of elders hardly changes. Consequently, the ratio of the working-age population to the dependent age groups (children and older adults) grows substantially. This growth in the support ratio (number in the working ages divided by number in dependent ages) is referred to as the "demographic dividend," because it provides an opportunity for less spending on dependents and more savings to foster economic growth (Lee and Mason, 2006).

China provides a clear example of how the support ratio changes with a decline in fertility. Between 1950 and 2015, the ratio of the population ages 15 to 64 to the population younger than age 15 and older than age 65 increased from 1.6 to 2.7. But moving forward, this demographic dividend will disappear as the proportion of elders grows at the expense of the working-age population. By 2060, the support ratio will be only 1.3. All countries can expect this pattern of growth, followed by a decline of the support ratio, during the demographic transition, although the speed of change is variable and depends on how rapidly the fertility decline occurs.

The hope is that countries will take advantage of the demographic dividend to make investments that accelerate economic growth and establish an infrastructure that will provide long-term economic benefits. In the long run, countries must be prepared for much older populations and lower support ratios.

Business will need to adapt to the new demographic reality of older populations. Up to now, ageism in the business sector has presented an obstacle to constructive response to aging populations. Such ageism has led both to discrimination against older workers and to the neglect of older adults as a market. But change in the business sector is happening and will likely accelerate in coming decades.

> **The challenge for the global community is to champion social change that capitalizes on the worth of an increasing older population.**

Business must re-evaluate the potential for older workers to make productive contributions. Empirical research challenges the stereotype that older workers are unhealthy, unable to learn, and too expensive (Biggs, Carstensen, and Hogan, 2012; Seiko, Biggs, and Sargent, 2012). In developed countries, cohorts reaching age 65 are increasingly composed of individuals who are well-educated and healthy, and who expect to live for another twenty to thirty years. To take advantage of older workers' potential, several straightforward responses by business are needed. The workplace can be made friendlier to older workers by increasing flexibility—offering gradual retirement, part-time work, and flexible hours. Employers can help workers avoid becoming obsolete by providing lifelong education and physical fitness programs. The linear career plan can be replaced with one that allows the transfer of older workers into less demanding jobs at lower salaries. Such adaptation by organizations can both improve the quality of life for older people and reduce the economic burden of population aging.

Recognition of the older population as a major market for business is beginning, as evidenced by an increasing number of articles about the "silver market." Because a great deal of wealth is held by the older population and the number of elders is increasing relative to other age groups, it makes sense for business to design products appealing to the older market, and to direct advertising to them. Consumption by the older population can stimulate the economy. The economic power of older adults also can act as a force to change the ageist stereotypes often perpetuated by advertising.

Finally, the way in which people age and the cultural meaning of old age can change. As sociologists put it, aging is to a large extent socially constructed. Social institutions can (and do) change over time, so the implications of a large portion of the population cresting age 65 are not static. As noted above, the way work is organized can change to take advantage of older workers' potential. Education can change to foster lifelong learning. Healthcare can move toward an emphasis on preserving good health and promoting healthy lifestyles that reduce disabilities and dependency in later life. New technology can be developed that enables people in later life to experience fewer limitations. Public policy can change to provide incentives for volunteering in later life. Religious organizations can move beyond seeing older people merely as a group in need of help to seeing them as a resource for ministry.

Little good comes from viewing population aging as the "gray peril." Large-scale population aging will inevitably occur in all countries around the world, and the challenge for the global community is to champion social change that capitalizes on the worth of an increasing older population. There is vast potential for improving and enhancing opportunity and incentive structures for people in later life. If we do this, we can help forge a future that includes a more balanced view of aging—one in which we collectively view older people more as a valuable resource than as a burden.

References

Albertini, M., Kohli, M., and Vogel, C. 2007. "Intergenerational Transfers of Time and Money in European Families: Common Patterns—Different Regimes?" *Journal of European Social Policy* 17(4): 319–34.

Biggs, S., Carstensen, L., and Hogan, P. 2012. "Social Capital, Lifelong Learning and Social Innovation." In Beard, J. R., et al., eds. *Global Population Ageing: Peril or Promise?* (pp. 39–41). Geneva, Switzerland: World Economic Forum. www3.weforum.org/docs/WEF_GAC_GlobalPopulationAgeing_Report_2012.pdf. Retrieved January 8, 2013.

Chen, F., and Liu, G. 2009. "Population Aging in China." In Uhlenberg, P., ed. *International Handbook of Population Aging* (pp. 157–72). Dordrecht, the Netherlands: Springer.

Houser, A., Gibson, M. J., and Redfoot, D. L. 2010. *Trends in Family Caregiving and Paid Home Care for Older People with Disabilities in the Community: Data from the National Long-Term Care Survey.* AARP Public Policy Institute Research Report 2010-09. Washington, DC: AARP Public Policy Institute.

Keely, C. B. 2009. "Replacement Migration." In Uhlenberg, P., ed. *International Handbook of Population Aging* (pp. 395–405). Dordrecht, the Netherlands: Springer.

Lee, R., and Mason, A. 2006. "What Is the Demographic Dividend?" *Finance and Development* 43(3). www.imf.org/external/pubs/ft/fandd/2006/09/basics.htm#author. Retrieved September 12, 2012.

Seiko, A., Biggs, S., and Sargent, L. 2012. "Organizational, Adaptation and Human Resource Needs for an Aging Population." In Beard, J. R., et al., eds. *Global Population Ageing: Peril or Promise* (pp. 46–50). Geneva, Switzerland: World Economic Forum. www3.weforum.org/docs/WEF_GAC_GlobalPopulationAgeing_Report_2012.pdf.

Sundstrom, G. 2009. "Demography of Aging in the Nordic Countries." In Uhlenberg, P., ed. *International Handbook of Population Aging* (pp. 91–111). Dordrecht, the Netherlands: Springer.

Uhlenberg, P. 2009. "Children in an Aging Society." *The Journals of Gerontology: Social Sciences* 64B (4): 489–96.

United Nations Department of Economic and Social Affairs (UN DESA), Population Division. 2011. *World Population Prospects:*

The 2010 Revision, Volume I: Comprehensive Tables. ST/ESA/ SER.A/313.esa.un.org/unpd/wpp/unpp/panel_indicators.htm. Retrieved September 12, 2012.

United States Census Bureau. 1996. *Population Projections of the United States by Age, Sex, Race, and Hispanic Origin: 1995 to 2050.* Current Population Reports P25–1130. census.gov/prod/1/ pop/p25-1130.pdf. Retrieved September 12, 2012.

Critical Thinking

1. What are the global effects of an aging population?

2. How does an aging population affect healthcare resources globally?

Internet References

National Council on Aging
   www.ncoa.org

World Health Organization: Aging and Life Course
   www.who.int/ageing/en

PETER UHLENBERG, PH.D., is professor of sociology and a Fellow of the Carolina Population Center at the University of North Carolina at Chapel Hill, North Carolina.

Article   Prepared by: Elaina Osterbur, *Saint Louis University*

Supporting the Entry of Older Adult Students into College Classrooms

QUINTANA CLARK AND LEVON T. ESTERS

Learning Outcomes

After reading this article, you will be able to:

- Explain the reasons older adults are entering college.

- Understand the support mechanisms needed for older adult success in the classroom.

- Identify the motivating factors that attract older adults to higher education.

Doretha Daniels witnessed many key moments in history, such as voting rights granted to White women, the Great Depression, both world wars, the Civil Rights Movement, the lunar landing and more. By the time she turned 50, she and other Black women in the U.S. were finally granted their right to vote in 1965.

Although Daniels has experienced more life than most, there was still something she had been longing to achieve. In 2015, at the age of 99, Daniels earned her college degree. She is the oldest of a new minority of students who are earning their college degrees much later in life.

For example, at 97, Allen Stewart received his master's in clinical science. At 95, Nola Ochs received her bachelor's in history. At 89, Mary Fasano attended Harvard University to receive a degree in liberal arts. At 67, Carol Mobley received her bachelor's in sociology and continued on to pursue a master's in social work. At 60, Helen White received her master's in sports management. And at 52, Bridgetta Cottingham received her bachelor's in human development gerontology.

The list of college graduates over the age of 50 is growing, as is their proportion of the world population. In 2011, the National Center for Education Statistics documented that there were more than one-half million students over the age of 50 enrolled in degree-granting institutions.

Some questions that naturally arise are: Are there any cognitive advantages for older students? What motivates older people to further their education? What issues do older students face when pursuing a college degree? What type of support is there for older students to return to college?

The good news is that scientific evidence disproves ill-conceived notions that older students might be burdened with cognitive disadvantages. For instance, Roger Gould, a New York psychiatrist, says an aging brain has variations much like that of a school-aged child.

"If you and your brain are healthy," Gould asserts, "the only limitations to learning new mental skills and information are your motivation and natural intelligence."

Dr. James Fallon, a neuroscientist at University of California, Irvine says that people reach their maximum cognitive abilities in their 60s, which is the ideal time to balance executive functions with intellectual techniques. Fallon, who is 66, says, "I have never been more creative and productive."

A Seattle Longitudinal Study of Adult Cognitive Development tracked the cognitive abilities of thousands of adults over the age of 50 and found that middle-aged adults performed better academically then they did as young adults. Furthermore, psychologist Timothy Salthouse at the University of Virginia recently completed a study that examined the consequence of age-related cognitive declines and found that there is no evidence that cognitive ability declines with age.

What motivates individuals who continue their education after 50 varies widely. Later in life, there can be differences in an individual's economic status, social status, personal and family obligations, identity or mental clarity that drive them to want what a higher degree can offer.

Forbes magazine highlighted that some individuals desire to achieve a sense of accomplishment and feeling of pride. There are also better job prospects for those who choose to re-invent themselves by obtaining an advanced degree. Still others want to continue to grow intellectually. Other motivations for returning to college later in life might be that middle-age students have a greater defined academic purpose and focus and are thus better situated to capitalize on the myriad of experiences college offers.

For retirees, getting involved in the bustling and stimulating environment of college can keep them mentally active on a much deeper level than traveling, golf or television.

Attending college later in life is not without its challenges. For example, issues that students age 50 and over face are more likely to be related to competing family demands such as managing the household or financial obligations. Other issues that students above 50 may experience include generational differences that exist when interacting with traditionally aged undergraduate and graduate students and the unfortunate possibility of ageism (implicit age discrimination).

Additionally, some students over 50 may experience a stressful adjustment period related to juggling a full-time schedule of course work, contributing to group research projects, attending conferences and maintaining a healthy balance between one's own academic load and supporting fellow peers. Fortunately, for older students, these types of newfound responsibilities are often welcomed.

The bottom line is that by 2030, more than 20 percent of the U.S. population will be age 65 or older. This fact alone will create a need for higher education institutions to examine how they can best serve a growing middle-age student population.

One suggestion might be to create networking events for middle-age students and newly degreed middle-age faculty. This will give middle-age students an opportunity to interact with like-minded students and faculty members. Faculty members might also consider adjusting their pedagogical techniques to reflect core principles of andragogy. This is especially important since adult education theories of learning imply that older students favor self-directed learning, share an immense reservoir of experiences and knowledge, demonstrate enthusiasm to learn, place emphasis on task- or problem-centered learning and possess a high degree of intrinsic motivation. Integrating adult education instruction into lesson plans could be a win-win situation for adult students as well as traditional students.

Middle-age college students bring a wealth of life experiences, knowledge and professionalism to classrooms and research groups. Not only are older students' contributions in classrooms being recognized, a growing number of higher education institutions have recognized that the middle-age college student numbers will continue to grow, and these schools and are now offering programs to students age 55 and over.

For example, California's 23 state universities offer tuition-free classes to students 60 years and older, Texas public colleges and universities have tuition reduction programs for students 55 years and older and Pennsylvania State University's Go-60 program offers tuition-free enrollment to students 60 years and older.

In addition, organizations such as Barclays, Goldman Sachs, Encore.org and others have programs in place to attract the ever-growing numbers of college-educated, middle-age people entering the workforce. Finally, there are several organizations that offer scholarships to women over the age of 50.

With the growing trend of middle-age students pursuing postsecondary education degrees, colleges and universities should continue to evolve in ways that meet these students' needs, thus helping to ensure that they obtain successful careers upon graduation.

Moreover, for institutions that may not know where to start in developing the types of adult education and training programs needed for middle-age students, there are a myriad of resources such as The Council of Adult and Experiential Learning (CAEL) and the American Association for Adult and Continuing Education (AAACE) that can help.

Critical Thinking

1. If you lived in the cultural climate that some older adults lived, what would your chances be of going to college?

2. Thirty or more years from now do you think you will want to reinvent yourself? What would it take?

3. Do you have an older adult in your life that has returned or wants to return to the classroom?

Internet References

Association of American Colleges and Universities
   https://www.aacu.org/

Distance Education
   http://www.distance-education.org/

Older Adults Technology Service
   https://oats.org/

QUINTANA "QUINCY" CLARK is a Ph.D. student at Purdue University. Dr. Levon T. Esters is an associate professor at Purdue University whose research focuses on the STEM career development of students of color and mentoring of women and graduate students of color in STEM.

Article

Prepared by: Elaina Osterbur, *Saint Louis University*

The First Person to Live to 150 Has Already Been Born—Revisited!

JOHN NOSTA

Learning Outcomes

After reading this article, you will be able to:

- Identify innovations that have led to the increase in average life span.
- Identify research that suggest we can delay aging.

Living Forever—Two Bold, Yet Different Perspectives

You might have heard this quote by Aubry de Grey. It's nothing new . . . and I wonder just how much closer to 150 that person might already be. But I got to thinking, what would be the impact of technology and specifically that of digital health.

Longevity—The Physiologic Basis

But first it might be interesting to review some of de Grey's thinking about regarding the nature of aging. He calls them "The Seven Deadly Things."

- **Mutations—in chromosomes causing cancer due to nuclear mutations/epimutations:**

  These are changes to the nuclear DNA (nDNA), the molecule that contains our genetic information, or to proteins which bind to the nDNA. Certain mutations can lead to cancer, and according to de Grey, noncancerous mutations and epimutations do not contribute to aging within a normal life span, so cancer is the only end point of these types of damage that must be addressed.

- **Mutations—in Mitochondria:**

  Mitochondria are components in our cells that are important for energy production. They contain their own genetic material, and mutations to their DNA can affect a cell's ability to function properly. Indirectly, these mutations may accelerate many aspects of aging.

- **Junk—inside of cells, aka intracellular aggregates:**

  Our cells are constantly breaking down proteins and other molecules that are no longer useful or which can be harmful. Those molecules which can't be digested simply accumulate as junk inside our cells. Atherosclerosis, macular degeneration, and all kinds of neurodegenerative diseases (such as Alzheimer's disease) are associated with this problem.

- **Junk—outside of cells, aka extracellular aggregates:**

  Harmful junk protein can also accumulate outside of our cells. The amyloid senile plaque seen in the brains of Alzheimer's patients is one example.

- **Cells—too few, aka cellular loss:**

  Some of the cells in our bodies cannot be replaced, or can only be replaced very slowly—more slowly than they die. This decrease in cell number causes the heart to become weaker with age, and it also causes Parkinson's disease and impairs the immune system.

- **Cells—too many, aka cell senescence:**

  This is a phenomenon where the cells are no longer able to divide, but also do not die and let others divide. They may also do other things that they're not supposed to, like secreting proteins that could be harmful. Cell senescence has been proposed as cause or consequence of type 2 diabetes. Immune senescence is also caused by this.

- **Extracellular protein cross-links:**

   Cells are held together by special linking proteins. When too many cross-links form between cells in a tissue, the tissue can lose its elasticity and cause problems, including arteriosclerosis and presbyopia.

So, I got to ask Dr. de Grey some questions to get a more up-to-date sense of his thinking. Here are some of his thoughts on longevity in the context of today's changing technological and medical enviormnent [environment].

Q: *Do you see the convergence of technology and health as a significant event with regard to longevity?*

A: I wouldn't say I really regard it as an "event" at all. I think medicine is best viewed as simply a subset of technology—technology for restoring or maintaining people's health. There is a continuing process of interchange and cross-fertilization between different branches of technology, and that includes things like the development of nonbiological approaches to medical problems, but I don't see any real sea change.

Q: *How does your background as a software engineer impact your thinking today?*

A: Quite a lot—and it especially impacted my thinking in the first several years of my time as a biomedical gerontologist. It let me look at the problem of aging somewhat differently than lifelong biologists had been doing.

Q: *Please comment on the myth of aging how we need not accept it as "just part of getting old."*

A: It's always been a mystery to me why this isn't totally obvious to everyone. Do we let cars fall apart when they get old?—yes in general, but not if we really want them not to—that's why we have 50-year-old VW Beetles driving around, and even vintage cars. It's bizarre that people don't see that the exact same thing is true of the machine we call the human body, just that that machine is a lot more complicated so the development of sufficiently comprehensive preventative maintenance is a lot more challenging.

Q: *Could you briefly explain the nature of free radicals and the role in aging?*

A: Free radicals come in a lot of flavors, and a number of them are created by the body. Some of them are good for us, but others are harmful, because they react with and damage molecules that we need for survival, such as our DNA. The body has a massive array of defenses against these problems, which can be grouped into four categories—tricks to minimize the rate at which these toxic free radicals come into existence in the first place, enzymes and compounds that react harmlessly with them before they can react harmfully with something

else, chemical tricks that make the harmful reactions happen less easily, and systems that repair the resulting damage after it's occurred—but those tricks are not completely comprehensive, so some damage still occurs and accumulates throughout life. We'd like to stop that happening, and we could theoretically do it by enhancing to perfection any one (or more) of those four types of defense. My view is that the last one, repairing damage post hoc, is the most practical. Eliminating free radical production would involve completely redesigning aspects of our metabolism, especially the way we use oxygen to extract energy from food. It would also have the problem that even the bad free radicals are also good in some ways, so we actually need them around somewhat; this is also the problem with perfecting the elimination of free radicals via harmless reactions. Ramifying our cells so that the reactions just don't occur is also tantamount to completely redesigning the body, So we're left with perfecting repair.

Q: *The digital health and quantified self-movement are increasingly gaining steam. Do you see this an a critical step forward in the quest for longevity?*

A: Not really, no. It's valuable, but only temporarily. That's because all personalized medicine is only valuable temporarily, while the treatments for such-and-such a condition are only modestly effective and can thereby be made more effective by being tuned to the specifics of the patient. We don't have personalized polio vaccines, because we don't need them—the same vaccine just works perfectly, on everyone.

Q: *Your famous quote, "the first person to live to 150 has already been born" really caught my eye. Is this a guess or do you have some data to support this?*

A: First, I've always been fastidious in only saying that the first such person is PROBABLY alive today. I would estimate the chance at 90 percent, though that could fall as low as 70 percent if funding for the relevant research in the coming decade or two is not sharply increased. No, no data—just informed intuition as to how much progress remains to be made to develop therapies that will work well enough to make that happen.

Q: *Cognition and Alzheimer's disease is a critical issue in a aging population. Are there emerging or current strategies to help reduce or eliminate its incidence?*

A: Absolutely—but there's still a long way to go. Alzheimer's is a very complex disease, involving the accumulation of a few different types of molecular and cellular damage, all of which we'll need to repair. There's very promising progress in using vaccines to stimulate the immune system to repair some types, and other types may yield to stem cell therapy, but a cure is not going to appear next year.

Q: *Do you personally use any technology or device to help in wellness is disease management?*

A: No.

Q: *Does the wait for "extensive data" and "controlled trials" adversely impact innovation in aging research?*

A: Yes, but it adversely impacts innovation across all medical research. There's a huge need for greater creativity in the regulatory process and that's coming: "adaptive licensing" is a big theme in that area right now.

Q: *What are some of your expectations for the future? Any bold predictions that might catch up off guard?*

A: I think my longevity predictions are quite bold enough!

Longevity—A Technological Perspective

The other resonant voice in the longevity discussion is Ray Kurzweil. His take on life extension, while inclusive of physiology, is very much focused on the role of technology and [how] it can impact many facets of life—from diagnosis to organ replacement. His bio—taken from his website—brings his expertise into perspective.

Ray Kurzweil has been described as "the restless genius" by *The Wall Street Journal*, and "the ultimate thinking machine" by *Forbes Inc.* magazine ranked him #8 among entrepreneurs in the United States, calling him the "rightful heir to Thomas Edison," and PBS included Ray as one of 16 "revolutionaries who made America," along with other inventors of the past two centuries.

But what I found interesting is that Dr. Kurzweil has made an interesting and bold prediction—we will live forever! In his recent interview in *The New York Times*, he established the techno-future where nanobots zoomed through our arteries and veins acting a vigilant seekers of disease and insult.

His vision of immortality is bold and makes living to 150 seem like being a kid!

He's stated that Moore's Law will no longer be applicable to our world and that new technologies will—like those little creatures humming around your blood vessels—change the game. Robotics, nanotechnology, and high-speed computational neuroscience will become the new reality. And with it, comes a new version of the something between 150 years old and infinity. Here's a glimpse into that future:

Within a quarter century, nonbiological intelligence will match the range and subtlety of human intelligence. It will then soar past it because of the continuing acceleration of information-based technologies, as well as the ability of machines to instantly share their knowledge. Intelligent nanorobots will be deeply integrated in our bodies, our brains, and our environment, overcoming pollution and poverty, providing vastly extended longevity, full-immersion virtual reality incorporating all of the senses (like *The Matrix*), "experience beaming" (like "Being John Malkovich"), and vastly enhanced human intelligence. The result will be an intimate merger between the technology-creating species and the technological evolutionary process it spawned.

Maybe Mel Brooks and Carl Reiner weren't that far off with their famous persona from the comedy skit—The Two Thousand Year Old Man?

Critical Thinking

1. Would you want to live to 150 years old?

2. Most research has been done using mice as research subjects. Would you consider becoming part of a human research trial?

3. How would the impact of living to 150 affect society?

Internet References

Institute for Aging Research
   http://www.instituteforagingresearch.org
National Institute on Aging
   http://www.nia.nih.gov
The Aging Research Centre
   http://www.arclab.org

Article   Prepared by: Elaina Osterbur, *Saint Louis University*

Living Long: 100 Years Is a Real Possibility

MARK HAGER

Learning Outcomes

After reading this article, you will be able to:

- Identify global statistics on aging.
- Understand health behaviors that contribute to increased life span.

You regularly hear in the news about people who are living long lives. Not a month goes by that you don't hear about people all over the world living to be 100 years old.

It is still neat to hear about them, the lives they've led, and the "secrets" they have to long-life.

However, centenarians (people who live to 100 years old) have been rare in the past . . . but, not in the coming years. We're going to see a *massive* increase in the number of people across the globe living to the age of 100 and beyond.

What's the Secret to Living Long?

We're not doctors. But, we're going to guess that healthy choices in lifestyle, diet, and exercise play a part in living long. Friendships, family, and other close relationships most likely do as well.

We're already seeing the results of how better health-care affects our life span. That will continue to drive our ability to live longer lives.

Not enough can be said for taking care of yourself . . . every part of yourself . . . mentally, physically, emotionally, and spiritually. Be good to you; it's the best way to set yourself up for success.

A Special Note

This is an interesting and fun topic. (That's one of the reasons we created this infographic.) Also, it's timely. *We're on the cusp of a health-care revolution that is going to make living to 100 more commonplace.*

We're going to guess you wouldn't mind being one of those people. (We would like to be, too!)

So, please, share this infographic. Help us spread a little fun information, and get people thinking about living a really long time. We want people to plan properly for their later life . . . so the later years can be as amazing and enjoyable as possible.

Critical Thinking

1. The article suggests being "on the cusp of a health-care revolution," what does this mean?
2. How does living longer affect health-care policies, such as Social Security and Medicare?

Internet References

Aging in Place
  http://www.ageinplace.com
Prevention
  http://www.prevention.org

MARK HAGER is an aging in place thought leader and advocate. He is the founder of AgeInPlace.com, the CEO of Age in Place Networks, a leading authority in the aging in place niche, and a trusted voice for both consumers and business owners serving older consumers. Over the years, Mark has provided help for thousands of consumers, organizations, and small businesses.

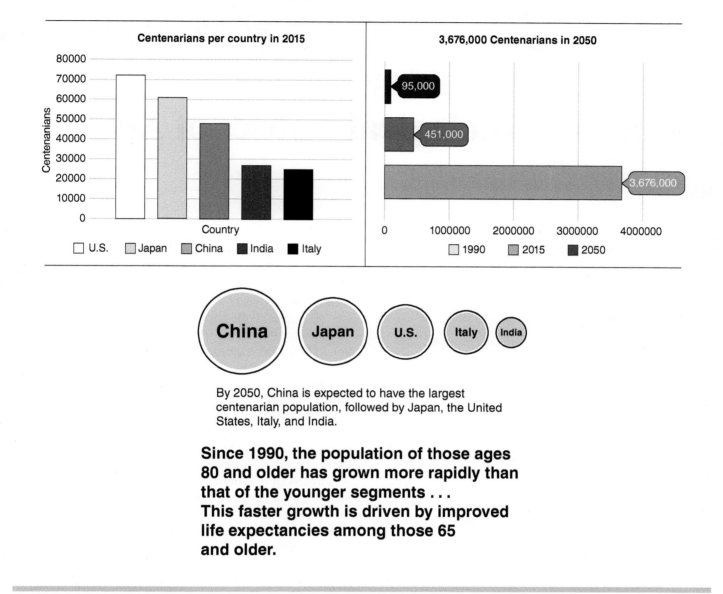

By 2050, China is expected to have the largest centenarian population, followed by Japan, the United States, Italy, and India.

Since 1990, the population of those ages 80 and older has grown more rapidly than that of the younger segments . . .
This faster growth is driven by improved life expectancies among those 65 and older.

Article   Prepared by: Elaina Osterbur, *Saint Louis University*

Aging 101: Biological Causes of Aging

H<small>ADRIEN</small> V<small>IELLE</small>

Learning Outcomes

After reading this article, you will be able to:

- Understand the biological causes of aging.
- Explain the genome and its relationship to DNA.
- Explain the effects of telomere shortening on aging.
- Identify the epigenetics and cellular senescence of aging.

Introduction

Aging can be defined as the sum of all the mechanisms that alter the functions of a living thing, prevents it from maintaining physiological balance and eventually leads to the death of said organism. In the human body and most other living things, the process is complex, gradual and depends on many biological factors. This natural process can be amplified by external factors throughout a lifetime (pollution, food, smoking…).

Scientists have taken a specific interest in aging during these past 30 years. Thanks to new technological breakthroughs, we have been able to conduct a closer study of the phenomenon. Studies have shown that aging is controlled, somehow, by genetic factors and biological processes inherent to humankind.

In order to slow down this natural process and prolong our life expectancy, the first step is to understand the causes of aging: how it works on living organisms, and what different factors determine life expectancy.

This article will be looking at the different causes of aging. The 7 main reasons are: genome damage, epigenetic factors, telomere shortening, unfolded protein response, mitochondrial dysfunction, cellular senescence and stem cell exhaustion. You will learn how these processes impact our cells and organs, and with what consequences.

DNA Repair: A Cause of Aging

Genome: the genome is the sum of the genetic information of a person or species. The information is mostly stored in the cell's nucleus, and the genome is the map to build the whole organism. It contains all the information that allow our cells to build and maintain our bodies, which is stored as DNA. Every fraction of DNA represents a specific characteristic of an individual (a gene). The human genome contains between 25,000 and 30,000 genes. The DNA contained in the nucleus is wrapped around proteins called histones. It is the combination of histones and DNA that makes up chromosomes. The chromosomes contain all of our genetic information and are replicated with every cell division in order to transmit the information to the newly created daughter cell.

Throughout life, our cells get to divide a great number of times. In older people, genetic anomalies can be observed [1]. Those mutations mostly happen during DNA replication and can affect important genes, or cause genetic transcription issues. These mutations cause the cell to malfunction and can affect the remaining tissue if the cell isn't eliminated through apoptosis (cellular death) or through senescence (degradation of the cell's functions).

Recent studies have shown that the DNA repair system could play a part in the aging process. A control system is in place to repair DNA that was modified during replication. The system uses proteins and enzymes in order to reprogram the modified cell. On top of correcting the corrupted DNA, these proteins have other effects, such as NAD+ consumption (see definition) and links to the mitochondrial functions [2]. Studies have shown that more DNA-repairing proteins (PARP) can be found in aged subjects [3]. Too much activation leads to the exhaustion of NAD+ stocks (although is it necessary to activate many NAD-dependent molecules such as sirtuins), and can induce cell apoptosis (death of the cell) if the DNA damage is too serious [4]. With age, there is an increase in the number of dead cells and in senescence, which can explain the degradation of organs.

Another part of the cell control system can have a negative effect over time: the protein P53 is responsible for elimination of carcinogenic cells, and allows to prolong the life of the organs by preventing the development of cancerous cells. However, the more that protein gets activated, the more it accelerates the aging process. Too many cells get destroyed and the tissues lose homogeneity[4]. Activation of the PARP enzyme can induce overexpression of the protein P53[5].

Both processes are beneficial to the body, but as the body ages, their action becomes detrimental.

One interpretation is that the damage sustained by the DNA can grow exponentially because of the mutations that can affect the genes responsible for replication, or the DNA repair system. PARP activation protects the body from DNA damage within the cells, and is linked to the exhaustion of NAD+ in cells. The coenzyme NAD+ is needed to activate all NAD-dependent enzymes (sirtuins). That exhaustion causes cells to dysfunction.

Telomere Shortening: Linked to Life Expectancy and Aging

Chromosomes are located in the nucleus of the cell, and carry genetic material. They have at their ends an area called telomere which contains no genetic information. Studies have shown that the length of the telomeres slowly reduced with age and that it was linked to a higher risk of age-related diseases – pulmonary fibrosis, degenerative diseases… [6][7][8].

Mechanisms of Telomere Shortening

During the cell cycle (all the steps in the life of a cell), a cell divides and replicates its DNA in order to transfer the genetic information to the newly created cell. During that replication process, a modification automatically happens: the non-replication of a portion of one end of the chromosome (telomere). This leads to a gradual shortening of the telomeres with each cell division. One enzyme called telomerase allows the full replication of a telomere. It is only found with stem cells, embryonic cells and cancer cells. It allows the full replication of a telomere which can remain sound throughout cell division. Presence of this enzyme in cancer cells explains why they are immortal: they can divide infinitely, without being stopped by their "biological clock". The workings of this enzyme is then very interesting to scientists – however, activating it could be linked to an onset of cancer.

The Effects of Telomere Shortening on Aging

Telomeres have a protecting effect on DNA. They are the portion of the chromosome that contains no genetic information, and erode throughout life with each replication until they almost disappear to leave the DNA information bare. DNA is no longer protected when it replicates, critical information get "chewed out" and it can lead to cell apoptosis (death of the cell) or change the cellular cycle by creating cancer cells.

A Harvard study genetically modified old and weak mice in order to activate the genes in charge of telomerase production: the mice were rejuvenated and damaged tissue even regenerated [9].

Another study was conducted on skin cells. Cultivated cells can divide about 40 to 60 times in their lifetime before beginning their aging process. By genetically modifying them in order to activate telomerase production, those same cells could divide 300 times.

Both experiments show the importance of telomeres in the life expectancy of a cell. However, adding telomerase or activating its production is not a viable solution to aging as of now, because of its link with cancer.

Telomere shortening can be seen as a biological clock which activates cell senescence as soon as its time is up. This mechanism limits the life expectancy of our cells, which is why it is central to all current research on aging.

The Epigenetics of Aging

Epigenetics are the study of the mechanisms managing the expression of the gene pool. Genetics are about genes, when epigenetics are about the use of those genes. This subject area shows how the expression of a gene can vary (activated or not) depending on the environment. Organs show this variability: each cell has a similar genetic information but different functions, which shows the difference in gene expression depending on the environment. One way to understand the phenomenon is to look at bees: one larva can become a queen or a worker depending on how it feeds. This is a very good example of an epigenetic phenomenon: one information can be expressed as two very different results. This subject area is very interesting to understand aging because it describes the evolution of cellular activity through time and gene expression.

Different Factors can Affect Gene Reading

Gene methylation: methylation is the epigenetic phenomenon through which some genes can be modified by adding or suppressing a methyl group. This can modify or inhibit gene expression, increase the chances of mutation… Methylation can affect many more or less important genes: estrogen receptors, tumor suppressors… Epigenetic modifications linked to methylation grow with age and can lead to serious health issues [9] (cholesterol, heart disease…).

Chromatin remodeling: in the nucleus, DNA takes the form of chromatin and allows the packaging of DNA with **proteins**. With age, chromatin remodeling decreases which can affect chromosome stability[10]. Studies have shown that chromatin regulation plays an important part in determining the length of telomeres. This epigenetic alteration can trigger accelerated aging by shortening the telomeres (see telomere shortening.)

Histone modification: histones are **proteins** around which the DNA wraps itself. They make up the most of a chromosome. Any modification in the histone components (acetyl group) can sensibly affect the body and change gene expression. For instance, suppressing acetyl groups on an histone in vertebrates can increase their life expectancy[11]. Some hormones are responsible for the addition or suppression of histone components (sirtuins, NF-kB) and affect **genome** stability[12]. Histone modification thus affects life expectancy through modifications of the expression of some genes.

The study of epigenetic alteration is at the core of the aging process. It describes changes in cell activity through time. Gene methylation and modification of histone proteins are responsible for changes in genome expression, and chromatin remodeling affects genome stability. The alterations are linked to age-related diseases like cancer, atherosclerosis and dementia.

Unfolded Protein Response: A Cause of Aging

Protein: proteins play a major role in many cellular mechanisms. They are the building blocks of our bodies and structure our cells. Inside the body, they can act as antibodies or hormones, and carry messages between our cells.

Amino acid: the building blocks of life. They make up proteins. Each amino acid bestows specific chemical properties to the protein, and its function depends on its place in the sequence.

Protein Folding

Proteins mostly work due to their shape which allows them to be identified and to perform their function. Protein folding allows them to take up their effective shape. This is a physical process through which a protein becomes functional by getting into the right shape. Each **protein** has a specific unfolded shape – a linear chain of amino acids – in which it is not functional. The

chemical properties of each amino acid shape each protein into the shape that allows it to perform its function within the cell.

Studies have shown that many age-related diseases, especially neuro-degenerative diseases (Alzheimer's disease, Parkinson's…) are due to the buildup of unfolded proteins inside the cell, causing it to malfunction[13].

Chaperon Proteins

Chaperon proteins are in charge of assembling, transporting and destroying other proteins. Their function is vital for the body to work[14]. Aging reduces the activity and synthesis of chaperon proteins which leads to issues in protein management [15] (buildup of defective proteins inside the cells, folding of denatured proteins…). The possible cause of chaperon proteins malfunction is a low supply of **ATP**, an energy source for the human body (see mitochondrial dysfunction), or a modification of its "sensor" which can prevent the chaperon protein from identifying its target[16].

In order to prevent accumulation of unfolded or partly folded proteins, the nucleus and the mitochondria communicate to destroy defective proteins. Communication degrades with aging (see mitochondrial dysfunction) which leads to a non-functional proteins buildup in the cells.

The dysfunction of proteins is one of the main causes of aging because of their essential role in our bodies (communication, antibodies, hormones…) Chaperon proteins and nucleus-mitochondria communication rule the behavior of proteins. Protein deterioration causes aging.

Mitochondrial Dysfunction and Aging

Mitochondria are organelles (constituents of the cell: nucleus, mitochondria…) in the cells. They maintain cellular respiration and **ATP** creation – an energy source vital to all mechanisms of the human body. They are the power source of all living things; their function is vital and dysfunctional mitochondria can lead to the death of the cell.

mtADN

Mitochondria are the only organelles (components of the cell) with their own DNA, called mtDNA.

Studies conducted on the evolution of mitochondrial function throughout their lives showed that mitochondrial dysfunction is a reliable indicator of aging. These studies have shown that mitochondrial dysfunction happened even without significant changes of mtDNA, which suggests that age-related dysfunction of mitochondria is not triggered by mtDNA mutation but by one or more other factors.

Oxidative Stress

Oxidative stress: oxidative stress is caused by the oxidation of the many elements of our cells (oxygen-related electron loss). Free radicals are the molecules responsible for oxidation, and come from the oxygen contained in the air we breathe.

Oxidative stress has long been studied as a potential cause of mitochondrial dysfunction. Aging was attributed for a long time to the wear induced by oxidative species (free radicals). It seems like the understanding of the phenomenon was only partial. Conversely, studies have shown that an increase in anti-oxidants had no effect on life expectancy, whereas an increase in the levels of free radicals led to longer life expectancy [17] [18]. The precise role of free radicals is not yet clear to science.

Cell-Mitochondria Communication

Cell-mitochondria communication is another possible cause of dysfunction [19]. These communications are necessary in order to replicate mitochondria, which makes them essential to the cell. They degrade with age, the necessary **protein** regulation decreases, leading to communication problems between the cell and mitochondria. It is a possible cause of mitochondrial deterioration that can lead to tissue aging.

Mitochondrial alteration is a complex phenomenon. Because of the many interactions between this organelle and the rest of the cell, many causes have been studied. Degradation could be induced by the alteration of communication between the nucleus and mitochondria. The dysfunction is a major cause of aging due to the vital role of mitochondria in our cells (cellular respiration, ATP production...)

Cellular Senescence and Aging

Cellular senescence happens when the cell ages and its function decreases. It stops dividing and changes activity (i.e.: secretion of inflammatory molecules[20]). Senescent cells can be seen at all stages of life. They can be caused by DNA modification (see genome damage), cancer occurrence... Senescent cells accumulate in some tissues with age and cause heterogeneity[21].

Senescence is useful in terms of limiting cancerous cells proliferation. Dead cells are destroyed (phagocytosis) which calls for an efficient immune system. However, with age, the immune system loses efficiency as the number of senescent cells increases, which leads to an accumulation of senescent cells in some tissues.

Therefore, this mechanism is beneficial during youth. It protects the body against cancerous cells proliferation, but relies on an efficient immune system to eliminate senescent cells. With aging, senescent cells accumulate because of the lack of stem cells renewal and of a less efficient immune system.

Stem Cell Exhaustion: An Aging Cause

Stem cell: Stem cells are undifferentiated cells, they belong to no specific organ, and can generate specialized cells through "cellular differentiation". The mechanisms allows stem cells to develop characteristics specific to one type of cell. The stem cells of an adult cannot end up with any type of cell (i.e.: red blood cells and T and B lymphocytes all come from the same undifferentiated cells, hematopoietic stem cells. They cannot end up as muscle cells, neuron cells...). Some organs already consist in specialized stem cells (unipotent stem cells) such as the skin, liver, intestinal lining, which ensures fast cell renewal.

Exhausted Stem Cells: A Link to Longevity

Stem cells allow the renewal of cells in an organ, they are stored in the body and used when needed. Some cells age and die on a regular basis and need to be replaced. A red blood cell lasts for an average of 120 days. Other organs can grow and demand more tissue (such as the uterus during pregnancy) and some animals' cells allow them to regenerate limbs (i.e.: lizards). Some organs have no stem cells and therefore cannot be renewed when damaged (heart, pancreas).

With aging, tissues don't regenerate as well due to the slow-down of cell division and the lack of stem cells replacement. This behavior can be explained by the overexpression of **proteins** blocking the cellular cycle, or the accumulation of DNA damage on stem cells[22][23]. This increases the number of senescent cells in tissues and can lead to an array of problems depending on which organ is affected. In the case of hematopoietic stem cells, exhaustion of stem cells can lead to immunodeficiency (T and B lymphocytes play a role in the immune system). The same can happen with muscles, brain, bones... On top of stem cell production going down, DNA mutations can occur and trigger cellular death with some cells, or modify the genetic information as well as increase resistance and replication speed, which leads to an increase of defective (or pre-cancerous) cells.

Exhaustion of stem cells is one of the main causes of aging since it prevents cell renewal and leads to the aging of organs. Understanding the workings of stem cells will be vital for regenerative medicine in the future.

Conclusion

Here were presented 7 causes of aging. These causes are potentially responsible for the alteration of the functions of the body. Some of them are at the very core of beneficial mechanisms which become detrimental with age, as it is the case with cellular senescence and the DNA repair system. The mechanisms prevent cancer from developing, but as their activity grows too strong or malfunctions, the degeneration of the body speeds up.

Other causes are simple mechanisms that slowly degrade through time (mitochondrial dysfunction, telomere shortening...). It is necessary to understand them if we ever want to work on it in order to potentially slow down aging and lengthen human life expectancy.

Definitions

Genome: the genome is the sum of the genetic information of a person or species. The information is mostly stored in the cell's nucleus, and the genome is the map to build the whole organism. It contains all the information that allow our cells to build and maintain our bodies, which is stored as DNA. Every fraction of DNA represents a specific characteristic of an individual (a gene). The human genome contains between 25,000 and 30,000 genes. The DNA contained in the nucleus is wrapped around proteins called histones. It is the combination of histone and DNA that makes up chromosomes. The chromosomes contain all of our genetic information and are replicated with every cell division in order to transmit the information to the newly created daughter cell.

Mitochondria are organelles (constituents of the cell: nucleus, mitochondria...) in the cells. They maintain cellular respiration and **ATP** creation – an energy source vital to all mechanisms of the human body. They are the power source of all living things; their function is vital and dysfunctional mitochondria can lead to the death of the cell.

Protein: proteins play a major role in many cellular mechanisms. They are the building blocks of our bodies and structure our cells. Inside the body, they can act as antibodies or hormones, and carry messages between our cells.

Amino acid: the building blocks of life. They make up proteins. Each amino acid bestows specific chemical properties to the protein, and its function depends on its place in the sequence.

Antibodies: protein used by the immune system to detect and neutralize pathogens.

Hormone: Chemical substance acting through the blood system by transmitting information in chemical form so it can be read by receptors.

Stem cell: Stem cells are undifferentiated cells, they belong to no specific organ, and can generate specialized cells through "cellular differentiation." The mechanisms allows stem cells to develop characteristics specific to one type of cell. The stem cells of an adult cannot end up with any type of cell (i.e.: red blood cells and T and B lymphocytes all come from the same undifferentiated cells, hematopoietic cells. They cannot end up as muscle cells, neuron cells...) Some organs already consist in specialized stem cells (unipotent stem cells) such as the skin, liver, intestinal lining, which ensures fast cell renewal.

NAD: nicotinamide adenine dinucleotide is a coenzyme that can be found in all living cells. It is used for many things such as ATP synthesis, mitochondrial function... NAD stocks decrease with age and affect the mechanisms for which this coenzyme is relevant.

Sirtuin: sirtuins are a class of NAD-dependent enzymes that play a role in the aging process. They play a vital part in controlling longevity.

ATP: the adenosine triphosphate molecule, or ATP, can be found in all living things. It supplies the energy necessary for the chemical reactions of the metabolism, during locomotion, cellular division...

Références

[1] Alexey A. Moskalev et al., "The Role of DNA Damage and Repair in Aging through the Prism of Koch-like Criteria," *Ageing Research Reviews* 12, no. 2 (March 2013): 661–84, doi:10.1016/j.arr.2012.02.001.

[2] Péter Bai and Carles Cantó, "The Role of PARP-1 and PARP-2 Enzymes in Metabolic Regulation and Disease," *Cell Metabolism* 16, no. 3 (September 5, 2012): 290–95, doi:10.1016/j.cmet.2012.06.016.

[3] Nady Braidy et al., "Age Related Changes in NAD+ Metabolism Oxidative Stress and Sirt1 Activity in Wistar Rats," *PLOS ONE* 6, no. 4 (avr 2011): e19194, doi:10.1371/journal.pone.0019194.

[4] Weihai Ying et al., "NAD+ as a Metabolic Link between DNA Damage and Cell Death," *Journal of Neuroscience Research* 79, no. 1–2 (January 1, 2005): 216–23, doi:10.1002/jnr.20289.

[5] Judith Campisi, "Senescent Cells, Tumor Suppression, and Organismal Aging: Good Citizens, Bad Neighbors," *Cell* 120, no. 4 (February 25, 2005): 513–22, doi:10.1016/j.cell.2005.02.003.

[6] Braidy et al., "Age Related Changes in NAD+ Metabolism Oxidative Stress and Sirt1 Activity in Wistar Rats."

[7] Elizabeth H. Blackburn, Carol W. Greider, and Jack W. Szostak, "Telomeres and Telomerase: The Path from Maize,

Tetrahymena and Yeast to Human Cancer and Aging," Nature Medicine 12, no. 10 (October 2006): 1133–38, doi:10.1038/nm1006-1133.

[8] *Jerry W. Shay and Woodring E. Wright, "Senescence and Immortalization: Role of Telomeres and Telomerase," Carcinogenesis 26, no. 5 (May 1, 2005): 867–74, doi:10.1093/carcin/bgh296.*

[9] *Mary Armanios and Elizabeth H. Blackburn, "The Telomere Syndromes," Nature Reviews. Genetics 13, no. 10 (October 2012): 693–704, doi:10.1038/nrg3246.*

[10] *"Partial Reversal of Aging Achieved in Mice," Harvard Gazette, accessed September 2, 2016, http://news.harvard.edu/gazette/story/2010/11/partial-reversal-of-aging-achieved-in-mice/.*

[11] *S. Sayols-Baixeras et al., "Identification and Validation of Seven New Loci Showing Differential DNA Methylation Related to Serum Lipid Profile: An Epigenome-Wide Approach. The REGICOR Study," Human Molecular Genetics, September 15, 2016, doi:10.1093/hmg/ddw285.*

[12] *Gianluca Pegoraro et al., "Aging-Related Chromatin Defects via Loss of the NURD Complex," Nature Cell Biology 11, no. 10 (October 2009): 1261–67, doi:10.1038/ncb1971.*

[13] *Chunyu Jin et al., "Histone Demethylase UTX-1 Regulates C. Elegans Life Span by Targeting the insulin/IGF-1 Signaling Pathway," Cell Metabolism 14, no. 2 (August 3, 2011): 161–72, doi:10.1016/j.cmet.2011.07.001.*

[14] *Ibid.*

[15] *Susmita Kaushik and Ana Maria Cuervo, "Proteostasis and Aging," Nature Medicine 21, no. 12 (December 2015): 1406–15, doi:10.1038/nm.4001.*

[16] *D. E. Feldman and J. Frydman, "Protein Folding in Vivo: The Importance of Molecular Chaperones," Current Opinion in Structural Biology 10, no. 1 (February 2000): 26–33.*

[17] *Stuart K. Calderwood, Ayesha Murshid, and Thomas Prince, "The Shock of Aging: Molecular Chaperones and the Heat Shock Response in Longevity and Aging – A Mini-Review," Gerontology 55, no. 5 (September 2009): 550–58, doi:10.1159/000225957.*

[18] *"Protein Modification and Maintenance Systems as Biomarkers of Ageing," n.d.*

[19] *Ryan Doonan et al., "Against the Oxidative Damage Theory of Aging: Superoxide Dismutases Protect against Oxidative Stress but Have Little or No Effect on Life Span in Caenorhabditis Elegans," Genes & Development 22, no. 23 (December 1, 2008): 3236–41, doi:10.1101/gad.504808.*

[20] *Ana Mesquita et al., "Caloric Restriction or Catalase Inactivation Extends Yeast Chronological Lifespan by Inducing H2O2 and Superoxide Dismutase Activity," Proceedings of the National Academy of Sciences of the United States of America*

107, no. 34 (August 24, 2010): 15123–28, doi:10.1073/pnas.1004432107.

[21] *Michael T. Ryan and Nicholas J. Hoogenraad, "Mitochondrial-Nuclear Communications," Annual Review of Biochemistry 76 (2007): 701–22, doi:10.1146/annurev.biochem.76.052305.091720.*

[22] *Tamara Tchkonia et al., "Cellular Senescence and the Senescent Secretory Phenotype: Therapeutic Opportunities," Journal of Clinical Investigation 123, no. 3 (March 1, 2013): 966–72, doi:10.1172/JCI64098.*

[23] *Chunfang Wang et al., "DNA Damage Response and Cellular Senescence in Tissues of Aging Mice," Aging Cell 8, no. 3 (June 2009): 311–23, doi:10.1111/j.1474-9726.2009.00481.x.*

[24] *Isabel Beerman et al., "Proliferation-Dependent Alterations of the DNA Methylation Landscape Underlie Hematopoietic Stem Cell Aging," Cell Stem Cell 12, no. 4 (April 4, 2013): 413–25, doi:10.1016/j.stem.2013.01.017.*

[25] *Claudia E. Rübe et al., "Accumulation of DNA Damage in Hematopoietic Stem and Progenitor Cells during Human Aging," PLoS ONE 6, no. 3 (March 7, 2011), doi:10.1371/journal.pone.0017487.*

Critical Thinking

1. What if a treatment were available that preserves telomeres by preventing their ability to shorten, prevents cancer, increases life expectancy, and is a relatively inexpensive treatment, how would this treatment affect the social welfare system?

2. Based on your personal family history, does this article explain common disease phenomena among family members?

3. How will knowing the biology of aging affect your health behavior?

Internet References

American Federation for Aging Research
https://www.afar.org/

Digital Aging Atlas
http://ageing-map.org/

Longevity Map
http://genomics.senescence.info/longevity//

HADRIEN VIELLE is an engineer and was trained in biology, physics and bio-engineering at the École Polytechnique féminine in Paris.

Unit 2

UNIT

Prepared by: Elaina Osterbur, *Saint Louis University*

The Quality of Later Life

Although it is true that one ages from the moment of conception to the moment of death, children are usually considered to be "growing and developing," but adults are often thought of as "aging." Having accepted this assumption, most biologists concerned with the problems of aging focus their attention on what happens to individuals after they reach maturity. Moreover, most of the biological and medical research dealing with the aging process focuses on the later part of the mature adult's life cycle. A commonly used definition of senescence is "the changes that occur generally in the post-reproductive period and that result in decreased survival capacity on the part of the individual organism" (B.L. Shrehler, *Time, Cells and Aging*, New York: Academic Press, 1977).

As a person ages, physiological changes take place. The skin loses it elasticity, becomes more pigmented, and bruises more easily. Joints stiffen, and the bone structure becomes less firm. Muscles lose their strength. The respiratory system becomes less efficient. The individual's metabolism changes thus requiring changes in dietary demands. Bowel and bladder movements are more difficult to regulate. Visual acuity diminishes, hearing declines, and the entire system is less able to resist environmental stresses and strains.

Increased medical technologies will probably increase the life expectancy for the 65-and-over population, resulting in longer life for the next generation. Although people 65 years of age today are living only slightly longer than 65-year-olds did in 1900, the quality of their later years has greatly improved. Economically, Social Security and a multitude of private retirement programs have given most older persons a more secure retirement. Physically, many people remain active, mobile, and independent throughout their retirement years. Socially, most older persons are married, involved in community activities, and leading productive lives. Many older adults are able to live independently, live in their own homes, direct their own lives, and involve themselves in activities they enjoy.

Although more people survive till age 65 today, many will live with at least one disabling chronic disease such as diabetes, arthritis, heart disease, effects of stroke, and cancer. These are the most common, costly, and preventable of all health problems according to the Center for Disease Control. The articles in this section attempt to explain how the older adults can improve the quality of their lives with or without chronic disease through nutrition, exercise, creativity, social activity, and other activities that bring happiness and purpose to the lives of older adults.

Article

Prepared by: Elaina Osterbur, *Saint Louis University*

Measuring and Improving Quality of Life in Older Adults with Special Needs

CRYSTAL MCGAHA

Learning Outcomes

After reading this article, you will be able to:

- Define quality of life.
- Understand medical conditions that affect quality of life.
- Identify strategies to improve quality of life.

Quality of life is defined by personal feelings, details, outlook, and day-to-day experiences—how happy and positive one feels, how comfortable and secure, how productive and desired, how healthy and free an individual considers themselves, etc. Professionals in aging must seek to assess quality of life through determination of individual meaning associated with various elements of quality of life, as best as possible. Positive outlook and quality of life in older adults may not always mean an individual is healthy mentally or physically, although positive outlook and presence of hope often encourages improved outcomes.

Physical and mental impairments have been known to significantly decrease quality of life in older adults, as many lose hope, become isolated or depressed, lose faith, and struggle to feel joy in everyday life. When care professionals identify factors such as depression, social isolation, or chronic medical illness in a client, immediate measures should be taken to address what can be done to improve quality of life; interventions to improve comfort level, happiness, social immersion, access to care, resources, support systems, etc., need to be explored.

Absence of hope, loneliness, lack of desire, negative reflection upon life, pessimistic personality, lack of control, and lack of satisfaction often dramatically decrease quality of life. Factors that negatively impact quality of life may include chronic mental and physical diseases, physical, mental, or spiritual decline, emotional setbacks, physical setbacks, inability, loss, negative affectivity, negative or debilitating symptoms, absence of successful intervention, fatigue, pain, fear, depression, absence of attention, absence of love, feeling unwanted, feeling inadequate, feeling unsuccessful, general insecurity, poor self-esteem, obesity, weight loss, etc.

Minute details can make major differences in quality of life and comfort level, such as food selections to meet personal preference and to encourage comfort and well-being; décor to meet personal preference and to encourage happiness and relaxation; spa accessibility (such as hair, skin, nails, and massage) to improve outward appearance, sense of well-being, and happiness; and improvements to overall living environment to promote comfort, healing, and well-being. Professionals in aging can use results from quality of life assessments to identify and target problem areas that damage quality of life, create positive interventions, sustain and encourage positive contributing factors to quality of life, further develop individual sense of purpose, stimulate learning and self-expression, promote dignity, build connection with others, and encourage overall health and well-being.

Beyond formal quality of life assessment, quality of life can be measured through identification of what the "ideal life" consists of in the hearts and minds of the clients you are caring for and making decisions for. Guiding conversation to discover what matters and is important to your clients, identifying what is fulfilling to them, and recognizing areas in which you can build individual self-esteem is important for quality of life improvement. Just as important, if not more important than written questionnaires, verbal communication is a wonderful, effective way to assess quality of life and to determine areas that can be improved upon; the approach to quality of life assessment can and should be individualized, according to personality, ability, and preference.

In assessing quality of life, seek to determine whether or not your client is afraid of anything and attempt to work through their fears with them. Some older adults regularly struggle with feelings of impending doom or fear of the unknown; encouraging communication and exploration of fears while seeking to address fears can improve quality of life. While older adults with physical and mental limitations, chronic illness or disease, and disabilities may not have the same possibilities as other individuals with full capacity, help them to identify what is possible—possibilities beyond their imagination that they *are* capable of. Extending life seems to be a common goal for researchers and medical providers, although just as important, if not more so, researchers and care providers should seek to improve the "life" in those years. Sadly, when quality of life is rapidly declining, many older adults—especially those suffering from chronic pain, physical and mental illness, and disability—do not have the desire to live longer.

Further elements to consider when assessing and seeking to improve quality of life in older adults include sexual health and activity, sleep patterns, dietary habits and nutritional needs, exercise levels and capability, hearing, vision, retirement status, and financial grounding. Dealing with gradual loss of hearing or vision that may occur with age or trauma, for example, can be a very difficult process both physically and emotionally. As an individual experiences gradual loss of ability or sensation in any aspect, regular communication and assistance from loved ones can make a world of difference. Those who experience loss of ability or sensation (in any form) may feel embarrassment, confusion, anxiety, fear, loneliness, etc. Professionals in aging can encourage methods of coping and connect clients with others who are going through some of the same experiences. Equipping clients with stress management tactics and guided techniques for handling stress and coping with depression is important for improved quality of life in older age—in particular, for clients dealing with mentally, emotionally, and physically altering conditions.

Professionals in aging must attempt to recognize unspoken signals, read body language, relate to, and understand clients as they assess quality of life and seek to make positive interventions. For example, not all responses in conversation or through written questionnaires will be truthful and accurate due to uncomfortable subject matter, feelings of embarrassment, hurt, fear, or denial. Professionals in aging must demonstrate sensitivity and the ability to identify specific, individual areas of emotional pain, hurt, fear, discomfort, avoidance, etc. Individual quality of life can be significantly improved when a care professional can effectively identify unspoken, unaddressed areas of need. While older adults with physical and mental limitations, chronic illness or disease, and disabilities may not have the same possibilities as other individuals with full capacity, professionals in aging can help clients to identify what *is* possible and how purpose, meaning, dignity, and fulfillment can be found.

Critical Thinking

1. Discuss professionalism in aging.
2. Discuss strategies to improve quality of life among persons with chronic disease or mental illness.

Internet References

Administration on Intellectual and Developmental Disabilities
   http://www.acl.gov/Programs/AIDD

American Society on Aging
   http://www.asaging.org

National Institute on Aging
   http://www.nia.nih.org

Article

Prepared by: Elaina Osterbur, *Saint Louis University*

Population Health and Older Adults: A Public Health Issue that is Coming of Age

Kathryn Kietzman

Learning Outcomes

After reading this article, you will be able to:

- Identify how public health has improved population health.

- Understand the importance of public health prevention measures that have increased longevity.

The field of public health in the United States has evolved from an industrial era focus on sanitation and housing reforms to today's more comprehensive approach that includes epidemiology, maternal and child health, environmental health, occupational health, and global health. Aging cuts across all 21st century public health concerns including bioterrorism, natural disasters, climate change, and infectious diseases—but has the public health field come of age? While trends suggest the demographic imperative of population aging is finally capturing the attention of policymakers and planners, is it too little, too late?

Public Health Tools Don't Necessarily Reach All Populations

The success of early public health interventions has contributed greatly to reductions in morbidity and premature mortality, in turn, increasing population longevity. These advancements are the result of a range of effectively implemented public health tools, including population surveillance and monitoring, health protection through environmental, occupational, and food safety, health promotion, and disease prevention. But it is important to note that not all older members of our society reap the benefits.

There are notable and egregious disparities in the health and well-being of our aging population. In 2015, the National Academies of Science, Engineering, and Medicine released a disturbing report providing evidence that disparities in life expectancy are increasing in the United States. Between 1980 and 2010, researchers found a 12.7-year difference in life expectancy between the wealthiest and poorest men in our society, with the wealthiest men living to 89, and the poorest living only to 76. Disparities between women were even greater: the wealthiest women lived to 92, while the poorest lived to 78.

These glaring disparities indicate that a 21st century public health response requires increased attention to social determinants of health, including race, ethnicity, gender, and class, which affect health outcomes throughout the life course. As noted by Steven P. Wallace in 2014, such inequities are avoidable and disparities could be reduced by taking a more upstream approach to health care, before the onset of disease or disability. The good news is that our public health delivery system is set up to do just that.

Prevention Efforts Must Include Elders

Public health is rooted in primary, secondary, and tertiary prevention efforts that significantly contribute to increased longevity. Primary prevention aims to prevent injury or disease, through, say, immunizations. Secondary prevention aims to detect and treat an injury or disease early on, slow its progression, or prevent recurrence. Tertiary prevention aims to ease the impact of long-term chronic disease or disability by optimizing function, quality of life, and life expectancy. Yet many disease prevention and health promotion efforts have not been designed to reach the most disadvantaged and vulnerable older adults. And, while investments in younger populations and primary prevention activities are essential to the health of all, additional investments in secondary and tertiary prevention efforts with middle- and older-age populations are crucial.

Chronic disease and disability have tremendous implications for population health—not only for those directly affected but also for those providing care: family caregivers, health and social service professionals, provider systems, and local, state, and federal governments. Consider the prevalence of Alzheimer's disease and other dementias—a public health crisis affecting a sizeable segment of our population and projected to grow exponentially. This disease's trajectory has profound effects on family members. In response, the clarion call for public health now extends beyond the primary prevention of disease, disability, and premature death to include the development and testing of population- and systems-level interventions that have the potential to better manage chronic disease and disability and improve quality of life.

As the implications of population aging become clear, public health professionals are beginning to identify places where public health intersects with aging. Federally Qualified Health Centers, which emerged in the mid-1960s, were intended to ensure that underserved communities would have access to health care and social services. While these safety net providers have traditionally focused on the acute health-care needs of children and young families, many are beginning to respond to the reality that their patients are living longer, with increased disability and multiple chronic conditions.

Another example of public health and aging intersecting is more livable and "age-friendly" communities. We now know Zip Code more accurately predicts health than genetic code. In response, public health is investing heavily in addressing these geographic disparities. Many of these efforts include the concerns of older adults, who benefit from physical environments that facilitate walking and social engagement, through design that accommodates mobility limitations and optimizes access to opportunities for social and civic engagement.

New Narratives Needed

However, the predominant narratives emerging from public health's increased awareness of the significance of population aging tend to skew from one extreme to another. One narrative construes population aging as largely positive—preventive interventions early in life lead to healthy aging and opportunities to contribute to population health and wellness through continued productivity. The opposite narrative portrays aging as a time of increasing deficit and decline—while living longer, we are more likely to be living with multiple chronic conditions and disability, to be a burden to our families and to society, and to become dependent on under-resourced and ill-prepared public programs.

While both are valid constructions for portions of the aging population, most aging adults fall in between. A more nuanced narrative would better help to advance public policy that addresses the needs of an aging population, one in which aging is presented as the "new normal" from which the field of public health can craft a more reasoned response to the diversity inherent in any definition of population aging.

So, does our 21st century reality demand a recalibration, a new definition of public health? Perhaps not. If the principles and the practice of primary, secondary, and tertiary prevention are more fully exploited, and effective interventions are designed to be appropriate for, and accessible to, all segments of the population, we can better serve an aging population and achieve better outcomes. One major hurdle is getting the public health community—and better yet, society at large—to dispel its inherent ageism and embrace the notion of prevention at any age and at every stage. The Leaders of Aging Organizations provides some hope through its recent launch of a robust, long-term effort to examine ageism and reframe the narrative perpetuated by the media, advocacy organizations, experts in aging and the general public.

Another hurdle is getting policymakers and program planners to take a longer view and recognize the payoff that will come from investing resources in multiple stages of prevention across the life course, resulting in reduced rates of morbidity, improved quality of life, and healthier and more productive communities. One important step is the implementation of multisectoral and evidence-based collaboration models, such as Sickness Prevention Achieved through Regional Collaboration (SPARC), that leverage existing community resources to build robust networks organized around specific prevention efforts.

As noted by Lynda Anderson and colleagues, opportunities to address the health and social care needs of an aging population abound, especially through evidence-based community programs that improve function and quality of life. But we still have work to do. Prohaska and colleagues identify a need to increase efforts to translate research about effective interventions into community-based programs. They also recommend additional research that better represents minority and disadvantaged older populations.

With a little tweaking, the tried and true tools of public health should work just fine. We just need to ensure that the tools are appropriate and made accessible to all members of our increasingly diverse aging population.

Critical Thinking

1. Discuss public health initiatives to address population aging.
2. How do policies fit in with an aging population, increased life expectancy, and chronic disease?

Internet References

American Public Health Association
http://www.apha.org

American Society on Aging
http://www.asaging.org

ASA Board member, **KATHRYN G. KIETZMAN**, PhD, MSW, is a research scientist at the UCLA Center for Health Policy Research in Los Angeles.

Unit 3

UNIT

Prepared by: Elaina Osterbur, *Saint Louis University*

Societal Attitudes Toward Old Age

There is a wide range of beliefs regarding the social position and status of aging American's today. Some people believe that the best way to understand the problems of older adults is to regard them as a minority group faced with difficulties similar to those of other minority groups. Discrimination against older people, like racial discrimination, is believed to be based on a bias against visible physical traits. Because the aging process is viewed negatively, it is natural that many older adults may try to appear and act younger. Some spend a tremendous amount of money trying to make themselves look and feel younger so they can blend in more readily with younger adults. Other older adults accept their position in an ageist society.

One theory suggests that older people are a weak minority group. However, this theory is questionable because too many circumstances prove otherwise. The U.S. Congress, for example, favors its senior members and delegates power to them by bestowing considerable prestige on them. Older adults vote and respect their position and rights as American citizens. Furthermore, leadership roles in religious organizations are often held by older persons. Many older Americans are in good health,

have comfortable incomes, and are treated with respect by friends and associates.

Perhaps the most realistic way to view people who are aged is as a status group, like other status groups in society. Every society has some method of "age grading" by which it groups together individuals of roughly similar age. ("Preteens" and "senior citizens" are some of the age-grade labels in U.S. society.) Because it is a labeling process, age grading causes members of the age group to be perceived by themselves as well as others in terms of the connotations of the label. Unfortunately, the tag "old age" often has negative connotations in U.S. society. Many of society's typical assumptions about the limitations of old age have been refuted. A major force behind this reassessment of the elderly is that so many people are living longer and healthier lives, and in consequence, playing more of a role in all aspects of our society. Older people can remain productive members of society for many more years than has been traditionally assumed.

The articles in this section attempt to explain a variety of social attitudes toward older adults such as biases and stereotypes, as well as social and health disparities.

Article   Prepared by: Elaina Osterbur, *Saint Louis University*

Social and Health Disparities in Aging: Gender Inequities in Long-term Care

Our society must learn to value caregiving—or existing health and financial inequities among paid and unpaid caregivers will remain.

NANCY R. HOOYMAN

Learning Outcomes

After reading this article, you will be able to:

- Identify health disparities based on gender.

- Understand the economic value of family caregiving.

- Identify strategies to decrease social and health disparities in aging.

To address escalating health and long-term care costs, the locus of care for older adults and persons with disabilities is shifting from institutional to community-based settings. The Affordable Care Act's (ACA) goals to reduce care costs through decreased hospital admissions and readmissions, emergency room use, and reliance on long-term care facilities rely, to a large extent, upon women's long hours serving as underpaid direct care staff and as unpaid family caregivers. Both the ACA and the 2008 Institute of Medicine report recognize that direct care workers and family caregivers are central members of the eldercare workforce and vital to the quality of long-term services and supports (LTSS) (Institute of Medicine [IOM], 2008).

Formal paid chronic care is the exception, not the rule, with families and direct care staff assuming higher levels of care for longer periods of time than in the past (Feinberg, 2014). More than 80 percent of older adults requiring LTSS are able to live in the community, primarily because of informal assistance by women, who comprise approximately 66 percent of family caregivers and provide more hours than their male counterparts

of the most difficult care tasks (Calasanti, 2009; Family Caregiver Alliance, 2012). Moreover, 90 percent of direct care workers—nursing assistants, home health aides, and personal care aides—are women (Direct Care Alliance, 2012). When women assume primary responsibility for these underpaid and unpaid caring roles, their health and well-being often suffer.

Despite greater attention by policymakers, caregiving remains undervalued in our society, partly because of intersecting inequities experienced by women as caregivers and care recipients; these disparities are reinforced by social institutions of the family (e.g., norms regarding who should provide care) and the labor market (e.g., formal mechanisms such as the Social Security benefit formula) (Calasanti, 2009, 2010). Feminist gerontology recognizes that gender, race, and social class are primary variables upon which individuals' lives pivot, limiting women's choices, whether as caregivers or as care recipients, and predetermining their place in the social order (Cruikshank, 2013; Freixas, Luque, and Reina, 2012).

This article also adds age and disability to these intersecting variables. Calasanti (2009) theorizes that being old in and of itself confers a loss of power, which is exacerbated by illness, disability, race, and gender. Those who care for the old, sick, and disabled (i.e., the powerless) may themselves experience loss of power, status, and respect, resulting in financial and subsequent health disparities across the life course and into old age. From a feminist perspective, it is essential to address the interconnections among women as unpaid and underpaid caregivers and with women as recipients of care. The ways in which these intersections shape women's aging and physical well-being are embedded in our society's undervaluing of paid work.

Gender-based Health Disparities

Calasanti (2010) posits that to theorize about gender gives us a framework for understanding not only why gender differences occur but also why and how they matter. Gender matters in long-term care because of the inequities experienced by women as givers and recipients of care—women who face poorer health status and higher rates of chronic illness in old age than men. Older women experience more non-fatal chronic conditions and higher prevalence of functional limitations, disabilities, and comorbidities than men, and this gender gap is exacerbated as they age (Freixas, Luque, and Reina, 2012). Social determinants of poverty, caregiving, and widowhood—not biology or individual health behaviors—contribute to older women's higher rates of illness and functional impairment (Cruikshank, 2013; Harrington-Meyer and Herd, 2007).

Race intersects with gender; as African American, Latina, and Native American women age, they experience disproportionately higher rates and earlier occurrence than whites of disabling conditions, particularly diabetes, heart disease, hypertension, and certain cancers (Centers for Disease Control and Prevention, 2010; Kerby, 2012). Additionally, inadequate health care and limited access to services earlier in life negatively impact the health of older women of color.

Accordingly, women are the primary LTSS recipients: 73 percent of nursing home residents and 67 percent of home healthcare users. It is estimated that 79 percent of women, compared to 60 percent of men, older than age 65 will need long-term care during their lifetime and on average, for 3.7 years, compared to 2.2 years for men (AARP, 2011). Older women's higher utilization of LTSS is associated at least in part with their lower socioeconomic status and greater likelihood of living alone than men. As the primary recipients of LTSS, older women, typically widowed or divorced, increasingly are cared for in both institutional and community-based settings by underpaid young women of color, many of whom are immigrants, and by unpaid female relatives.

Similarly, women comprise the majority of those covered by Medicare and Medicaid. Women on Medicare have higher rates of illness and spend more on healthcare then men; at the same time, Medicare does not cover what older women with chronic illnesses most need—home- and community-based care (Cruikshank, 2013; Kaiser Family Foundation, 2012). Two-thirds of Medicaid beneficiaries are women, who are disproportionately more likely to be poor, persons of color, in ill health, and have lower educational levels compared to the general population. Not surprisingly, women also form the majority of the dual eligibles, who are poorer and sicker than other populations. Women dependent upon Medicaid rely on clinics and hospital outpatient departments for much of their care, with less access to specialists than their higher income counterparts;

although the ACA's temporary payment increases to primary care providers of Medicaid recipients will partially mitigate this inequity (Kaiser Family Foundation, 2012; Ranji et al., 2013).

To summarize, caregiving's low status in our society perpetuates gender-based health disparities across the life course. Moreover, ageism means that caring for those who are old, sick, or disabled brings neither financial nor status rewards. In short, older women, who are more likely to be of lower income than older men, largely are cared for by young women who are typically low income and low status.

Next, this article examines how the unpaid nature of family care undergirds gender-based health inequities among the givers and receivers of informal care.

Gender Inequities in Family Care

The economic value contributed to our society by family caregivers is estimated to be $450 billion, far more than the total expenditures for formal services; yet their contributions are still largely unsupported, creating a "shadow workforce" in long-term care (Feinberg et al., 2011; Gonyea, 2008). To some extent, this relative invisibility reflects the intersection of gender with age. Caring for older relatives is what one does out of love for someone who is "dependent" (and, therefore, of lower status), and thus not viewed as "real" work to be compensated financially or with status (Calasanti, 2009; Cruikshank, 2013). Although the number of male caregivers is increasing, family caregiver remains a euphemism for one primary caregiver, who typically is female (Gonyea, 2008).

Women predominate not simply because they are more likely to be socialized to be caring. They predominate because of underlying power differentials created by gender-based workforce inequities that create their poorer financial status and resultant low power. When women earn less than men, often in service occupations associated with domestic work, they tend to be viewed as more expendable. They are assumed to be able to give up or cut back on their poorly paid employment to provide care without compensation, an assumption that decisively and permanently affects women in terms of financial and health disparities (Allen, 1993; Calasanti, 2010; Calasanti and Slevin, 2006; Freixas, Luque, and Reina, 2012). When women's responsibility for undervalued family care work limits their paid labor force participation, their earnings and retirement income are lowered, compared to men.

Such inequitable divisions of labor and status—and subsequent lost opportunity costs—shape women's experiences across the life course, resulting in their higher poverty rate in old age. As noted by Malveaux (1993), the economic status of old women is a "map or mirror" of their past lives. Moreover, African American and Latina older women are the poorest groups in our society, reflecting the intersections of age, gender, race, and immigrant status.

Poverty also increases the likelihood of chronic illness and disability. As posited by Freixas and colleagues (2012), poverty and poor quality of life in old age are the price women pay for other people's dependence upon them. Unpaid family care carries health and financial costs. Health problems affect 25 percent to 30 percent of informal caregivers, particularly those who are African American, female, unemployed, middle-aged, and who are providing highest levels of care (Family Caregiver Alliance, 2012; Haley et al., 2010; Schulz and Sherwood, 2008). Poor physical health and low physical stamina are, in turn, associated with increased emotional distress and mental health problems. Women caregivers report higher levels of depression, anxiety, psychiatric symptomatology, and lower life satisfaction than males (Family Caregiver Alliance, 2012; Pinquart and Sorensen, 2006).

Racial inequities typically intensify health disparities. Although findings regarding burden among caregivers of color are mixed, both African American and Latina caregivers tend to experience more physical health problems than whites (Pinquart and Sorenson, 2003, 2005; Weiss et al., 2005). African American caregivers often provide higher levels of care to relatives and friends with multiple illnesses and are more economically disadvantaged than whites. Latinos generally experience greater burden, role, and personal strain, rates of depression, and less positive appraisals and feelings of competence than white or African American caregivers (Cox and Monk, 1996; Dilworth-Anderson, Williams, and Gibson, 2002). Such disparities may be exacerbated by Latinos' high rates of poverty. For immigrants, limited access to insurance and healthcare across the life course exacerbates disparities. If caregivers of color, because of lifetime disadvantage, bring long-term health risks to the caregiving situation, their physical health as caregivers and into old age is likely to be further compromised (Adams et al., 2002; Dilworth-Anderson et al., 2002; Magana, 2006).

Family caregivers and low-income paid staff are interdependent. Women's unpaid caregiving intersects with their underpaid care, and with the line between formal and informal gender-based patterns of care increasingly blurred, the situation results in financial and health costs for both underpaid caregivers and their care recipients.

Gender Inequities: Underpaid Caregivers

Age, race, and gender inequities shape the lives of direct care workers, who comprise the majority of paid (albeit underpaid) caregivers, providing 70 percent to 80 percent of institutional and home-based personal assistance to older adults and persons with disabilities. Direct care staff account for 30 percent of the health-care workforce, more than any other worker category (PHI, 2013). As the "hands, voice, and face" of LTSS, they give "high touch," intimate, personal care primarily to older women. Similar to family caregivers, they are expected to be compassionate hands-on providers of physically and emotionally challenging care, yet often do not feel prepared, respected, or valued (Seavey, 2011).

The intersections of gender, race, and immigration status are reflected in the defining characteristics of direct care workers. Ninety percent are women, typically they are single mothers with minimal education who frequently hold more than one job to survive financially, but who are still living in poverty or near poverty. They struggle to support themselves and their families on a median wage of little more than $10 an hour, well below the $16 an hour wage for all workers. Their earnings are more than 30 percent lower than that of the overall female workforce. Moreover, 50 percent are so poorly paid that they qualify for public assistance, which is essential to supplementing their income. Additionally, their jobs frequently are part time or temporary, with limited or no benefits (Direct Care Alliance, 2012; Seavey, 2011).

Low-income young women of color often provide hands-on care for low-income white older women. Racial inequities, in terms of education and employment opportunities across the life course, partially explain the predominance (51 percent) of African American, Asian, and Latina women among direct care staff, many of whom are immigrants. Foreign-born women comprise 20 percent to 25 percent of the direct care workforce, with the highest rates coming from Mexico, Haiti, Puerto Rico, Jamaica, and the Philippines. Immigrant women are especially vulnerable to financial exploitation when they are paid under the table and when labor laws are not enforced (Hess and Henrici, 2013; Polson, 2013; Stone, 2011).

Our society's failure to value the socially and economically essential work of caregiving is, in turn, reflected in direct care workers' difficult working conditions. These include lack of respect and feeling undervalued by their employers and immediate supervisors; inadequate training and supervision; unpredictable hours; a heavy workload of repetitive tasks; and, risks to personal safety and health from physical work. Workers of color and immigrant women may be treated disrespectfully (e.g., called "girl" or "maid" by older care recipients). And few incentives exist for direct care workers to obtain more training or education (IOM, 2008). Not surprisingly, turnover rates are high—up to 66 percent in some categories in nursing homes and 40 percent to 60 percent in homecare. This "workforce churning" disrupts continuity and quality of care, negatively impacting the physical and mental well-being of the low-income women who provide care and the older women receiving it (Stone, 2011; Wiener et al., 2009).

Direct care workers in 2010 were nearly twice as likely as the overall population to lack health insurance and paid sick days, with less than half having employer-sponsored health insurance and 30 percent without any insurance. Fortunately, the ACA expands insurance to low-income families, but the extent to which direct care workers have obtained such coverage is unclear. While the majority of nursing assistants in skilled nursing facilities are entitled to paid sick leave, only half of home health aides working for agencies receive any sick leave benefit, and even more who work informally lack paid leave (PHI, 2013; Direct Care Alliance, 2012, 2014). Such coverage is crucial because direct care workers have above average rates of chronic conditions, such as diabetes and asthma, which, if untreated, can worsen. The stressful nature of hands-on care also may underlie higher than average rates of depression among personal care workers. High rates of work-related job injuries—sprains, fractures, and chronic injury—also threaten direct care workers' physical and mental well-being. If they are unable to pay for treatment or take time off to recover, healing is slowed and the effects of their illness or injury may be long term.

Lack of paid sick leave affects not only direct care workers and their families but also care recipients who may be put at risk. As noted by a personal care attendant, "I have been caring for people with disabilities for over 24 years. I have never had a paid sick day. I have gone to work sick on too many occasions, once even with pneumonia" (Direct Care Alliance, 2012).

Decades of inequities based on race, class, or gender exact a serious toll on direct care workers' health (Cruikshank, 2013). Low socioeconomic status and the conditions associated with it are more fundamental causes of poor health than individual lifestyle choices. Additionally, poor health threatens the economic resources accumulated over a lifetime. If direct care staff can retire, they enter retirement with a higher likelihood of disability and functional limitations and fewer resources for their own care than those who held higher wage jobs (Cruikshank, 2013; Herd, Robert, and House, 2011).

The intersections between women who are informal and formal caregivers and their care recipients mean that the low societal value placed on caregiving is problematic not only for workers, but also for older adults, family members, and other formal providers of care. Quality of care is diminished when direct care staff morale is low, turnover is high, and labor shortages plague the long-term care system. Adverse work environments faced by their low-income female caregivers most often negatively impact older women, who are the predominant long-term care recipients and often of low income.

Moving Toward Gender Justice

Admittedly, the primary strategy for reducing health disparities and making healthy aging a reality for more women is to eradicate poverty, thereby increasing the income and educational levels of those who are disadvantaged by gender, race,

functional ability, or age (Cruikshank, 2013; Herd, Robert, and House, 2011). Because this is unlikely in the near future, other solutions to reduce financial and health disparities among older women must take into account the power differentials faced by women as unpaid and underpaid caregivers. As long as caregiving is seen as a private duty rather than a service with "public value," the economic disadvantage of women who do this work will continue (Hooyman, 1999). Addressing such inequities within LTSS is central to improving women's well-being across the life course and into old age.

Calasanti (2010) argues that in our market-based society, the way to increase the value of any form of labor is to pay for it, including paying relatives to provide care. Such payment through Medicaid Home- and Community-Based Care often is justified in terms of savings for states or allowing consumer choice, not as a way to support informal caregivers. In contrast, attendant allowances for family caregivers of dependents in Western European countries legitimize the socially essential work of care with public resources. Such allowances are strategies to prevent reduced labor market participation and poverty as outcomes from care provision (Glendinning, 2009). In the United States, modifications in Social Security and other pension systems, such as care credits, are needed to recognize the years spent out of the labor force by many female family caregivers. Similarly, higher wages, guaranteed benefits (including paid sick leave), and opportunities for career advancement are central to reducing direct care workers' poverty, enhancing their health, and ensuring their ability to provide quality LTSS.

Fortunately, the media, policymakers, care providers, and families increasingly are calling for creative solutions to the long-term care dilemma. Caring across Generations, an advocacy group for older adults, people with disabilities, workers, and families, is circulating petitions to put long-term care on the agenda at the 2015 White House Conference on Aging, arguing that, as a society, we must find ways to ensure quality care. The 2014 first White House Summit on Working Families highlighted public- and private-sector options to create a better workplace for all Americans who face dependent care responsibilities. Such national initiatives must make explicit that public supports for women as unpaid and underpaid caregivers are central to the well-being of the givers and receivers of care, and to the quality of LTSS.

Professional organizations, unions, advocates for older adults, and federal and state policy makers must address the gender inequities inherent in how direct care work is structured. Without monetary and other public supports of informal and formal care providers, the well-being of women as caregivers and as older care recipients remains at risk. From a feminist and social justice perspective, caregiving values ultimately must become public rather than individual values divided along economic, racial, and gender lines.

References

AARP. 2011. "Long-term Care: A Women's Issue." www.aarp.org/content/dam/aarp/relationships/caregiving/2011-09/Long-Term-Care-A-Womens-Issue.pdf. Retrieved November 9, 2014.

Adams, B., et al. 2002. "Ethnic and Gender Differences in Distress Among Anglo-American, African American, Japanese American and Mexican American Spousal Caregivers of Persons with Dementia." *Journal of Clinical Geropsychology* 8(4): 279–301.

Allen, J. 1993. "Caring Work and Gender Equity in an Aging Society." In J. Allen and A. Piper, eds., *Women on the Front Line.* Washington, DC: The Urban Institute.

Calasanti, T. 2009. "Theorizing Feminist Gerontology, Sexuality and Beyond: An Intersectional Approach." In V. Bengtson et al., eds., *Handbook of Theories of Aging* (2nd ed.). New York: Springer.

Calasanti, T. 2010. "Gender Relations and Applied Research on Aging." *The Gerontologist* 50(6): 720–34.

Calasanti, T. M., and Slevin, K. F. 2006. *Age Matters: Realigning Feminist Thinking.* New York: Routledge/Taylor and Francis Group.

Centers for Disease Control and Prevention. 2010. "REACH U.S: Finding Solutions to Health Disparities: At a Glance, 2010." www.cdc.gov/chronicdisease/resources/publications/AAG/reach.htm. Retrieved September 15, 2013.

Cox, C., and Monk, A. 1996. "Strain Among Caregivers: Comparing African American and Hispanic Caregivers of Alzheimer's Relatives." *International Ageing and Human Development* 43(2): 93–105.

Cruikshank, M. 2013. *Learning to Be Old: Gender, Culture and Aging* (3rd ed.). New York: Rowman & Littlefield Publishers.

Dilworth-Anderson, P., Williams, I. C., and Gibson, B. E. 2002. "Issues of Race, Ethnicity, and Culture in Caregiving Research: A 20-year Review." *The Gerontologist* 42(2): 237–72.

Direct Care Alliance. 2012. "Fair Pay for Quality Care." www.directcarealliance.org/index.cfm?pageId=538. Retrieved January 2, 2013.

Direct Care Alliance. 2014. "Direct Care Workers Help Lead Movement for Paid Sick Days." http://blog.directcarealliance.org/2012/08/direct-care-workers-help-lead-movement-to-earn-paid-sick-days/. Retrieved June 16, 2014.

Family Caregiver Alliance. 2012. *Fact Sheet: Selected Caregiver Statistics.* San Francisco, CA: Family Caregiver Alliance.

Feinberg, L. F. 2014. "Family Caregiving: There's Nothing Informal About It." http://blog.aarp.org. Retrieved May 1, 2014.

Feinberg, L. F., et al. 2011. *Valuing the Invaluable: 2011 Update—The Growing Contributions and Costs of Family Caregiving.* Washington, DC: AARP Public Policy Institute.

Freixas, A., Luque, B., and Reina, A. 2012. "Critical Feminist Gerontology: In the Back Room of Research." *Journal of Women & Aging* 24(16): 44–58.

Glendinning, C. 2009. "Cash for Care: Implications for Carers." *Geneva Association of Health and Aging Newsletter* 21: 3–6.

Gonyea, J. 2008. "Foreword: America's Aging Workforce: A Critical Business Issue." *Journal of Workplace Behavioral Health* 23(1/2): 1–14.

Haley, W. E., et al. 2010. "Caregiving Strain and Estimated Risk for Stroke and Coronary Heart Disease Among Spousal Caregivers." *Stroke* 41(2): 331–6.

Harrington-Meyer, M., and Herd, P. 2007. *Market Friendly or Family Friendly? The State and Gender Inequality in Old Age.* New York: Russell Sage.

Herd, P., Robert, S. A., and House, J. S. 2011. "Health Disparities Among Older Adults: Life Course Influences and Policy Solutions." In R. H. Binstock and L. K. George, eds., *Handbook of Aging and the Social Sciences.* Amsterdam: Elsevier.

Hess, C., and Henrici, J. M., 2013. *Increasing Pathways to Legal Status for Immigrant In-Home Care Workers.* Washington, DC: Institute for Women's Policy Research.

Hooyman, N. 1999. "Research on Older Women: Where Is Feminism?" *The Gerontologist* 39(1): 115–18.

Institute of Medicine (IOM). 2008. *Retooling for an Aging America: Building the Health Care Workforce.* Washington, DC: The National Academies Press.

Kaiser Family Foundation. 2012. "Medicaid's Role for Women Across the Lifespan: Current Issues and the Impact of the Affordable Care Act." http://kff.org/healthreform/issue-brief/health-reform-implications-for-womens-accessto-2/. Retrieved June 16, 2014.

Kerby, S. 2012. "The State of Women of Color in the United States." http://americanprogress.org/issues/race/report/2012/07/17/11923/the-state-of-women-of-color-in-the-united-states/. Retrieved June 17, 2014.

Magana, S. 2006. "Older Latino Family Caregivers." In B. Berkman, ed., *Handbook of Social Work in Health and Aging.* New York: Oxford University Press.

Malveaux, J. 1993. "Race, Poverty and Women's Aging." In J. Allen and J. Pifer, eds., *Women on the Front Lines.* Washington, DC: The Urban Institute.

PHI. 2013. *FACTS 3: America's Direct Care Workforce.* http://phinational.org/fact-sheets/facts-3-americas-direct-care-work force. Retrieved June 16, 2014.

Pinquart, M., and Sorenson, S. 2003. "Differences Between Caregivers and Non-caregivers in Psychological Health and Physical Health: A Meta-analysis." *Psychology & Aging* 18(2): 250–67.

Pinquart, M., and Sorensen, S. 2006. "Gender Differences in Caregiver Stressors, Social Resources, and Health: An Updated Meta-analysis." *Journals of Gerontology, Series B: Psychological Sciences and Social Sciences* 61(1): 33–45.

Polson, D. 2013. *By Our Sides: The Vital Work of Immigrant Direct Care Workers.* Washington, DC: The Direct Care Alliance.

Ranji, U., et al. 2013. "The Role of Medicaid and Medicare in Women's Health Care." *Journal of the American Medical Association* 309(19): 1984.

Schulz, R., and Sherwood, P. R. 2008. "Physical and Mental Health Effects of Family Caregiving." *Journal of Social Work Education* 44(3): 105–13.

Seavey, D. 2011. "Caregivers on the Front Line: Building a Better Direct Care Workforce." *Generations* 34(4): 27–35.

Stone, R. I. 2011. "Long-Term-Care Policy: Yesterday, Today, and Tomorrow." Testimony presented at Aging in America: Future Challenges, Promise and Potential Forum convened by the Senate Special Committee on Aging, Washington, DC. http://aging.senate.gov/events/hr241rs.pdf. Retrieved February 12, 2014.

Weiss, C., et al. 2005. "Differences in the Amount of Informal Care Received by Non-Hispanic Whites and Latinos in a Nationally Representative Sample of Older Americans." *Journal of the American Geriatrics Society* 53(1): 146–51.

Wiener, J. M., et al. 2009. "Why Do They Stay? Job Tenure Among Certified Nursing Assistants in Nursing Homes." *The Gerontologist* 49(2): 198–210.

Critical Thinking

1. What are the demographics of both formal and informal caregivers?
2. Discuss both the physical and emotional burden of caregiving.
3. Discuss potential support systems for both male and female family caregivers.

Internet References

AARP
http://www.aarp.org
Family Caregiver Alliance
http://www.caregiver.org

NANCY R. HOOYMAN, MSW, PhD, holds the Hooyman Professor of Gerontology and is dean emeritus at the University of Washington School of Social Work in Seattle.

Article

Prepared by: Elaina Osterbur, *Saint Louis University*

The Public Policies We Need to Redress Ageism

ROBERT B. BLANCATO AND MEREDITH PONDER

Learning Outcomes

After reading this article, you will be able to:

- Define ageism.
- Offer solutions to ageist problems.

In our nation, not every person will be a victim of racism. Not every person will be a victim of sexism. However, virtually everyone will have the chance to be a victim of ageism. Now that the youngest baby boomer has reached age 50 and the oldest is about to reach age 70, leading by 2030 to a doubling of our aging population, we need to reexamine federal policies and programs through the lens of ageism. Some programs, including those whose milestone anniversaries we celebrate in 2015, were developed for a different group of older adults than exist today. Adapting to changing times, instead of working off of old stereotypes about older adults, is critical to their success.

Areas of concern include the chronic shortage of providers trained in geriatric care, the caregiving challenge of grandparents raising grandchildren, ageism that exists in Social Security policies, access to benefits, elder justice, employment discrimination, and the digital divide.

This article explores current policies that may help to foster ageism and offers solutions that could potentially end ageism in America.

Ageism Abounds: The Realities, Some Solutions

In this year, we celebrate the anniversaries of Medicare, Medicaid, and the Older Americans Act, all of which have improved the quality of life for older Americans. Though these programs have been largely successful for older Americans, ageism issues remain within health care, and should be redressed.

An important trend that shows promise is ongoing efforts to rebalance how federal health-care funds are directed. The trend in recent years has been away from institutional care (where fewer than 5 percent of older persons live) to home- and community-based care (Administration for Community Living, 2015). If this trend is to continue and expand, it would show we recognize that remaining at home and in the community for as long as possible is key to an older person's quality of life.

There is an element of ageism in the failure of any comprehensive federal response to America's growing caregiving/caregiver challenge. First, it is time to update the Family and Medical Leave Act to allow benefits to help those caring for an older relative. This otherwise progressive law is behind the times. However, older adults also can be caregivers. Today, nearly 5 million grandparents are providing primary care to grandchildren (Makin, 2014). Yet they receive only 10 percent of the funds from the sole federal program that specifically helps family caregivers—the National Family Caregiver Support Program in the Older Americans Act (Butts, 2010). This translates into roughly $15 million a year. These grandparents' circumstances are unique, and they deserve more federal support. Ignoring the realities of caregiving provided by and for older adults is discriminatory.

Our nation also must adopt a long-term care policy to address the largest unfunded liability of the Baby Boom Generation as they age. According to the Associated Press–NORC Center for Public Affairs Research, about half of Americans older than age 40 believe "almost everyone" is likely to require long-term care as they age, but only about 25 percent believe they will fall into that category (Kane, 2013). In reality, 70 percent of Americans older than age 65 will need some form of long-term care (Kane, 2013). This denial of the need for care is largely why there is no real funding for long-term care. To further deny the need for a comprehensive public–private partnership in long-term care is to perpetuate ageism—denial of growing old is ageist.

Greater attention than ever before is being focused on end-of-life decisions and care. We must ensure that policies respect the wishes of older persons. Medicare should provide reimbursements for end-of-life consultations with patients, and the Centers for Medicare & Medicaid Services (CMS) has proposed a new rule that would reimburse physicians for time spent with Medicare beneficiaries discussing advance-care planning (Belluck, 2015). Practices such as providing unwanted medical treatment must cease, and those who do not respect the wishes of beneficiaries should be sanctioned.

Other emerging health priorities to redress ageism should include having more older persons involved in research studies, when appropriate. We should also ensure that electronic health records are accessible and understandable to older adults. Further, we should fully fund the **Brain Research through Advancing Innovative Neurotechnologies (BRAIN) Initiative**, as proposed in 2013 by President Obama, to invest more in brain health as people age.

Finally, as America ages, we should recognize that geriatric health-care needs are distinct and warrant special training. We are entering our fourth decade with an acute shortage of health-care personnel trained in geriatrics. The impact on the quality of healthcare to older adults is real, and to perpetuate this further constitutes a distinct form of ageism.

More Ageism: Issues of Economic (In)Security

Social Security has succeeded in keeping millions of older adults out of poverty. However, this is a "double jeopardy" program with long-standing ageist and sexist policies. The benefit disparity between men and women has to disappear in the future. According to the Social Security Administration, a typical working woman receives $800 to $900 in benefits per month when she retires, but the typical man receives $1,500 per month (Caplinger, 2014). One way to lower this disparity would be to allow women to continue to earn credits when they leave the paid labor force to care for family members of any age.

A law enacted by Congress in 1983 included a provision to raise the retirement age to age 67 over an extended period of time. This policy did not take into account that certain older adults, especially minorities and those with lower average incomes, have shorter life expectancies.

According to the Centers for Disease Control and Prevention (Cook, 2015), the average African American man lives five years less than the average white man. The average man with lower income lives almost six years less than the average man with higher income (Waldron, 2007). Discussions continue about a further increase in the retirement age for the future. We must resist such an increase because it could result in fewer years of benefits for individuals who may need them the most.

Before many older adults become eligible for Social Security, they can encounter age-based discrimination in the workplace. Among the top categories of discrimination addressed by the federal Equal Employment Opportunity Commission each year is age discrimination, making up almost 25 percent of their caseload (U.S. Equal Employment Opportunity Commission, 2015). People who are working, but not provided with updated training for advancement, are victims of age discrimination.

Older adults who want to work but are unable to get jobs also are victims of discrimination. A recent AARP study showed that older workers during the current recession and recovery period suffered the longest duration of unemployment and, when they returned to the workforce, it was to jobs with much lower pay (Koenig, Trawinski, and Rix, 2015). Also, an increase in the minimum wage must be adopted for all workers, including (and especially) older workers.

We should be alarmed at the rising rate of hunger, food insecurity, and malnutrition among older adults, and seek solutions tailored to this constituency. Since 2001, the number of food insecure older adults has doubled, rising from 2.3 million to 4.8 million, according to the National Council on Aging (2015). In 2012, one in five older adults living with grandchildren was food insecure (National Council on Aging, 2015). Federal policies of the future must be more age conscious in offering solutions to this alarming trend.

One of the most insidious forms of ageism is the failure of older persons who qualify for federal benefits to obtain them. This often affects the most vulnerable older adults. It has long been estimated that less than 1/3 of those older adults who are eligible for the Supplemental Nutrition Assistance Program (SNAP) receive this benefit (National Council on Aging, 2015). Better access to benefit programs is a positive sign to help redress this form of ageism, and must be expanded in the future.

Congressional (In)Action

In recent years, Congress's inaction on two initiatives important to older adults may be indicative of ageism. The first is the failure to renew the Older Americans Act, the only comprehensive federal program specifically for those ages 60 and older. On July 16, 2015, the Senate unanimously approved S.192, the Older Americans Act Reauthorization Act of 2015, a three-year reauthorization bill, but the House has taken no action this Congress, despite the fact that the Older Americans Act is five years late in being renewed. The Act is a proven program that operates in virtually all congressional districts and has a proud history. The trend in Washington, however, is to elect new members of the House who have no history with, or knowledge of, these programs. One solution is for advocates to educate their Representatives about this program, how it benefits older people, and how it saves Medicaid and Medicare real dollars.

The second is the failure to fund the Elder Justice Act of 2010. This landmark law represented the most comprehensive federal response to the problem of elder abuse, which affects one out of every ten people older than age 60. By contrast, in 1974, child abuse legislation was enacted, and in the 1980s and 1990s, family violence acts and the Violence Against Women Act were enacted; all have received hundreds of millions of dollars in funding each year (Laney, 2010). After five years, the Elder Justice Act has received one direct appropriation of $4 million (Elder Justice Coalition, 2014). This could be a reflection of ageism in either not accepting—or denying— the fact that elder abuse exists. Preventing abuse, neglect, and exploitation should be advocated across the life span, but today, elder abuse is the final frontier, which policymakers cannot seem to get to.

Other Issues and Challenges

We must have a national strategy to promote aging in place, as this is the preference of so many older adults. We need to accelerate federal support for accessible housing and transportation, and revisions in the tax code, to incentivize aging in place. The ability to develop and implement a national aging in place strategy will do much to redress ageism at the local level—keeping older adults visible and active in the community is important to keeping them front and center in policy making.

The very real digital divide and the extent to which it includes older adults must be seen as ageist. Those in the divide often are the poorest and most vulnerable, unable to access technology. However, they often are most in need of the information and services the Internet provides—they may be in rural areas or homebound and socially isolated, they may need to sign up for benefits, and they may need to bank online or manage their Social Security accounts now that field offices are closing. We cannot be swayed to inaction by false stereotypes that older adults lack technological knowledge and therefore choose not to provide access. The Federal Communications Commission is working to modernize the Lifeline program, which currently pays a small monthly subsidy to low-income consumers to help them pay for telephone service (Federal Communications Commission, 2015). This must be modified to allow these consumers to pay for broadband Internet access with Lifeline funds.

Last, but as critical as anything else, is to make sure all future federal policies for older adults recognize that cultural competency must be at the core of how programs and services are conceived, developed, and delivered. One in three older persons in 2030 will be minorities (Administration for Community Living, 2015), and our society has growing numbers of LGBT older adults who face "triple jeopardy" discrimination challenges (age, race, and sexual orientation) unless policies to prevent this are adopted.

Conclusion

In this historic year, as we celebrate many anniversaries and have held the sixth White House Conference on Aging, it is fitting to confront ageism in a real way. President Obama, though he did not address ageism by name in his address to the Conference, highlighted some of the key policy points necessary for its redress, such as an emphasis on retirement security and on elder justice. However, his pinpointing of ageism by name would have been noteworthy and, in fact, no one at the Conference mentioned this topic. Advocates who work on behalf of older adults must add combating ageism to their agendas as the overarching issue it is.

Because politics and policies intersect, let us be vigilant in not allowing ageism to creep into the 2016 presidential race. Already some attacks against Hillary Clinton have ageist overtones, with code words and phrases such as "we need a new generation," "let's not go back to tired ideas of the past," etc. As voters and advocates for older adults, we cannot let any candidate from either side run a negative ageist campaign. We must be citizen watchdogs on this.

The older adults of today and tomorrow are the engines that will drive our economy and social capital of the future. The actions we take today and tomorrow are critical, as the population of those ages 65 and older is larger than at any time in history. A national advocacy agenda of the future must include the recognition that ageism exists and policies and programs must be evaluated from the context of reducing or furthering ageism. Changes that are proposed can either be small and incremental, or large and landmark in scope. We are a nation built on opportunity and progress. Ageism represses both and thus must be addressed for us to be a better society for all.

References

Administration for Community Living. 2015. **Profile of Older Americans 2013: Future Growth**. Retrieved April 14, 2015.

Belluck, P. 2015. "**Medicare Plans to Pay Doctors for Counseling on End of Life**." *The New York Times,* July 8. Retrieved July 22, 2015.

Butts, D. 2010. "**Written Testimony to the House Ways and Means Committee, Subcommittee on Human Resources**." Retrieved June 12, 2015.

Caplinger, D. 2014. "**Social Security Benefits: The Striking Gap Between Women and Men**." Retrieved April 14, 2015.

Cook, L. 2015. "**Why Black Americans Die Younger**." Retrieved April 14, 2015.

Elder Justice Coalition. 2014. "**EJC Hails Final Passage of Elder Justice Funding Bill**." Retrieved April 14, 2015.

Federal Communications Commission. 2015. "**Lifeline Program for Low-income Consumers**." Retrieved June 12, 2015.

Kane, J. 2013. "**Americans Seriously Unprepared for Long-term Care, Survey Finds**." Retrieved June 12, 2015.

Koenig, G., Trawinski, L., and Rix, S. 2015. "**The Long Road Back: Struggling to Find Work After Unemployment**." *AARP Public Policy Institute Future of Work @50+, Insight on the Issues.* Retrieved April 14, 2015.

Laney, G. 2010. "**Violence Against Women Act: History and Federal Funding**." Retrieved June 12, 2015.

Makin, C. 2014. "**More Grandparents Raising their Grandkids**." *USA Today*, July 27. Retrieved April 14, 2015.

National Council on Aging. 2015. "**Facts about SNAP and Senior Hunger**." Retrieved April 14, 2015.

U.S. Equal Employment Opportunity Commission. 2015. "**Charge Statistics**." Retrieved April 14, 2015.

Waldron, H. 2007. "**Trends in Mortality Differentials and Life Expectancy for Male Social Security–Covered Workers, by Average Relative Earnings**." Retrieved July 22, 2015.

Critical Thinking

1. Discuss how federal programs currently address ageism.
2. What other federal policies need to redress ageism aside from the ones mentioned in the article?

Internet References

American Society on Aging
http://www.asaging.org

National Council on Aging
http://www.ncoa.org

ROBERT B. BLANCATO, MPA, is president of Matz, Blancato, & Associates in Washington, DC.

MEREDITH PONDER, JD, is a senior associate at Matz, Blancato, & Associates.

Health Disparities among Lesbian, Gay, and Bisexual Older Adults by Karen Fredriksen-Goldsen et al.

51

Article

Prepared by: Elaina Osterbur, *Saint Louis University*

Health Disparities among Lesbian, Gay, and Bisexual Older Adults: Results from a Population-Based Study

KAREN I. FREDRIKSEN-GOLDSEN, ET AL.

Learning Outcomes

After reading this article, you will be able to:

- Discuss the health outcomes of lesbian, gay, and bisexual older adults.

- Identify the health disparities among lesbian, gay, and bisexual older adults.

- Identify the methods to learn more about the health needs in the lesbian, gay, and bisexual communities.

Changing demographics will make population aging a defining feature of the 21st century. Not only is the population older, it is becoming increasingly diverse.[1] Existing research illustrates that older adults from socially and economically disadvantaged populations are at high risk of poor health and premature death.[2] A commitment of the National Institutes of Health is to reduce and eliminate health disparities,[3] which have been defined as differences in health outcomes for communities that have encountered systematic obstacles to health as a result of social, economic, and environmental disadvantage.[4]

Social determinants of health disparities among older adults include age, race/ethnicity, and socioeconomic status.[5] Centers for Disease Control and Prevention (CDC) and *Healthy People* 2020 identify health disparities related to sexual orientation as one of the main gaps in current health research.[6] The Institute of Medicine identifies lesbian, gay, and bisexual (LGB) older adults as a population whose health needs are understudied.[7]

The institute has called for population-based studies to better assess the impact of background characteristics such as age on health outcomes among LGB adults. A review of 25 years of literature on LGB aging found that health research is glaringly sparse for this population and that most aging-related studies have used small, non-population-based samples.[8]

Several important studies have begun to document health disparities by sexual orientation in population-based data and have revealed important differences in health between LGB adults and their heterosexual counterparts, including higher risks of poor mental health, smoking, and limitations in activities.[9,10] Studies have found higher rates of excessive drinking among lesbians and bisexual women[9,10] and higher rates of obesity among lesbians[10,11] than among heterosexual women; bisexual men and women are at higher risk of limited health care access than are heterosexuals. In addition, important subgroup differences in health are beginning to be documented among LGB adults. For example, bisexual women are at higher risk than lesbians for mental distress and poor general health.[12] A primary limitation of most existing population-based research is a failure to identify the specific health needs of LGB older adults. Most studies to date address the health needs of LGB adults aged 18 years and older[9] or those younger than 65 years.[10] This lack of attention to older adult health leaves unclear whether disparities diminish or persist or even become more pronounced in later life.

A few studies have begun to examine health disparities among LGB adults aged 50 years and older.[13,14] Wallace et al. analyzed data from the California Health Interview Survey and found that LGB adults aged 50 to 70 years report higher rates of mental distress, physical limitations, and poor general health than do their heterosexual counterparts. The researchers also found that older gay and bisexual men report higher rates of hypertension and diabetes than do heterosexual men.[14] To better address the needs of an increasingly diverse older adult population and to develop responsive interventions and public health policies, health disparities research is needed for this at-risk group.

Examining to what extent sexual orientation is related to health disparities among LGB older adults is a first step toward developing a more comprehensive understanding of their health and aging needs. We analyzed population-based data from the Washington State Behavioral Risk Factor Surveillance System (WA-BRFSS) to compare lesbians and bisexual women and gay and bisexual men with their heterosexual counterparts aged 50 years and older on key health indicators: outcomes, chronic conditions, access to care, behaviors, and screening. We also compared subgroups to identify differences in health disparities by sexual orientation among LGB older adults.

Methods

The BRFSS is an annual random-digit-dialed telephone survey of noninstitutionalized adults conducted by each US state. Each year, disproportionate stratified random sampling is used to select eligible households, and from each selected household 1 adult is randomly selected as the respondent.[15] Washington State began including a measure of sexual orientation in 2003. We aggregated the WA-BRFSS data collected from 2003 to 2010 for respondents aged 50 years and older (n = 96 992) and stratified by gender for further analyses. We selected 50 years as the lower age limit to be consistent with previous health studies focusing on sexual minority older adults,[13,14] as well as research addressing specific chronic health conditions[16,17] and older adult health and well-being, such as the Health and Retirement Study and other population-based studies.[18–20] Annual response rates to the WA-BRFSS range from 43% to 50%, calculated according to Council of American Survey and Research Organizations methods.[21] To adjust for unequal probabilities of selection resulting from nonresponse, sample design, and households without telephones, we applied sample weights provided by the WA-BRFSS.

According to weighted estimation, among women aged 50 years and older (n = 58 319), 1.03% (n = 562) identified as lesbian and 0.54% (n = 291) as bisexual; among men aged 50 years and older (n = 37 820), 1.28% (n = 463) identified as gay and 0.51% (n = 215) as bisexual. The age range in the sample for LGB older adults was 50 to 98 years (50–94 years for women and 50–98 years for men).

Measures

To measure sexual orientation, survey respondents were asked to select 1 of the following: heterosexual or straight, homosexual (gay or lesbian), bisexual, or something else. About 0.2% (n = 266) of the sample selected something else, and we excluded them from our analyses.

The background characteristics in this study were as follows: age, household income ($\leq$ 200% vs > 200% of the federal poverty level), education ($\leq$ high school vs $\geq$ some college), employment (part time or full time vs other), race/ethnicity (non-Hispanic White vs other), living arrangement (living alone vs other), and number of children in household. We categorized relationship status as married versus partnered (a member of an unmarried couple) versus other (divorced, widowed, separated, or never married).

Health outcomes (recommended and validated by CDC) in our study were poor physical health, disability, and poor mental health.[22] We defined poor physical health as 14 or more days of poor physical health during the previous 30 days and poor mental health as 14 or more days of poor mental health during the previous 30 days.[22] We defined disability as limitations in any activities because of physical, mental, or emotional problems or any health problem that required the use of special equipment, as recommended by *Healthy People 2020.*[4]

The BRFSS asked respondents whether they had ever been told by a health professional they had arthritis, asthma, diabetes (not included if prediabetes or gestational diabetes alone), high blood pressure (not included if borderline or during pregnancy alone), or high cholesterol. As recommended by other health studies, we designated cardiovascular disease (CVD) as diagnosis by a physician of a heart attack, angina, or stroke.[23,24] We defined obesity as a body mass index score (defined as weight in kilograms divided by height in meters squared) of 30 or higher, as recommended by CDC.[25] The BRFSS measured health care access by asking whether respondents had insurance coverage, a personal doctor or provider, or a financial barrier to seeing a doctor in the past 12 months.

Health behaviors were (1) current smoking (defined, as suggested by CDC, as having ever smoked $\geq$ 100 cigarettes and currently smoking every day or some days),[26] (2) excessive drinking (defined, as suggested by National Institute of Alcohol Abuse and Alcoholism, as women having $\geq$ 4 and men having $\geq$ 5 drinks on 1 occasion during the past month),[27] and (3) physical activity (defined, as suggested by the US Department of Health and Human Services, as $\geq$ 30 minutes of moderate-intensity activity $\geq$ 5 days/week or $\geq$ 20 minutes of vigorous-intensity activity $\geq$ 3 days/week).[28] The BRFSS measured health screening, according to public health guidelines for older adults, by whether respondents received a flu shot in the past year,[29] an HIV test ever, a mammogram (for women) in the past 2 years,[30] and a prostate-specific antigen test (for men) in the past year.[31]

Statistical Analysis

We conducted analyses separately by gender. First, we described the weighted distribution of background characteristics by sexual orientation, comparing lesbians and bisexual women with heterosexual women aged 50 years and older and gay and bisexual men with heterosexual men aged 50 years and older, applying t tests or χ^2 tests as appropriate. We also tested statistical significance of differences in background characteristics between lesbians and bisexual women and between gay and bisexual men.

We then estimated weighted prevalence rates of health indicators, which were health outcomes, chronic conditions, access to care, behaviors, and screening, by sexual orientation (lesbian and bisexual vs heterosexual women; gay and bisexual vs heterosexual men). We conducted a series of adjusted logistic regressions, with control for sociodemographic characteristics (age, income, and education), to test associations between health-related indicators and sexual orientation. We also conducted adjusted logistic regression analyses to examine health disparities between lesbian and bisexual women and between gay and bisexual men. We used Stata version 11 (StataCorp LP, College Station, TX) for data analyses.

Results

Table 1 illustrates the weighted prevalence of background characteristics by sexual orientation among older adults. Lesbians and bisexual women were younger, had more education, and had higher rates of employment than did heterosexual women; income levels were similar. Lesbians and bisexual women were less likely to be married and more likely to be partnered than were their heterosexual counterparts, but the average number of children in the household and the likelihood of living alone were similar. Lesbians were more likely than bisexual women to be employed ($P = .019$) and less likely to be married, but more likely to be partnered ($P < .001$). We found no differences in other background characteristics.

Table 1 Background Characteristics of Respondents Aged 50 Years and Older, by Sexual Orientation: Washington State Behavioral Risk Factor Surveillance System, 2003–2010

	Women				Men			
		Lesbian and Bisexual				Gay and Bisexual		
Characteristic	Heterosexual, % or Mean (SD)	Total, % or Mean (SD)	Lesbian, % or Mean (SD)	Bisexual, % or Mean (SD)	Heterosexual, % or Mean (SD)	Total, % or Mean (SD)	Gay, % or Mean (SD)	Bisexual, % or Mean (SD)
Age, y	63.82 (0.06)	58.63*** (0.37)	58.09 (0.40)	59.67 (0.78)	62.35 (0.07)	59.54*** (0.39)	59.26 (0.45)	60.22 (0.75)
≤ 200% poverty level	27.38	27.12	26.47	28.43	20.85	24.79	25.45	23.18
≤ high school	30.18	13.44***	13.83	12.69	24.96	14.57***	12.34	20.09
Employed	39.97	59.31***	63.07	52.08	51.17	55.30	55.25	55.43
Non-Hispanic White	91.79	90.31	89.86	91.23	90.40	93.22*	92.85	94.18
Relationship status								
Married	61.67	20.15***	9.57	40.44	77.60	20.83***	8.16	52.07
Partnered	1.59	27.83	36.96	10.31	1.50	20.27	27.30	2.96
Other	36.74	52.02	53.47	49.25	20.90	58.90	64.55	44.97
Children in household, no.	0.15 (0.00)	0.20 (0.04)	0.18 (0.05)	0.24 (0.06)	0.22 (0.00)	0.07*** (0.02)	0.03 (0.01)	0.15 (0.05)
Living alone	26.24	29.43	29.65	28.99	15.15	38.34***	40.66	32.59

Note. Estimates were weighted; significance tests were conducted to examine the association between background characteristics and sexual orientation (lesbians and bisexual women vs heterosexual women; gay and bisexual men vs heterosexual men).

*P < .05; ***P < .001.

Gay and bisexual men were significantly younger and more highly educated than were heterosexual men; income levels and employment rates were similar. Gay and bisexual men were less likely than heterosexual men to be married but more likely to be partnered; they also had fewer children in the household, were more likely to live alone, and were more likely to be non-Hispanic Whites. Gay men had more education ($P = .037$), were less likely to be married and more likely to be partnered ($P < .001$), and had fewer children in the household ($P = .017$) than did bisexual men.

Health Outcomes

Lesbians and bisexual women had higher odds than heterosexual women for disability (adjusted odds ratio [AOR] = 1.47) and poor mental health (AOR = 1.40), but not for poor physical health, after adjustment for age, income, and education (Table 2). Lesbians and bisexual women had similar rates of poor physical health, disability, and poor mental health.

In adjusted analyses, gay and bisexual men were more likely than heterosexual men to have poor physical health (AOR = 1.38), disability (AOR = 1.26), and poor mental health (AOR = 1.77). Although the unadjusted prevalence rates of disability were similar between sexual minority and heterosexual men, the analyses with adjustment for sociodemographic characteristics showed that gay and bisexual men were more likely than their heterosexual counterparts to have a disability. We did not observe differences in health outcomes between gay and bisexual men.

Chronic Conditions

Lesbians and bisexual women had greater adjusted odds of obesity (AOR = 1.42) relative to heterosexual women. Unadjusted odds of CVD were similar for sexual minority and heterosexual women, but after adjustment for sociodemographic characteristics, lesbians and bisexual women had significantly greater risk (AOR = 1.37). The unadjusted odds of asthma for lesbians and bisexual women were significantly higher than for heterosexual women, but the difference did not remain significant when the analyses adjusted for sociodemographic differences. We observed no significant differences in chronic conditions between lesbians and bisexual women in the adjusted analyses.

Gay and bisexual men had significantly lower odds of obesity than did heterosexual men (AOR = 0.72), after adjustment for sociodemographic factors. The unadjusted odds of asthma for gay and bisexual men were higher than for heterosexual men (OR = 1.41), but the difference did not remain significant after

Table 2   Weighted Prevalence Rates and Regression Analyses of Health Outcomes and Chronic Conditions among Respondents Aged 50 Years and Older: Washington State Behavioral Risk Factor Surveillance System, 2003–2010

	Women				Men			
	Heterosexual,	Lesbian and Bisexual			Heterosexual,	Gay and Bisexual		
Health Outcomes/ Conditions	%	%	OR (95% CI)	AOR (95% CI)	%	%	OR (95% CI)	AOR (95% CI)
Frequent poor physical health	15.47	15.79	1.02 (0.81, 1.30)	1.02 (0.80, 1.30)	12.88	16.79	1.36* (1.05, 1.78)	1.38* (1.04, 1.83)
Disability	36.87	44.27	1.36** (1.14, 1.62)	1.47*** (1.22, 1.77)	33.96	38.27	1.21 (0.98, 1.48)	1.26* (1.02, 1.56)
Frequent poor mental health	9.36	15.92	1.83*** (1.42, 2.37)	1.40* (1.07, 1.81)	6.88	13.09	2.04*** (1.51, 2.76)	1.77** (1.28, 2.45)
Obesity	25.93	36.27	1.63*** (1.36, 1.95)	1.42*** (1.18, 1.71)	27.07	22.57	0.79* (0.62, 0.99)	0.72* (0.56, 0.93)
Arthritis[a]	52.24	53.70	1.06 (0.83, 1.36)	1.29 (0.99, 1.67)	39.25	41.85	1.11 (0.84, 1.48)	1.19 (0.89, 1.60)
Asthma	15.89	20.57	1.37** (1.10, 1.70)	1.20 (0.96, 1.49)	11.56	15.52	1.41* (1.07, 1.85)	1.28 (0.95, 1.71)
Diabetes	11.87	13.59	1.17 (0.91, 1.51)	1.25 (0.96, 1.64)	13.96	12.44	0.88 (0.66, 1.17)	0.92 (0.67, 1.25)
High blood pressure[b]	43.33	36.02	0.74 (0.54, 1.00)	0.86 (0.62, 1.20)	44.35	40.59	0.86 (0.61, 1.21)	0.88 (0.61, 1.26)
High cholesterol[a]	47.13	44.10	0.88 (0.69, 1.14)	1.00 (0.77, 1.30)	50.21	51.66	1.06 (0.79, 1.42)	1.08 (0.80, 1.46)
Cardiovascular disease[c]	10.71	10.51	0.98 (0.73, 1.31)	1.37* (1.00, 1.86)	16.49	14.11	0.83 (0.62, 1.12)	1.04 (0.76, 1.43)

Note. AOR = adjusted odds ratio; CI = confidence interval; OR = odds ratio. Adjusted logistic regression models controlled for age, income, and education; heterosexuals were coded as the reference group.
[a]Questions were asked in 2003, 2005, 2007, and 2009.
[b]Question was asked in 2003, 2005, and 2009.
[c]Questions were asked in 2004 through 2010.
*$P < .05$; **$P < .01$; ***$P < .001$.

adjustment. The adjusted odds of diabetes were significantly higher for bisexual men (19.74%) than for gay men (9.50%; AOR = 2.33; $P < .01$). We detected no other significant differences in chronic conditions between gay and bisexual men.

Access to Care

As shown in Table 3, although we found no significant difference in the prevalence of having a health care provider, lesbians and bisexual women were less likely than heterosexual women to have health insurance coverage and more likely to experience financial barriers to health care. These differences, however, did not remain significant after adjustment for sociodemographic characteristics. We detected no significant differences in health care access indicators between lesbians and bisexual women.

In the unadjusted analyses, gay and bisexual men were less likely than heterosexual men to have health insurance coverage, but the difference did not remain significant after adjustment. No significant differences appeared in the indicators of health care access between gay and bisexual men.

Health Behaviors

Prevalence rates of physical activity were similar among all female respondents, but lesbians and bisexual women were more likely than heterosexual women to smoke (AOR = 1.57) and to drink excessively (AOR = 1.43; Table 3). Lesbians (9.95%) were significantly more likely than bisexual women (3.90%; AOR = 0.40) to drink excessively ($P < .05$).

Gay and bisexual men had higher adjusted odds of smoking (AOR = 1.52) and excessive drinking (AOR = 1.47) than did heterosexual men; prevalence rates of physical activities were similar. We observed no differences in health behaviors between gay and bisexual men.

Health Screening

Sexual minority women were significantly less likely than heterosexual women to have had a mammogram (AOR = 0.71), more likely to have been tested for HIV (AOR = 1.80), and equally likely to have received a flu shot. We observed no

Table 3 Weighted Prevalence Rates and Regression Analyses of Health Indicators among Respondents Aged 50 Years and Older: Washington State Behavioral Risk Factor Surveillance System, 2003–2010

| | | Women | | | | Men | | |
| | | Lesbian and Bisexual | | | | Gay and Bisexual | | |
Health Indicator	Heterosexual, %	%	OR (95% CI)	AOR (95% CI)	Heterosexual, %	%	OR (95% CI)	AOR (95% CI)
Access to care								
Insurance	94.56	91.24	0.60*** (0.44, 0.82)	0.79 (0.55, 1.13)	93.36	89.42	0.60** (0.43, 0.84)	0.71 (0.48, 1.04)
Financial barrier	8.26	13.05	1.67*** (1.29, 2.16)	1.25 (0.97, 1.62)	6.81	8.43	1.26 (0.86, 1.84)	0.97 (0.63, 1.50)
Personal provider	92.41	93.09	1.11 (0.76, 1.60)	1.43 (0.97, 2.11)	88.57	88.41	0.98 (0.73, 1.33)	1.16 (0.84, 1.60)
Behavior								
Smoking	11.61	18.33	1.71*** (1.36, 2.15)	1.57*** (1.22, 2.00)	13.15	20.04	1.66*** (1.30, 2.11)	1.52** (1.18, 1.96)
Excessive drinking	4.61	7.88	1.77** (1.27, 2.47)	1.43* (1.02, 2.00)	11.12	17.13	1.65** (1.24, 2.20)	1.47* (1.09, 1.98)
Physical activity[a]	49.02	51.92	1.12 (0.88, 1.01)	1.01 (0.78, 1.31)	51.23	53.04	1.08 (0.81, 1.43)	1.04 (0.78, 1.40)
Screening								
Flu shot	55.07	52.99	0.92 (0.77, 1.10)	1.20 (1.00, 1.44)	50.40	54.87	1.20 (0.98, 1.46)	1.47*** (1.18, 1.82)
Mammogram[b]	79.77	74.16	0.73* (0.54, 0.98)	0.71* (0.52, 0.97)	...	...	...	...
PSA test[b]	...	...	...	...	49.85	40.67	0.69* (0.51, 0.93)	0.81 (0.59, 1.10)
HIV test[c]	23.89	40.80	2.20*** (1.79, 2.70)	1.80*** (1.46, 2.23)	28.31	76.47	8.23*** (6.22, 10.88)	7.91*** (5.94, 10.54)

Note. AOR = adjusted odds ratio; CI = confidence interval; OR = odds ratio; PSA = prostate-specific antigen. Adjusted logistic regression models controlled for age, income, and education; heterosexuals were coded as the reference group.

[a]Questions were asked in 2003, 2005, 2007, and 2009.
[b]Questions were asked in 2004, 2006, and 2008.
[c]Question was asked only of those younger than 65 years.
*$P < .05$; **$P < .01$; ***$P < .001$.

significant differences in health screenings between older lesbians and bisexual women.

The adjusted analyses indicated that gay and bisexual men were more likely than heterosexual men to have received a flu shot (AOR = 1.47) and an HIV test (AOR = 7.91). In the initial analyses, sexual minority men were significantly less likely than heterosexual men to receive a prostate-specific antigen test, but the difference was not significant after adjustment for sociodemographic characteristics. Although we found no significant differences between gay and bisexual men in the prevalence of receiving a flu shot or a prostate-specific antigen test, bisexual men (60.33%) were less likely than gay men (82.59%) to have been tested for HIV (AOR = 0.31; $P < .001$).

Discussion

We conducted one of the first studies to comprehensively examine leading CDC-defined health indicators among LGB older adults in population-based data. Contrary to the myth that older adults will not reveal their sexual orientation in public health surveys, in this population-based survey we found that approximately 2% of adults aged 50 years and older self-identified as lesbian, gay, or bisexual. The findings reveal significant health disparities among LGB older adults, with both strengths and gaps across the continuum of health indicators examined. Our results suggest that some health disparity patterns that have been found in LGB adults at younger ages[9,10] persist in later life, including higher likelihoods of disability, poor mental health, and smoking, and, among lesbians and bisexual women, excessive drinking and obesity. We also found some health disparities—heightened risks of CVD among lesbian and bisexual women and of poor physical health and excessive drinking among gay and bisexual men—that may emerge later in the life course. Such health disparities likely have detrimental consequences for the quality of life of these LGB older adults.[14,32,33]

According to the life course perspective, social context, cultural meaning, and structural location (in addition to time, period, and cohort) affect aging processes, including health.[34,35] Situating LGB older adults within the historical and social context of their lives may help us to better understand the health issues they face as they age.[36] LGB older adults came of age during a time when same-sex relationships were criminalized and severely stigmatized and same-sex identities were socially invisible.

Elevated risks of disability and poor mental health among LGB older adults may be linked with experiences of stigmatization[37-39] and victimization,[39;41] especially in light of the profound impact that events at a given stage of life can have on subsequent stages.[42] The social contexts in which they have lived may have exposed LGB older adults to multiple types of victimization and discrimination related to sexual orientation,

disability, age, gender, and race/ethnicity.[41] D'Augelli and Grossman, for example, argue that lifetime experiences of victimization among sexual minority older adults because of their sexual orientation affects mental health in later life.[40] The evidence of physiological impact of chronic stressors on health[43] suggests that lifetime experiences of victimization may partially account for higher rates of disability among LGB older adults. Although our study was designed to identify health disparities among LGB older adults, further research is needed to compare LGB age cohorts and health changes over time.

Heightened risks of disability and poor physical and mental health among older gay and bisexual men may also be related to HIV.[44] Lacking information on HIV status in our data set, we could not explore this issue, but the disparity may be related to the prevalence of HIV among gay and bisexual men. With the advances in antiretroviral therapies, more adults with HIV are living into old age,[45,46] and older adults living with HIV have been found to be at increased risk of disability and poor physical and mental health.

Elevated risks of smoking and excessive drinking are of major concern among LGB older adults. Although smoking and excessive drinking are leading causes of preventable morbidity and mortality,[47] most prevention campaigns target only younger populations.[48,49] Intervention strategies that both identify and address distinctive cultural factors that may promote smoking and drinking among LGB older adults are desperately needed. Previous research has found that LGB adults smoke at much higher rates than their heterosexual counterparts,[9,10,50] and our findings illustrate that such disparities persist among LGB older adults. We also found that older sexual minority women were more likely than older heterosexual women to drink excessively, which has also been documented in studies of younger sexual minority women.[9,10,50]

Existing research documents that drinking rates decline with age among older adults in general.[51] Although the prevalence rates of excessive drinking among younger gay, bisexual, and heterosexual adult men were similar in other population-based studies, we found higher rates among older gay and bisexual than heterosexual men. It may be that the rate of decline in drinking among older gay and bisexual men is slower than among older heterosexual men.[52] In addition, we found that older lesbians had higher rates of excessive drinking than did older bisexual women, which is also inconsistent with reports from population-based studies of younger lesbian and bisexual women.[10,50] A longitudinal study is warranted to better understand such changes in drinking behavior patterns among sexual minorities, and it will be important to examine how earlier experiences, such as frequent attendance at bars, clubs, and private house parties,[53] combined with minority stressors such as discrimination and victimization,[54] influence changes in drinking patterns over time among LGB older adults.

Older lesbians and bisexual women were more likely than their heterosexual counterparts to be obese and to have CVD; older gay and bisexual men were less likely than heterosexuals to be obese. The higher prevalence of obesity among lesbians and bisexual women than heterosexual women is well documented,[55] but increased risk of CVD has rarely been reported.[56] According to Conron et al., lesbian and bisexual adults may have a higher risk of CVD, possibly attributable to higher prevalence of obesity and smoking.[10] It is likely that disparities in obesity and smoking in early life influence disparities in CVD in later life among lesbians and bisexual women.[57,58]

Our subgroup analyses revealed that diabetes was more common in older bisexual than gay men, even though the obesity rates for the 2 groups were similar. The association between type 2 diabetes and obesity is well known.[59] Although previous studies found that among young adults, gay men were less likely to be obese than were heterosexual men, bisexual men were not.[10] Additional research is needed to investigate whether it is the duration of obesity among older bisexual men that increases their risk of diabetes,[60] as well as to further explore weight change and its impact on older gay men.

We observed some positive trends in preventive screenings, such as the higher likelihood of receiving a flu shot and an HIV test for gay and bisexual than for heterosexual men. Lesbians and bisexual women were more likely than their heterosexual peers to receive an HIV test. Yet we also found evidence of gaps and missed opportunities for prevention. For example, among sexual minority older men, bisexual men were less likely than gay men to obtain an HIV test. Older lesbians and bisexual women were less likely than heterosexual women to report having had a mammogram. Efforts to promote mammography screening among older lesbians and bisexual women is particularly important, because higher risks of breast cancer have been documented among sexual minority women, attributable to elevated prevalence of obesity, substance use, and nulliparity.[61–63] Hart and Bowen suggest that lack of knowledge regarding breast cancer and the benefits of mammography combined with reluctance to use health services because of stigma likely prevent lesbians and bisexual women from receiving mammography in a timely manner.[64]

We observed several important differences in background characteristics by sexual orientation. Contrary to existing stereotypes, despite higher levels of education among LGB older adults, and the higher likelihood of employment among lesbians and bisexual women, LGB older adults do not have higher incomes than do heterosexuals, as observed in other population-based data.[65] In addition, LGB older adults are less likely than heterosexuals to be married but more likely to be partnered, which may have implications for health care advocacy, caregiving, and the availability of financial resources as they age. A recent study found that for gay men, being legally married is

associated with mental health benefits.[38] Older gay and bisexual men have significantly fewer children in the household than do heterosexuals and are more likely to live alone, which corroborates findings in other population-based studies.[14] Higher rates of living alone may be related to the increased likelihood of the loss of a partner to AIDS.[66] It is also possible that structural factors do not support committed relationships or legal marriage among same-sex partners. LGB older adults who live alone are likely at risk for social isolation, which has been linked to poor mental and physical health, cognitive impairment, and premature morbidity and mortality in the general elderly population.[67]

Limitations

The cross-sectional nature of BRFSS data limits the ability to disentangle the temporal relationships between variables of interest. Although the purpose of the BRFSS is monitoring overall prevalence of health status, chronic conditions, and behaviors in the United States, and the measures are based on self-report, objective information such as symptoms and severity of health conditions is not available. We analyzed BRFSS data from only 1 state, limiting applicability to other state populations.

Our findings were limited with respect to the response rate of the BRFSS[68,69] and the self-identification of sexual orientation. The proportion of the older population that self-identified as sexual minorities in our data (~ 2%) was less than the 3.5% of adults aged 18 years and older who self-identified as LGB in most other population-based studies.[70] This may reflect the historical context in which today's LGB older adults came of age; these cohorts may be less likely than younger age groups to identify themselves as a sexual minority in a telephone-based survey.

Conclusions

More research with a life-course perspective is needed to examine how age and cohort effects may differentiate the experiences of younger and older LGB adults. Studies that examine the interplay between resilience and the stressors associated with aging and living as a sexual minority would likely help us better understand the mechanisms through which social contexts directly and indirectly affect the health of LGB older adults. Further research, especially a longitudinal study of health among LGB older adults that directly tests the relationships between transitions and trajectories through the life course and investigates the role of human agency in adapting to structural and legal constraints, would provide a greater understanding of how life experiences and shifting social contexts affect health outcomes in later life. Because LGB older adults may rely less on partners, spouses, and children, future research needs to investigate how differing types of social networks, support, and family structures influence health and aging experiences.[71] Although the sample size in our data did not allow for direct comparisons across different birth cohorts of LGB older adults, they are needed. The oldest-old LGB population, for example, may have experienced greater challenges in disclosing their sexual orientation; they may also have faced more barriers to social resources affecting health outcomes.

Our findings document population-based health disparities among LGB older adults. Early detection and identification of factors associated with such at-risk groups will enable public health initiatives to expand the reach of strategies and interventions to promote healthy communities. It is imperative that we understand the health needs of older sexual minorities in general as well as those specific to subgroups in this population to develop effective preventive interventions and services tailored to their unique needs. It is imperative that we begin to address healthy aging in our increasingly diverse society.

Human Participant Protection

The institutional review board of the University of Washington approved this study.

References

1. Vincent GA, Velkoff VA. *The Next Four Decades, The Older Population in the United States: 2010 to 2050.* Washington, DC: US Census Bureau; 2010.

2. Centers for Disease Control and Prevention, Merck Company Foundation. The state of aging and health in America. 2007. Available at: www.cdc.gov/aging/pdf/saha_2007.pdf. Accessed October 26, 2011.

3. *Biennial Report of the Director, National Institutes of Health, Fiscal Years 2008 & 2009.* Washington, DC: National Institutes of Health; 2010.

4. Disparities. HealthyPeople.gov. Available at: www. healthypeople.gov/2020/about/disparitiesAbout.aspx#six. Accessed October 26, 2011.

5. MacArthur Foundation Research Network on an Aging Society. Facts and fictions about an aging America. *Contexts.* 2009;8(4):16–21.

6. Truman BI, Smith KC, Roy K, et al. Rationale for regular reporting on health disparities and inequalities—United States. *MMWR Suveill Summ.* 2011;60(suppl):3–10.

7. Institute of Medicine. *The Health of Lesbian, Gay, Bisexual, and Transgender People: Building a Foundation for Better Understanding.* Washington, DC: National Academies Press; 2011.

8. Fredriksen-Goldsen KI, Muraco A. Aging and sexual orientation: a 25-year review of the literature. *Res Aging.* 2010;32(3):372–413.

9. Dilley JA, Simmons KW, Boysun MJ, Pizacani BA, Stark MJ. Demonstrating the importance and feasibility of including sexual orientation in public health surveys: health disparities in the Pacific Northwest. *Am J Public Health.* 2010;100(3):460–467.

10. Conron KJ, Mimiaga MJ, Landers SJ. A population-based study of sexual orientation identity and gender differences in adult health. *Am J Public Health.* 2010;100(10):1953–1960.

11. Boehmer U, Bowen DJ, Bauer GR. Overweight and obesity in sexual-minority women: evidence from population-based data. *Am J Public Health.* 2007;97(6):1134–1140.

12. Fredriksen-Goldsen KI, Kim H-J, Barkan SE, Balsam KF, Mincer S. Disparities in health-related quality of life: a comparison of lesbian and bisexual women. *Am J Public Health.* 2010;100(11):2255–2261.

13. Valanis BG, Bowen DJ, Bassford T, Whitlock E, Charney P, Carter RA. Sexual orientation and health: comparisons in the Women's Health Initiative sample. *Arch Fam Med.* 2000;9(9):843–853.

14. Wallace SP, Cochran SD, Durazo EM, Ford CL. *The Health of Aging Lesbian, Gay and Bisexual Adults in California.* Los Angeles: University of California, Los Angeles Center for Health Policy Research; 2011.

15. Centers for Disease Control and Prevention. Behavioral Risk Factor Surveillance System operational and user's guide. Available at: ftp://ftp.cdc.gov/pub/Data/Brfss/userguide.pdf. Accessed July 10, 2012.

16. Levin B, Lieberman DA, McFarland B, et al. Screening and surveillance for the early detection of colorectal cancer and adenomatous polyps, 2008: a joint guideline from the American Cancer Society, the US Multi-Society Task Force on Colorectal Cancer, and the American College of Radiology. *CA Cancer J Clin.* 2008;58(3):130–160.

17. AgePage. Menopause. National Institute on Aging. Available at: www.nia.nih.gov/healthinformation/publications/menopause .htm. Accessed June, 24, 2011.

18. Alexander CM, Landsman PB, Teutsch SM, Haffner SM, Third National Health and Nutrition Examination Survey (NHANES III), National Cholesterol Education Program (NCEP). NCEP-defined metabolic syndrome, diabetes, and prevalence of coronary heart disease among NHANES III participants age 50 years and older. *Diabetes.* 2003;52(5):1210–1214.

19. Office of Applied Studies. *The NSDUH Report—Serious Psychological Distress Among Adults Aged 50 or Older: 2005 and 2006.* Rockville, MD: Substance Abuse and Mental Health Services Administration; 2008.

20. Bowen ME, González HM. Racial/ethnic differences in the relationship between the use of health care services and functional disability: the health and retirement study (1992–2004). *Gerontologist.* 2008;48(5):659–667.

21. 2003–2010 Behavioral Risk Factor Surveillance System summary data quality reports. Centers for Disease Control and Prevention. Available at: www.cdc.gov/brfss/annual_data/ annual_data.htm#2001. Accessed July 10, 2012.

22. *Measuring Healthy Days.* Atlanta, GA: Centers for Disease Control and Prevention; 2000.

23. Fan AZ, Strine TW, Jiles R, Berry JT, Mokdad AH. Psychological distress, use of rehabilitation services, and disability status among noninstitutionalized US adults aged 35 years and older, who have cardiovascular conditions, 2007. *Int J Public Health. 2009;*54(suppl 1):100–105.

24. Shankar A, Syamala S, Kalidindi S. Insufficient rest or sleep and its relation to cardiovascular disease, diabetes and obesity in a national, multiethnic sample. *PLoS ONE.* 2010;5(11):e14189.

25. Overweight and obesity: defining overweight and obesity. Centers for Disease Control and Prevention. Available at: www.cdc.gov/obesity/defining.html. Accessed April 10, 2012.

26. Centers for Disease Control and Prevention. Vital signs: current cigarette smoking among adults aged ≥ 18 years–United States, 2005–2010. *MMWR Morb Mortal Wkly Rep.* 2011;60(35):1207–1212.

27. National Institute of Alcohol Abuse and Alcoholism. NIAAA council approves definition of binge drinking. *NIAAA Newsletter.* 2004;3:3.

28. Objectives 22-2 and 22-3. *Healthy People 2010* (conference ed, 2 vols). Washington, DC: US Department of Health and Human Services; 2000.

29. Key facts about seasonal flu vaccine. Centers for Disease Control and Prevention. Available at: www.cdc.gov/flu/protect/keyfacts.htm. Accessed December 13, 2011.

30. National Cancer Institute fact sheet: mammograms. National Cancer Institute. Available at: www.cancer.gov/cancertopics/factsheet/detection/mammograms. Accessed December 13, 2011.

31. National Cancer Institute fact sheet: prostate-specific antigen (PSA) test. National Cancer Institute. Available at: www.cancer.gov/cancertopics/factsheet/detection/PSA. Accessed December 13, 2011.

32. Fried LP, Guralnik JM. Disability in older adults: evidence regarding significance, etiology, and risk. *J Am Geriatr Soc.* 1997;45(1):92–100.

33. Fredriksen-Goldsen KI, Kim H-J, Emlet CA, et al. The aging and health report: disparities and resilience among lesbian, gay, bisexual, and transgender older adults. 2011 Available at: http://caringandaging.org. Accessed December 13, 2011.

34. Mayer KU. New directions in life course research. *Annu Rev Sociol.* 2009;35:413–433.

35. Elder GH., Jr. Time, human agency, and social change: perspectives on the life course. *Soc Psychol Q.* 1994;57(1):4–15.

36. Clunis DM, Fredriksen-Goldsen KI, Freeman PA, Nystrom N. *Lives of Lesbian Elders: Looking Back, Looking Forward.* Binghamton, NY: Haworth Press; 2005.

37. Meyer IH. Prejudice, social stress, and mental health in lesbian, gay, and bisexual populations: conceptual issues and research evidence. *Psychol Bull.* 2003;129(5):674–697.

38. Wight RG, LeBlanc AJ, de Vries B, Detels R. Stress and mental health among midlife and older gay-identified men. *Am J Public Health.* 2012;102(3):503–510.

39. Fredriksen-Goldsen KI, Emlet CA, Kim HJ, et al. The physical and mental health of lesbian, gay male, and bisexual (LGB) older adults: the role of key health indicators and risk and protective factors. *Gerontologist.* Epub ahead of print October 3, 2012.

40. D'Augelli AR, Grossman AH. Disclosure of sexual orientation, victimization, and mental health among lesbian, gay, and bisexual older adults. *J Interpers Violence.* 2001;16(10):1008–1027.

41. Fredriksen-Goldsen KI, Kim H-J, Muraco A, Mincer S. Chronically ill midlife and older lesbians, gay men, and bisexuals and their informal caregivers: the impact of the social context. *Sex Res Social Policy.* 2009;6(4):52–64.

42. Marmot MG, Wilkinson RG. *Social Determinants of Health.* 2nd ed. New York, NY: Oxford University Press; 2006.

43. Juster RP, McEwen BS, Lupien SJ. Allostatic load biomarkers of chronic stress and impact on health and cognition. *Neurosci Biobehav Rev.* 2010;35(1):2–16.

44. Jia H, Uphold CR, Zheng Y, et al. A further investigation of health-related quality of life over time among men with HIV infection in the HAART era. *Qual Life Res.* 2007;16(6):961–968.

45. Justice AC. HIV and aging: time for a new paradigm. *Curr HIV/AIDS Rep.* 2010;7(2):69–76.

46. Brennan DJ, Emlet CA, Eady A. HIV, sexual health, and psychosocial issues among older adults living with HIV in North America. *Ageing Int.* 2011;36(3):313–333.

47. Center for Substance Abuse Treatment. *Substance Abuse Among Older Adults.* Rockville, MD: Substance Abuse and Mental Health Services Administration; 1998. Treatment Improvement Protocol (TIP) Series 26.

48. Backinger CL, Fagan P, Matthews E, Grana R. Adolescent and young adult tobacco prevention and cessation: current status and future directions. *Tob Control.* 2003;12(suppl 4):iv46–iv53.

49. Wakefield MA, Loken B, Hornik RC. Use of mass media campaigns to change health behaviour. *Lancet.* 2010;376(9748): 1261–1271.

50. Burgard SA, Cochran SD, Mays VM. Alcohol and tobacco use patterns among heterosexually and homosexually experienced California women. *Drug Alcohol Depend.* 2005;77(1):61–70.

51. Kanny D, Liu Y, Brewer RD. Centers for Disease Control and Prevention. Binge drinking–United States, 2009. *MMWR Surveill Summ.* 2011;60(suppl):101–104.

52. Green KE, Feinstein BA. Substance use in lesbian, gay, and bisexual populations: an update on empirical research and implications for treatment. *Psychol Addict Behav.* 2012;26(2):265–278.

53. Trocki KF, Drabble L, Midanik L. Use of heavier drinking contexts among heterosexuals, homosexuals and bisexuals: results from a National Household Probability Survey. *J Stud Alcohol.* 2005;66(1):105–110.

54. Brubaker MD, Garrett MT, Dew BJ. Examining the relationship between internalized heterosexism and substance abuse among lesbian, gay, and bisexual individuals: a critical review. *J LGBT Issues Couns.* 2009;3(1):62–89.

55. Bowen DJ, Balsam KF, Ender SR. A review of obesity issues in sexual minority women. *Obesity (Silver Spring)* 2008;16(2):221–228.

56. Roberts SA, Dibble SL, Nussey B, Casey K. Cardiovascular disease risk in lesbian women. *Womens Health Issues.* 2003;13(4):167–174.

57. Hubert HB, Feinleib M, McNamara PM, Castelli WP. Obesity as an independent risk factor for cardiovascular disease: a 26-year follow-up of participants in the Framingham Heart Study. *Circulation.* 1983;67(5):968–977.

58. He J, Ogden LG, Bazzano LA, Vupputuri S, Loria C, Whelton PK. Risk factors for congestive heart failure in US men and women: NHANES I epidemiologic follow-up study. *Arch Intern Med.* 2001;161(7):996–1002.

59. Nguyen NT, Nguyen XM, Lane J, Wang P. Relationship between obesity and diabetes in a US adult population: findings from the National Health and Nutrition Examination Survey, 1999–2006. *Obes Surg.* 2011;21(3):351–355.

60. Lee JM, Gebremariam A, Vijan S, Gurney JG. Excess body mass index-years, a measure of degree and duration of excess weight, and risk for incident diabetes. *Arch Pediatr Adolesc Med.* 2012;166(1):42–48.

61. Case P, Austin SB, Hunter DJ, et al. Sexual orientation, health risk factors, and physical functioning in the Nurses' Health Study II. *J Womens Health (Larchmt)* 2004;13(9):1033–1047.

62. Cochran SD, Mays VM, Bowen D, et al. Cancerrelated risk indicators and preventive screening behaviors among lesbians and bisexual women. *Am J Public Health.* 2001;91(4):591–597.

63. Dibble SL, Roberts SA, Nussey B. Comparing breast cancer risk between lesbians and their heterosexual sisters. *Womens Health Issues.* 2004;14(2):60–68.

64. Hart SL, Bowen DJ. Sexual orientation and intentions to obtain breast cancer screening. *J Womens Health (Larchmt)* 2009;18(2):177–185.

65. Albelda R, Badgett MVL, Schneebaum A, Gates GJ. *Poverty in the Lesbian, Gay, and Bisexual Community.* Los Angeles, CA: Williams Institute; 2009.

66. Cochran SD, Mays V, Corliss H, Smith TW, Turner J. Self-reported altruistic and reciprocal behaviors among homosexually and heterosexually experienced adults: implications for HIV/AIDS service organizations. *AIDS Care.* 2009;21(6):675–682.

67. Cornwell EY, Waite LJ. Measuring social isolation among older adults using multiple indicators from the NSHAP Study. *J Gerontol B Psychol Sci Soc Sci.* 2009;64B(suppl 1):i38–i46.

68. Schneider KL, Clark MA, Rakowski W, Lapane KL. Evaluating the impact of non-response bias in the Behavioral Risk Factor Surveillance System (BRFSS). *J Epidemiol Community Health.* 2012;66(4):290–295.

69. Keeter S, Kennedy C, Dimock M, Best J, Craighill P. Gauging the impact of growing nonresponse on estimates from a national RDD telephone survey. *Public Opin Q.* 2006;70(5):759–779.

70. Gates GJ. *How Many People Are Lesbian, Gay, Bisexual, and Transgender?* Los Angeles, CA: Williams Institute; 2011.

71. Muraco A, Fredriksen-Goldsen K. "That's what friends do": informal caregiving for chronically ill lesbian, gay, and bisexual elders. *J Soc Pers Relat.* 2011;28(8):1073–1092.

Critical Thinking

1. Do you think that the attitudes of professionals and others influence service delivery to the lesbian, gay, and bisexual population?

2. How do you think some of the gaps in health disparities can be closed, or even shortened?

Internet References

The LGBT Aging Project
www.lgbtagingproject.org

National Resource Center on LGBT Aging
www.lgbtagingcenter.org

KAREN I. FREDRIKSEN-GOLDSEN, HYUN-JUN KIM, SUSAN E. BARKAN, AND CHARLES P. HOY-ELLIS are with the School of Social Work, University of Washington, Seattle. ANNA MURACO is with the Department of Sociology, Loyola Marymount University, Los Angeles.

Fredriksen-Goldsen, Karen et al., From *American Journal of Public Health*, October 2013, pp. 1802–1809. Copyright ©2013 by American Public Health Association. Reprinted by permission via Sheridan Reprints.

Article   Prepared by: Elaina Osterbur, *Saint Louis University*

Attitudes about Aging: A Global Perspective

In a Rapidly Graying World, Japanese Are Worried, Americans Aren't

PEW RESEARCH CENTER

Learning Outcomes

After reading this article, you will be able to:

- Explain why America is less worried about the increase in the aging population than Japan.

- Understand the impact of aging in a population.

- Identify the impact of fertility rates globally.

Overview

At a time when the global population of people ages 65 and older is expected to triple to 1.5 billion by mid-century, public opinion on whether the growing number of older people is a problem varies dramatically around the world, according to a Pew Research Center survey.

Concern peaks in East Asia, where nearly nine-in-ten Japanese, eight-in-ten South Koreans and seven-in-ten Chinese describe aging as a major problem for their country. Europeans also display a relatively high level of concern with aging, with more than half of the public in Germany and Spain saying that it is a major problem. Americans are among the least concerned, with only one-in-four expressing this opinion.

These attitudes track the pattern of aging itself around the world. In Japan and South Korea, the majorities of the populations are projected to be older than 50 by 2050. China is one of most rapidly aging countries in the world. Germany and Spain, along with their European neighbors, are already among the countries with the oldest populations today, and their populations will only get older in the future. The U.S. population

is also expected to get older, but at a slower rate than in most other countries.

Public concern with the growing number of older people is lower outside of East Asia and Europe. In most of these countries, such as Indonesia and Egypt, the proportion of older people in the population is relatively moderate and is expected to remain so in the future.

Pakistan, Nigeria and other countries potentially stand to benefit from future demographic trends. These are countries that currently have large shares of children in their populations, and these children will age into the prime of their work lives in the future.

The Pew Research survey also finds a wide divergence in people's confidence that they will have an adequate standard of living in their old age. Confidence in one's standard of living in old age appears to be related to the rate at which a country is aging and its economic vitality. Confidence is lowest in Japan, Italy and Russia, countries that are aging and where economic growth has been anemic in recent years. In these three countries, less than one-third of people are confident about their old-age standard of living. Meanwhile, there is considerable optimism about the old-age standard of living among the public in countries whose populations are projected to be relatively young in the future or that have done well economically in recent years, such as in Nigeria, Kenya, South Africa and China.

When asked who should bear the greatest responsibility for the economic well-being of the elderly—their families, the government or the elderly themselves—the government tops the list in 13 of the 21 countries that were surveyed. However, many who name the government are less confident in their own standard of living in old age compared with those who name themselves or their families.

Rarely do people see retirement expenses as mainly a personal obligation. In only four countries—South Korea, the U.S., Germany and Britain—do more than one-third of the public say that the primary responsibility for the economic well-being of people in their old age rests with the elderly themselves.

American public opinion on aging differs dramatically from the views of the nation's major economic and political partners. Americans are less likely than most of the global public to view the growing number of older people as a major problem. They are more confident than Europeans that they will have an adequate standard of living in their old age. And the U.S. is one of very few countries where a large plurality of the public believes individuals are primarily responsible for their own well-being in old age.

This is not because the U.S. is perennially young. American baby boomers are aging, and one-in-five U.S. residents are expected to be 65 and older by mid-century, greater than the share of seniors in the population of Florida today.[1] It is also projected that the share of people 65 and older in the U.S. will eclipse the share of children younger than 15 by 2050.

But the U.S. is aging less rapidly than most of the other countries. In 2010, the global median age (29) was eight years lower than the U.S. median age (37).[2] By 2050, the difference in age is projected to narrow to only five years. Also, driven by immigration, the U.S. population is expected to increase by 89 million by mid-century even as the populations of Japan, China, South Korea, Germany, Russia, Italy and Spain are either at a standstill or decreasing. For these reasons, perhaps, the American public is more sanguine than most about aging.

The aging of populations does raise concerns at many levels for governments around the world. There is concern over the possibility that a shrinking proportion of working-age people (ages 15 to 64) in the population may lead to an economic slowdown. The smaller working-age populations must also support growing numbers of older dependents, possibly creating financial stress for social insurance systems and dimming the economic outlook for the elderly.

Graying populations will also fuel demands for changes in public investments, such as the reallocation of resources from the needs of children to the needs of seniors. At the more personal level, longer life spans may strain household finances, cause people to extend their working lives or rearrange family structures.[3] Perhaps not surprisingly, an aging China announced a relaxation of its one-child policy in November 2013.

This study reports on the findings from a Pew Research Center survey of publics in 21 countries. The surveys, conducted from March 3 to April 21, 2013, and totaling 22,425 respondents,[4] gauged public opinion on the challenges posed by aging

for the country and for the respondents personally. The report also examines trends in the aging of the global population, the U.S. population, and the populations in 22 other selected countries.[5] The focus is on changes from 2010 to 2050, as projected by the United Nations (UN) in its latest World Population Prospects, the 2012 revision, released in June 2013.[6]

Global Trends in Aging

The global population is on the brink of a remarkable transformation. Thanks to the aging of today's middle-aged demographic bulge and ongoing improvements in life expectancy, the population of seniors is projected to surge, increasing from 530.5 million in 2010 to 1.5 billion in 2050. The result will be a much older world, a future in which roughly one-in-six people is expected to be 65 and older by 2050, double the proportion today.

The population of children, meanwhile, will be at a virtual standstill due to long-term declines in birth rates around the world. The number of children younger than 15 is expected to increase by only 10%, from 1.8 billion in 2010 to 2 billion in 2050.[7] Consequently, the global share of the population that is 65 and older will double, from 8% in 2010 to 16% in 2050. And, more countries will find that they have more adults ages 65 and older than they have children younger than 15.

The graying of the world's population in the aggregate conceals some important variations. Japan, China, South Korea and many countries in Europe are expected to have greater numbers of people dependent on shrinking workforces, a potentially significant demographic challenge for economic growth. However, aging elsewhere, such as India and several African countries, mostly means the aging of children into the workforce. That is a potentially favorable demographic trend for economic growth. Thus, the coming changes in world demography conceivably could alter the distribution of global economic power over the coming decades.

For the United States, population trends may lead to greater opportunities in the global economy of the future. Although the U.S. population is anticipated to turn older and grow at a slower rate in the future, it is projected to increase at a faster pace and age less than the populations of most of the rest of the developed world. Thus, to the extent that demography is destiny, the U.S. may be in a position to experience a more robust economic future in comparison with other developed nations.

Aging in Major Regions of the World

In the future, aging and slower rates of growth are expected to characterize the populations of all major regions in the world.

Ranked by median age, Europe is currently the oldest region in the world and should retain that distinction in 2050. However, Latin America and Asia are projected to age the most rapidly through 2050. It is expected that the median age in Latin America, currently 10 years lower than the median age in North America, will match North America's age level by 2050. Africa will continue to have the youngest population in the world.

Africa is expected to be home to a greater share of the world's population in the future, 25% in 2050, up from 15% in 2010. The UN estimates that Africa's population should more than double from 2010 to 2050 with the addition of 1.4 billion people, greater than the increase of 1 billion expected in Asia & Oceania and the gain of just 0.3 billion expected for the Americas. In sharp contrast, Europe's population is expected to shrink by more than 30 million by the middle of the century.

Aging in the U.S. and Other Countries

Across the countries examined in this report, projections show that the U.S. population will grow at a faster rate than the populations of European and several East Asian and Latin American countries. Countries whose populations should grow at rates slower than in the U.S. include Brazil, Argentina, Britain, France, Spain, China, South Korea and South Africa. Some countries—Russia, Germany, Italy and Japan—are projected to experience reductions in their populations.

Nations expected to experience relatively rapid population growth are located mostly in Africa. Most notably, Nigeria's population is projected to nearly triple and to overtake the U.S. population by 2050. Kenya is expected to more than double its population from 2010 to 2050. Pakistan, Egypt and Israel are expected to grow at much faster rates than the U.S. The populations of Mexico, India, Indonesia and Iran should increase at rates that are slightly higher than in the U.S.

Regardless of their initial size or the rate of growth in their population, the countries covered by this study are all expected to turn grayer between now and 2050. The median age in the U.S. is projected to increase from 37 in 2010 to 41 in 2050. That will be less of an increase than in the rest of the world as the global median age is projected to increase from 29 in 2010 to 36 in 2050.

The median age and the share of the population ages 65 and older also is projected to increase in other countries, sharply in China, South Korea, Mexico and Brazil, among others. Also, the total dependency ratio—the size of the "dependent" population (those younger than 15 or older than 64) relative to the "working age" population (ages 15 to 64)—is projected to rise in most countries. This means that future demographic conditions may not support the same rates of economic growth experienced in those countries in the past.

A handful of countries, even as their populations age, are poised to experience a potential demographic boost to their economies. The total dependency ratios in Egypt, India, Pakistan, Nigeria, Kenya and South Africa should decrease in the future, a consequence of their currently large youth populations aging into the workforce. This demographic transition is potentially a boon for economic growth. But, because these countries will also experience rising proportions of seniors in their populations, they will not be entirely immune to the social and economic challenges posed by an aging citizenry.

Pension and Health Care Expenditures

With aging, it is not surprising that public expenditures on pensions and health care are generally projected to increase as a share of gross domestic product (GDP). Increases in pension expenditures are principally driven by aging. In response, many countries have implemented reforms, such as a rise in the retirement age, designed to decelerate the rate of increase. Nonetheless, public pension expenditures are expected to consume about 15% of GDP by 2050 in several European countries. Pension expenditures in the U.S. are projected to increase by less, from 6.8% of GDP in 2010 to 8.5% in 2050.

Larger concerns revolve around public health care expenditures, which are rising faster than pension expenditures in most countries. The reason is that health care expenditures are pushed up not just by aging but also by cost inflation. In the U.S., public health expenditures are projected to more than double, from 6.7% of GDP in 2010 to 14.9% in 2050. Similarly, large increases are expected in Japan and several countries in Europe, if current rates of cost inflation persist.[8]

1. The term "baby boomers" refers to the large cohort born in the U.S. from 1946 to 1964. The oldest members of this cohort started to turn 65 in 2011.

2. The median age divides the population into two equal parts, with 50% of the population older than the median age and 50% of the population younger than the median age.

3. See, for example, National Research Council (2012), OECD (2012), UNFPA and HelpAge International (2012), Clements et al. (2012), Gordon (2012), Bloom, Canning and Fink (2011), CIA (2001), Eberstadt (2011), Peterson (1999), and Beard et al. (2011).

4. See the Survey Methods section for more details on the surveys.

5. The two countries included in the demographic analysis but for which survey data are not presented are India, because of concerns about the survey's administration in the field, and Iran, where no survey was conducted.

6. Data from the 2012 revision are available at http://esa.un.org/unpd/wpp/index.htm. The UN reports four variants for population growth: high, medium, low, and constant-fertility. All estimates in this report are from the UN's medium variant.

7. Percentage changes are computed before numbers are rounded.

8. Projections of pension and health expenditures are subject to a great degree of uncertainty. That is because they depend not only on population projections but also on macroeconomic projections for GDP, assumptions about the labor force, policy parameters relating to eligibility ages and replacement rates, inflation in the cost of health care services, consumption of health care services and other factors.

Critical Thinking

1. How do you think the aging population will affect the health-care workforce?

2. Why are fertility rates so important when estimating the economic impact of aging on the population?

3. What is the global impact of aging?

Internet References

Pew Research Center
http://www.pewglobal.org/

The Oxford Institute of Population Aging
https://www.ageing.ox.ac.uk/

World Health Organization
http://www.who.int/

"Attitudes about Aging: A Global Perspective," *Pew Research Center*, January 30, 2014. Washington, D.C.: Pew Research Center, 2014.

Article

Prepared by: Elaina Osterbur, *Saint Louis University*

Sexual Orientation, Socioeconomic Status and Healthy Aging

BRIDGET K. GORMAN AND ZELMA OYARVIDE

Learning Outcomes

After reading this article, you will be able to:

- Discuss the impact of socioeconomic status on health.

- Identify the disadvantages experienced by bisexual elders compared to heterosexual, gay, or lesbian older adults.

- Explain the importance of sexual identity disclosure to medical professionals.

The older adult population in the United States is more diverse than ever before—including diversity based on sexual and gender minority status. Recent studies indicate that there are more than 2.4 million lesbian, gay, bisexual, and transgender (LGBT) adults ages 50 and older in the United States, and that this population will grow to more than 5 million by the year 2030 (Fredriksen-Goldsen et al., 2014). In recent years, LGBT older adults have been the focus of a small but growing body of research examining the characteristics and circumstances associated with their health and healthy aging (Institute of Medicine [IOM], 2011).

These studies paint a picture of a population that, on average, faces a variety of health challenges, including stigma, discrimination, and related stressors; barriers to receiving formal and informal healthcare services; and financial instability (Choi and Meyer, 2016). In this article, we discuss how sexual orientation relates to socioeconomic status (SES) among older adults, and the importance of SES differences for the health status and healthy aging trajectories of selected sexual minority (lesbian, gay, and bisexual) adults.

Socioeconomic Status, Sexual Orientation, and Health

While healthy aging relates to a variety of factors, socioeconomic resources loom large. Scholarship has firmly established the fundamental role of socioeconomic status for health (Link and Phelan, 1995). Socioeconomic differences in health impairment accumulate across the life course, and education is an especially important cause of healthy aging due to its key role in the acquisition of material assets (e.g., good jobs, health insurance, income, and wealth), as well as the development of health-related habits, skills, and abilities (Ross and Mirowsky, 2010). While education acts as an intrinsic resource that helps delay the onset of chronic health conditions and functional limitations, income operates more as a coping resource that helps slow the progression of health problems after they occur (Herd, Goesling, and House, 2007). Considered together, the education and income profile of older adults is a crucial factor shaping their likelihood of living a long life relatively free from disease and impairment.

Table 1   Education and Income Profile of Older U.S. Adults, by Gender, Sexual Orientation, and Age

	Completed Schooling		Annual Household Income	
	% Less than High School	% College Degree	% Less than $25,000	% $75,000 and higher
OLDER WOMEN				
Heterosexual				
50–64	10.1	30.1	24.5	33.8
65–79	12.6	22.0	35.2	15.3
80+	16.4	18.1	50.8	8.9
Lesbians				
50–64	2.3	48.3	23.8	45.0
65–79	6.6	45.7	27.8	28.1
80+	15.0	38.9	38.2	6.3
Bisexual				
50–64	15.8	31.8	35.5	28.0
65–79	22.4	33.0	53.9	12.7
80+	17.1	13.2	50.7	6.1
OLDER MEN				
Heterosexual				
50–64	12.7	30.8	21.8	38.4
65–79	14.5	28.4	24.6	24.4
80+	18.9	24.6	33.1	18.5
Gay				
50–64	5.4	41.3	28.5	37.9
65–79	7.9	50.9	23.1	24.9
80+	23.0	35.1	34.9	19.4
Bisexual				
50–64	18.8	34.7	46.6	25.7
65–79	12.6	25.4	48.4	17.2
80+	42.8	20.4	62.8	14.7

Source: Calculated by the authors based o Behavioral Risk Factor Surveillance System (BRFSS) data frorn 2011–2015 waves for the following 40 U.S. states (various years by state): AK, AZ, CA, CO, CT, DE, FL, GA, HI, ID, IL, IN, IA, KS, KY, LA, ME, MD, MA, MI, MN, MO, MT, NV, NM, NY, NC, ND, OH, OR, PA, RI, TX, UT, VT, VA, WA, WV, WI, and WY.

Due to the fundamental role of education, income, and other aspects of socioeconomic status for healthy aging, the wide disparities seen in SES across sociodemographic groups is troubling, especially for older adults. To illustrate, we calculated estimates for SES by gender, sexual orientation, and age using data from the 2011–2015 waves of the Behavioral Risk Factor Surveillance System. Table 1 shows how low education (less than a high school diploma) and high education (college degree or more), as well as low annual household income (less than $25,000) and higher income ($75,000 or more) differ by sexual orientation and gender among older adults in three age cohorts: ages 50 to 64, ages 65 to 79, and ages 80 and older. Overall, it shows that across groups, completed schooling and household income decline with increasing age.

Socioeconomic and Health Status of Bisexual Older Adults

Table 1 also highlights the socioeconomic disadvantages of bisexual older adults. Across age groups, bisexual elders have the lowest rates of completed schooling, and they live in lower-income households than do heterosexual, gay, or lesbian older adults. While the percentages of their disadvantage vary by gender and age cohort, SES disparities can be quite high. For example, among older women ages 65 to 70, 22.4 percent of bisexual women did not complete high school—this compares to 12.6 percent of heterosexual women, and just 6.6 percent of lesbians.

As another example, Table 1 shows that annual household income varies strongly among the oldest men; while about one-third of heterosexual and gay men ages 80 and older report an annual income of less than $25,000, this rate is almost double among bisexual men (62.8 percent). As recent assessments have concluded (Fredriksen-Goldsen and Muraco 2010; IOM, 2011), previous research on older adults has disproportionately focused on gay men and lesbians, while bisexuals and other sexual minority groups rarely were examined. Yet the data patterns in Table 1 illustrate the risks associated with only considering gay or lesbian adults (or lumping together subgroups into an umbrella "sexual minority" category). Doing so would obscure or ignore the poorer socioeconomic standing of bisexual older adults relative to their heterosexual and gay or lesbian peers—a key factor shaping health disparities across the life course that are based on sexual orientation.

A recent study by Fredriksen-Goldsen and colleagues (2016) concluded that the poorer socioeconomic standing of bisexual older adults operated as a strong explanatory mechanism for their poorer health reports, compared to heterosexual and gay or lesbian older adults. Recent reviews of LGBT aging issues have discussed how financial instability is a major concern for many sexual minority older adults (e.g., Movement Advancement Project [MAP] and Sage, 2010).

As summarized by Choi and Meyer (2016): "Lifetime disparities in earnings, employment, and opportunities to build savings, as well as discriminatory access to legal and social programs that are traditionally established to support aging adults, put LGBT older adults at greater financial risk than their non-LGBT peers." The findings shown in Table 1 and from previous scholarship indicate that financial stress may be especially high among bisexuals in later life.

This finding about financial stress more generally reflects a growing body of research documenting substantial financial and other health-related risks among bisexuals. Scholarship focused upon adults in general has shown that, compared to heterosexual and gay or lesbian adults, those who identify as bisexual report poorer socioeconomic circumstances, higher participation in health-damaging behaviors like smoking and heavy alcohol use, and poorer mental and physical health status (Conron, Mimiaga, and Landers, 2010; Gorman et al., 2015; Veenstra, 2011).

Bisexuals also report lower averages of life satisfaction and less emotional support than either gay or lesbian or heterosexual adults (Gorman et al., 2015). Additionally, Fredriksen-Goldsen and colleagues (2016) show that older bisexual adults report more internalized stigma as well as a lower sense of community belonging and perceived social supports than their gay or lesbian peers. This study also showed a lower rate of sexual identity disclosure among bisexuals—a finding that applies not only to friends, family, and co-workers, but also to medical care providers (see also IOM, 2011).

Considered together, these studies indicate that a variety of health-related risks—including economic vulnerability, participation in unhealthy behaviors (e.g., smoking), stress, and lower levels of social support—may be elevated among bisexual older adults. Furthermore, the lower rate of sexual identity disclosure to medical professionals among bisexuals is worrisome, because research on the medical experiences of sexual minorities highlights the importance of sexual identity disclosure for a positive medical encounter (Daley, 2012; Sherman et al., 2014).

Analyzing SES Similarities

Looking again at Table 1, it also shows more positive socioeconomic profiles for gay men and lesbian older adults relative to same-age heterosexuals. Depending upon the contrast, gay men and lesbians often report similar or better levels of completed schooling and annual household income. This is seen most strongly for education: with just one exception (among men ages 80 and older), gay men and lesbians report higher levels of completed schooling, on average, than their heterosexual peers. This educational advantage is especially stark when we look at the percentage with a college degree, where the proportion with a college degree is markedly higher among gay men and lesbians. For example, among adults ages 50 to 64, 48.3 percent of lesbians have a college degree, compared to 30.1 percent of heterosexual women. Among men ages 50 to 64, 41.3 percent of gay men have at least a college degree, compared to 30.8 percent of heterosexual men.

Looking at annual household income among older women, we see a more muted but generally similar pattern. The proportion of older women reporting a household income below $25,000 is lower among lesbians than heterosexuals in each age group, and (with the exception of women ages 80 and older) a higher proportion also report a household income of $75,000 or above.

Among older men, however, the proportion in either income group is very similar between gay and heterosexual men in most age groups. The biggest difference occurs among men ages 50 to 64, where a higher proportion of gay men (28.5 percent) report an annual household income of less than $25,000, compared to 21.8 percent of heterosexual men.

Previous studies also have found higher levels of educational achievement among gay men and lesbians in comparison to comparably aged heterosexual adults (IOM, 2011). Additionally, work by Fredriksen-Goldsen and colleagues (2013) found a similar pattern wherein gay and lesbian adults ages 50 and older report higher levels of education, but fairly equivalent rates of poverty in comparison to similar-age heterosexuals—a pattern they attribute to discrimination and blocked opportunities across the life course, which limited the ability of sexual minorities to fully capitalize on the economic benefits associated with their educational achievement. That we see this more strongly among older gay men than among lesbians (in Table 1) may relate to elevated experiences with stigma and discrimination among gay men. Herek (2002) has documented that U.S. adults (especially heterosexual men) hold more negative attitudes toward gay men than they do toward lesbians, and gay men experience substantially higher rates of harassment, verbal abuse, violence, and property crimes than either lesbians or bisexuals (Herek, 2009).

Healthy Aging Among Sexual Minorities

As detailed in Healthy People 2020, improving the health and well-being of sexual minorities is an important public health goal for the United States (U.S. Department of Health and Human Services, 2010). Existing health disparities research provides a framework for understanding how SES contributes to sexual orientation differences in health status, because SES often is implicated as one of the strongest contributors to health stratification (Link and Phelan, 1995). Overall, the poor health standing of bisexuals documented across an increasing number of studies may be due in large part to their lower socioeconomic standing, on average, than members of other sexual orientation groups.

In particular, our understanding of how education and income relate to disease onset and progression is important, because the poorer socioeconomic profile of bisexual older adults suggests that they may face particular hardships in navigating the health challenges associated with aging. Older sexual minority adults are more likely to be single, living alone, and without children than heterosexual elders, and they rely more on partners and friends to provide caregiving assistance (Fredriksen-Goldsen and Muraco, 2010; MAP and Sage, 2010).

The fact that bisexual older adults report elevated rates of low income and education indicates that they may face difficult challenges in securing quality housing and medical care services as they age. While survey data suggest that gay or lesbian adults do not experience the same education deficits as bisexuals, it appears that older lesbians and gay men especially have been less able to capitalize economically on their education. As such, policy makers and healthcare providers need to realize how financial stress and instability in later life may play a large role in shaping not only the health status of sexual minorities, but also how successful their management of health problems may be as they seek to maintain a high quality of life as they age.

References

Choi, S. K., and Meyer, I. H. 2016. LGBT Aging: A Review of Research Findings, Needs, and Policy Implications. Los Angeles: The Williams Institute.

Conron, K. J., Mimiaga, M., and Landers, S. 2010. "A Population-based Study of Sexual Orientation Identity and Gender Differences in Adult Health." American Journal of Public Health 100(10): 1953–60.

Daley, A. E. 2012. "Becoming Seen, Becoming Known: Lesbian Women's Self-disclosures of Sexual Orientation to Mental Health Service Providers." Journal of Gay & Lesbian Mental Health 16(3): 215–34.

Fredriksen-Goldsen, K. I., and Muraco, A. 2010. "Aging and Sexual Orientation: A 25-year Review of the Literature." Research on Aging 32(3): 372–413.

Fredriksen-Goldsen, K. I., et al. 2013. "Health Disparities Among Lesbian, Gay, and Bisexual Older Adults: Results from a Population-based Study." American Journal of Public Health 103(10): 1802–9.

Fredriksen-Goldsen, K. I., et al. 2014. "Successful Aging Among LGBT Older Adults: Physical and Mental Health-Related Quality of Life by Age Group." The Gerontologist 55(1): 154–68.

Fredriksen-Goldsen, K. I., et al. 2016. "Health Equity and Aging of Bisexual Older Adults: Pathways of Risk and Resilience." The Journals of Gerontology, Series B: Social Sciences 72(3): 468–78.

Gorman, B. K., et al. 2015. "A New Piece of the Puzzle: Gender, Health, and Sexual Orientation." Demography 52(4): 1357–82.

Herd, P., Goesling, B., and House, J. S. 2007. "Socioeconomic Position and Health: The Differential Effects of Education Versus Income on the Onset Versus Progression of Health Problems." Journal of Health and Social Behavior 48(3): 223–8.

Herek, G. M. 2002. "Gender Gaps in Public Opinion about Lesbians and Gay Men." Public Opinion Quarterly 66(1): 40–66.

Herek, G. M. 2009. "Hate Crimes and Stigma-related Experiences Among Sexual Minority Adults in the United States: Prevalence

Estimates from a National Probability Sample." *Journal of Interpersonal Violence* 24(1): 54–74.

Institute of Medicine (IOM). 2011. *The Health of Lesbian, Gay, Bisexual, and Transgender People: Building a Foundation for Better Understanding.* Washington, DC: National Institutes of Health.

Link, B. G., and Phelan, J. 1995. "Social Conditions as Fundamental Causes of Disease." *Journal of Health and Social Behavior* 35(extra issue): 80–94.

Movement Advancement Project (MAP) and SAGE. 2010. *Improving the Lives of LGBT Older Adults.* New York: MAP and SAGE.

Ross, C. E., and Mirowsky, J. 2010. "Why Education Is the Key to Socioeconomic Differentials in Health." In C. E. Bird et al., eds., *Handbook of Medical Sociology* (6th ed.). Nashville, TN: Vanderbilt University Press.

Sherman, M. D., et al. 2014. "Communication Between VA Providers and Sexual and Gender Minority Veterans: A Pilot Study." *Psychological Services* 11(2): 235–42.

U.S. Department of Health and Human Services. 2010. *Healthy People 2020.* goo.gl/zOJxmv. Retrieved July 1, 2016.

Veenstra, G. 2011. "Race, Gender, Class, and Sexual Orientation: Intersecting Axes of Inequality and Self-rated Health in Canada." *International Journal for Equity in Health* 10(3).

Critical Thinking

1. Imagine explaining to healthcare professionals your sexual orientation, what do you expect the response should be?

2. Do you think you could idenitfy discrimination—any kind of discrimination?

3. What would be your response to discrimination in health, education or workforce towards you or a loved one?

Internet References

American Psychological Association
   https://www.apa.org/

Aging Life Care Association
   https://www.aginglifecarejournal.org/

National Resource Center on LGBT Aging
   https://www.lgbtagingcenter.org/

Bridget K. Gorman, PhD, is professor and chair of Sociology at Rice University in Houston, Texas.

Zelma Oyarvide is a doctoral student in the Department of Sociology, and a research affiliate at the Kinder Institute for Urban Research, at Rice University.

Unit 4

UNIT

Prepared by: Elaina Osterbur, *Saint Louis University*

Problems and Potentials of Aging

Aging is part of every aspect of the life cycle. Aging begins from the day we are born. Every aspect of life-span transitions includes aging at its core. Theories abound within these transitions that help to explain the problems and potentials along the life span. Developmental psychologists and psychoanalysts explain the development of attachment, psychosexual development, cognitive development, and much more. Many of these theorists explain development from birth to death. Other theorists concentrate on biological aging.

American society is often concerned with the biology of aging because of the potential for disability at older ages. Diseases such as cancer and heart disease not only cause disability, but can also cause death. Stroke, diabetes, and arthritis are among the top 10 chronic diseases of aging. These diseases can cause disability that affects older adult's activities of daily living, as well as the instrumental activities of daily living. The prevention of chronic disease in older adults is a major priority of health-care systems and institutions.

The maintaining of health is also important to older adults as many older Americans try to remain masters of their own destinies for as long as possible. They fear dependence and try to avoid it. Many are successful at maintaining independence and the right to make their own decisions. Others are less successful and must depend on their families for care and to make critical decisions. However, some older people are able to overcome the difficulties of aging and to lead comfortable and enjoyable lives.

The articles in this section explain age-associated diseases and dysfunction, effects of healthy aging, children as caregivers, and the impact of aging on policy, medical technology, and population health.

Article Prepared by: Elaina Osterbur, *Saint Louis University*

Physician Supply and Demand Through 2025: Key Findings

ASSOCIATION OF AMERICAN MEDICAL COLLEGES

Learning Outcomes

After reading this article, you will be able to:

- Identify the issues that affect the supply and demand of physicians.
- Understand the impact of the growth in demand for physicians.
- Discuss the potential solutions to the shortage of physicians.

In April 2016, the economic modeling and forecasting firm IHS Inc. released *2016 Update: The Complexities of Physician Supply and Demand: Projections from 2014 to 2025*, a new study commissioned by the AAMC. Projections for individual specialties were aggregated for reporting into four broad categories: primary care, medical specialties, surgical specialties, and other specialties.[1] To reflect future uncertainties in health policy and patterns in care use and delivery, the study presents ranges for the projected shortages of physicians rather than specific shortage numbers.

Demand for physicians continues to grow faster than supply. Although physician supply is projected to increase modestly between 2014 and 2025, demand will grow more steeply.

- By 2025, demand for physicians will exceed supply by a range of 61,700 to 94,700. The lower estimate would represent more aggressive changes in care delivery patterns subsequent to the rapid growth in non-physician clinicians and widespread delayed retirement by currently practicing physicians.
- Total shortages in 2025 vary by specialty grouping and include:
  - A shortfall of between 14,900 and 35,600 primary care physicians.

- A shortfall of between 37,400 and 60,300 non-primary care physicians, including:
  - 3,600 to 10,200 medical specialists
  - 25,200 to 33,200 surgical specialists
  - 22,200 to 32,600 other specialists[2]
- Population growth and aging continue to be the primary drivers of increasing physician demand. By 2025, the U.S. population under age 18 is projected to grow by only 5%, while the population aged 65 and over is projected to grow by 41%. Because seniors have much higher per capita consumption of health care, the demand for physicians—especially specialty physicians—is projected to increase.

The total projected physician shortage persists under every likely scenario, including increased use of advanced practice

---

1 Primary care consists of family medicine, general internal medicine, general pediatrics, and geriatric medicine. Medical specialties consist of allergy & immunology, cardiology, critical care, dermatology, endocrinology, gastroenterology, hematology & oncology, infectious diseases, neonatal & perinatal medicine, nephrology, pulmonology, and rheumatology. Surgical specialties consist of general surgery, colorectal surgery, neurological surgery, obstetrics & gynecology, ophthalmology, orthopedic surgery, otolaryngology, plastic surgery, thoracic surgery, urology, vascular surgery and other surgical specialties. The other specialties category consists of anesthesiology, emergency medicine, neurology, pathology, physical medicine & rehabilitation, psychiatry, radiology, and all other specialties.

2 The range in the projected shortfall for total physicians is smaller than the sum of the ranges in the projected shortfalls for the specialty categories. The demand scenarios modeled project future demand for physician services, but scenarios can differ in terms of whether future demand will be provided by primary care or non-primary care physicians. Likewise, the range for total non-primary care is smaller than the sum of the ranges for the specialty categories.

nurses (APRNs) and physician assistants (PA), greater use of alternate settings such as retail clinics, delayed physician retirement, and rapid changes in payment and delivery (e.g., ACOs).

Addressing the shortage will require a multipronged approach, including innovation in delivery; greater use of technology; improved, efficient use of all health professionals on the care team; and an increase in federal support for residency training. The magnitude of the projected shortfalls is significant enough that no single solution will be sufficient on its own to resolve physician shortages.

Because physician training can take up to a decade, a physician shortage in 2025 is a problem that needs to be addressed in 2016.

The study is an update to last year's report. It incorporates the most current and best available evidence on health care delivery and responds to questions received after the release of the previous report. The AAMC has committed to updating the study annually to make use of new data and new analyses and take an active role in fostering the conversation around physician workforce projections modeling.

Critical Thinking

1. Discuss the result of the shortage of primary care physicians in the delivery of health care.
2. How do you think that medical technology could assist in easing the shortage of physicians?

Internet References

Association of American Medical Colleges
  http://www.aamc.org
Gerontological Society of America
  http://www.geron.org

Article Prepared by: Elaina Osterbur, *Saint Louis University*

Sexuality in Later Life

NATIONAL INSTITUTE ON AGING

Learning Outcomes

After reading this article, you will be able to:

- Explain the normal physical changes as we age that may impact the ability to have a healthy sex life.

- Discuss the potential problems experienced that can interfere with sexual activity.

- Identify strategies to compensate or accommodate sexual activity.

Many people want and need to be close to others as they grow older. For some, this includes the desire to continue an active, satisfying sex life. With aging, that may mean adapting sexual activity to accommodate physical, health, and other changes.

There are many different ways to have sex and be intimate—alone or with a partner. The expression of your sexuality could include many types of touch or stimulation. Some adults may choose not to engage in sexual activity, and that's also normal.

Here, we explore some of the common problems older adults may face with sex.

What are Normal Changes?

Normal aging brings physical changes in both men and women. These changes sometimes affect the ability to have and enjoy sex.

A woman may notice changes in her vagina. As a woman ages, her vagina can shorten and narrow. Her vaginal walls can become thinner and a little stiffer. Most women will have less vaginal lubrication, and it may take more time for the vagina to naturally lubricate itself. These changes could make certain types of sexual activity, such as vaginal penetration, painful or less desirable. If vaginal dryness is an issue, using water-based lubricating jelly or lubricated condoms may be more comfortable. If a woman is using hormone therapy to treat hot flashes or other menopausal symptoms, she may want to have sex more often than she did before hormone therapy.

As men get older, impotence (also called erectile dysfunction, or ED) becomes more common. ED is the loss of ability to have and keep an erection. ED may cause a man to take longer to have an erection. His erection may not be as firm or as large as it used to be. The loss of erection after orgasm may happen more quickly, or it may take longer before another erection is possible. ED is not a problem if it happens every now and then, but if it occurs often, talk with your doctor. Talk with your partner about these changes and how you are feeling. Your doctor may have suggestions to help make sex easier.

What Causes Sexual Problems?

Some illnesses, disabilities, medicines, and surgeries can affect your ability to have and enjoy sex.

Arthritis. Joint pain due to arthritis can make sexual contact uncomfortable. Exercise, drugs, and possibly joint replacement surgery may help relieve this pain. Rest, warm baths, and changing the position or timing of sexual activity can be helpful.

Chronic pain. Pain can interfere with intimacy between older people. Chronic pain does not have to be part of growing older and can often be treated. But, some pain medicines can interfere with sexual function. Always talk with your doctor if you have side effects from any medication.

Dementia. Some people with dementia show increased interest in sex and physical closeness, but they may not be able to judge what is appropriate sexual behavior. Those with severe dementia may not recognize their spouse or partner, but they still desire sexual contact and may seek it with someone else. It can be confusing and difficult to know how to handle this situation. Here, too, talking with a doctor, nurse, or social worker with training in dementia care may be helpful.

Diabetes. This is one of the illnesses that can cause ED in some men. In most cases, medical treatment can help. Less is known about how diabetes affects sexuality in older women. Women with diabetes are more likely to have vaginal yeast infections, which can cause itching and irritation and make sex uncomfortable or undesirable. Yeast infections can be treated.

Heart disease. Narrowing and hardening of the arteries can change blood vessels so that blood does not flow freely. As a result, men and women may have problems with orgasms. For both men and women, it may take longer to become aroused, and for some men, it may be difficult to have or maintain an erection. People who have had a heart attack, or their partners, may be afraid that having sex will cause another attack. Even though sexual activity is generally safe, always follow your doctor's advice. If your heart problems get worse and you have chest pain or shortness of breath even while resting, your doctor may want to change your treatment plan.

Incontinence. Loss of bladder control or leaking of urine is more common as people, especially women, grow older. Extra pressure on the belly during sex can cause loss of urine. This can be helped by changing positions or by emptying the bladder before and after sex. The good news is that incontinence can usually be treated.

Stroke. The ability to have sex is sometimes affected by a stroke. A change in positions or medical devices may help people with ongoing weakness or paralysis to have sex. Some people with paralysis from the waist down are still able to experience orgasm and pleasure.

Depression. Lack of interest in activities you used to enjoy, such as intimacy and sexual activity, can be a symptom of depression. It's sometimes hard to know if you're depressed. Talk with your doctor. Depression can be treated.

Surgery. Many of us worry about having any kind of surgery—it may be even more troubling when the breasts or genital area are involved. Most people do return to the kind of sex life they enjoyed before surgery.

Hysterectomy is surgery to remove a woman's uterus because of pain, bleeding, fibroids, or other reasons. Often, when an older woman has a hysterectomy, the ovaries are also removed. Deciding whether to have this surgery can leave both women and their partners worried about their future sex life. If you're concerned about any changes you might experience with a hysterectomy, talk with your gynecologist or surgeon.

Mastectomy is surgery to remove all or part of a woman's breast because of breast cancer. This surgery may cause some women to lose their sexual interest, or it may leave them feeling less desirable or attractive to their partners. In addition to talking with your doctor, sometimes it is useful to talk with other women who have had this surgery. Programs like the American Cancer Society's "Reach to Recovery" can

be helpful for both women and men. If you want your breast rebuilt (reconstruction), talk to your cancer doctor or surgeon.

Prostatectomy is surgery that removes all or part of a man's prostate because of cancer or an enlarged prostate. It may cause urinary incontinence or ED. If you need this operation, talk with your doctor before surgery about your concerns.

Medications. Some drugs can cause sexual problems. These include some blood pressure medicines, antihistamines, antidepressants, tranquilizers, Parkinson's disease or cancer medications, appetite suppressants, drugs for mental problems, and ulcer drugs. Some can lead to ED or make it hard for men to ejaculate. Some drugs can reduce a woman's sexual desire or cause vaginal dryness or difficulty with arousal and orgasm. Check with your doctor to see if there is a different drug without this side effect.

Alcohol. Too much alcohol can cause erection problems in men and delay orgasm in women.

Am I Too Old to Worry About Safe Sex?

Age does not protect you from sexually transmitted diseases. Older people who are sexually active may be at risk for diseases such as syphilis, gonorrhea, chlamydial infection, genital herpes, hepatitis B, genital warts, and trichomoniasis.

Almost anyone who is sexually active is also at risk of being infected with HIV, the virus that causes AIDS. The number of older people with HIV/AIDS is growing. You are at risk for HIV/AIDS if you or your partner has more than one sexual partner, if you are having unprotected sex, or if either you or your partner is sharing needles. To protect yourself, always use a condom during sex that involves vaginal or anal penetration. A man needs to have a full erection before putting on a condom.

Talk with your doctor about ways to protect yourself from all sexually transmitted diseases and infections. Go for regular checkups and testing. Talk with your partner. You are never too old to be at risk.

Can Emotions Play a Part?

Sexuality is often a delicate balance of emotional and physical issues. How you feel may affect what you are able to do and what you want to do. Many older couples find greater satisfaction in their sex lives than they did when they were younger. In many cases, they have fewer distractions, more time and privacy, no worries about getting pregnant, and greater intimacy with a lifelong partner.

As we age, our bodies change, including our weight, skin, and muscle tone, and some older adults don't feel as comfortable in their aging bodies. Older adults, men and women alike, may worry that their partners will no longer find them attractive. Aging-related sexual problems like the ones listed above can cause stress and worry. This worry can get in the way of enjoying a fulfilling sex life.

Older couples face the same daily stresses that affect people of any age. They may also have the added concerns of illness, retirement, and lifestyle changes, all of which may lead to sexual difficulties. Talk openly with your partner, and try not to blame yourself or your partner. You may also find it helpful to talk with a therapist, either alone or with your partner. Some therapists have special training in helping with sexual problems. If you sense changes in your partner's attitude toward sex, don't assume they are no longer interested in you or in an active sex life. Talk about it. Many of the things that cause sexual problems in older adults can be helped.

What Can I Do?

There are things you can do on your own for an active and enjoyable sex life. If you have a long-term partner, take time to enjoy each other and to understand the changes you both are facing.

Don't be afraid to talk with your doctor if you have a problem that affects your sex life. He or she may be able to suggest a treatment. For example, the most common sexual difficulty of older women is painful intercourse caused by vaginal dryness. Your doctor or a pharmacist can suggest over-the-counter vaginal lubricants or moisturizers to use. Water-based lubricants are helpful when needed to make sex more comfortable. Moisturizers are used on a regular basis, every 2 or 3 days. Or, your doctor might suggest a form of vaginal estrogen.

If ED is the problem, it can often be managed and perhaps even reversed with medication or other treatments. There are pills that can help. They should not be used by men taking medicines containing nitrates, such as nitroglycerin. The pills do have possible side effects. Be wary of any dietary or herbal supplements promising to treat ED. Always talk to your doctor before taking any herb or supplement.

Physical problems can change your sex life as you get older. If you are single, dating and meeting new people may be easier later in life when you're more sure of yourself and what you want. If you're in a relationship, you and your partner may discover new ways to be together as you get older. Talk to your partner or partners about your needs. You may find that affection—hugging, kissing, touching, and spending time together—can be just what you need, or a path to greater intimacy and sex.

Critical Thinking

1. What is the importance of sexual activity across the life span?
2. Discuss the positive and negative cultural aspects of sexuality in older adults.
3. How would you discuss your sexual health with your health-care provider?

Internet References

American Society on Aging
http://asaging.org/
Harvard Health Publishing
https://www.health.harvard.edu/
Next Avenue
https://www.nextavenue.org/

"AgePage Sexuality in Later Life," *National Institute on Aging*, November 2017.

Article   Prepared by: Elaina Osterbur, *Saint Louis University*

The Edinburgh Social Cognition Test (ESCoT): Examining the Effects of Age on a New Measure of Theory of Mind and Social Norm Understanding

R. ASAAD BAKSH, ET AL.

Learning Outcomes

After reading this article, you will be able to:

- Discuss the study of social cognition.
- Explain how Theory of Mind is tested and its importance in the study of social cognition.
- Discuss the importance of social norm understanding from intrapersonal and interpersonal perspectives.
- Discuss the quality of the ESCoT compared to other tests of social cognition.

Introduction

The study of social cognition is concerned with the higher-order cognitive processes that allow individuals to interpret the behaviors of others [1]. These abilities allow us to process and understand social information in order to respond appropriately in everyday interactions [2–5]. Social cognition includes abilities such as theory of mind (ToM; i.e., the ability to recognise other people's mental states to understand and predict their behavior), emotion recognition, empathy, moral judgments and the understanding of social norms [6, 7].

Healthy aging is associated with reliable improvement in emotional well-being [8] and social functioning [9]. Although social network size decreases with age, older adults' social interactions with individuals who remain within their social networks are rated as being more satisfying [10]. Life experience is thought to influence how people process and respond to social information (e.g., [11]). For example, older adults are thought to be more receptive to emotional cues when making social judgements compared to younger adults (see [12]). Yet, some studies examining individuals' ability to understand and evaluate relevant social information have reported poorer performance in healthy older adults compared to younger adults [13, 14].

One of the most extensively studied aspects of social cognition in healthy aging is ToM [14]. More recently, it has been argued that ToM is not a one-dimensional concept, but processes differ based on whether they refer to cognitive or affective judgements [15]. Cognitive ToM is defined as the ability to make inferences about the thoughts, intentions and beliefs of another individual. Affective ToM refers to the ability to make inferences about what another individual is feeling [15–17]. Age-related differences have been found where older adults perform more poorly compared to their younger counterparts on tests such as Reading the Mind in the Eyes (RME) [18], Faux Pas stories (a verbal story based test that requires participants to make ToM inferences from short interactions involving social norms violations and non-social norm violations) [19] and Happé's Strange Stories, among others [20–29]. Yet, other studies have found age-related improvements in favour of older adults such as Happé et al. [29] or equivalent performance between younger and older adults [25, 30–35]. Potentially, age-related differences may be related to one aspect of ToM but not the other, for example cognitive ToM but not affective ToM. However, research into possible dissociations between cognitive and affective ToM has yielded mixed findings. In perspective taking tests which assess cognitive ToM, older adults perform more poorly than younger adults [20, 22, 23, 26, 30, 36–38]. Nonetheless, other authors have failed to find age-related differences in cognitive ToM [30, 31]. Affective ToM has been examined using tests such as the RME [18] where individuals are required to make inferences from the eye region of photographs. Older adults have been found to perform significantly more poorly than younger adults [20, 21, 36, 39, 40]. Video based ToM tests have also shown that older adults perform significantly more poorly than younger adults [28, 40]. However, Castelli et al. [30] and Li et al. [32] have both reported comparable performance between younger and older adults on the RME. Moreover, story-based affective ToM tests such as the Faux Pas test [19] have less consistently reported age-related differences with some studies reporting poorer performance with age [35] but others not reporting age-related differences [33]. Overall, it is unclear how social cognitive abilities, specifically cognitive and affective ToM abilities are affected by aging when the performance of older adults is compared to younger adults. A possible reason for the inconsistencies in the literature could be related to the way in which researchers assess ToM [13].

The aging literature has tended to assess the influence of age on the distinct components of ToM using different tests (e.g., [36]), and these paradigms vary in both their stimuli type and level of difficulty. For example, affective ToM has been examined using tests involving visual-static stimuli such as Tom's taste test [23] and the RME [39]. In contrast, cognitive ToM has been examined using verbal vignettes [41] and visual-dynamic false belief story tests [20]. Existing tests of social cognition have been criticised as they require participants to read factual or fictional information regarding multiple characters and process mental state information. Poor performance could be a secondary consequence of broader cognitive difficulties [42]. Moreover, few aging studies have compared affective and cognitive ToM within the same test, making it difficult to contrast the influence of age on tests that are not directly comparable. Recently, Bottiroli et al. [22] attempted to measure cognitive and affective ToM using the Faux Pas test. They demonstrated that compared to younger adults, older adults performed poorer on cognitive ToM, but showed intact affective ToM abilities. Yet, some authors have argued that the Faux Pas imposes demands on both cognitive and affective ToM [13]. This test was designed before researchers explicitly regarded ToM as a multidimensional process and so there is no clear distinction between cognitive and affective ToM. Moreover, we would argue that the Faux Pas is a measure of affective ToM, as well as social norm understanding, since it primarily requires the participant to understand that a protagonist's feelings have been hurt by a social norm violation.

One important aspect of social cognition which has not typically been assessed in the aging literature is the ability to understand social norms from interpersonal and intrapersonal perspectives. While intrapersonal understanding of social norms has been explored in studies of dementia [43], adults with Autism Spectrum Disorders (ASD) [7] and patients with schizophrenia and bipolar disorder [6], few studies have examined this ability in healthy aging. In one of the only studies exploring interpersonal understanding of social norms in healthy aging, Halberstadt, Ruffman, Murray, Taumoepeau and Ryan [44] found that older adults were poorer at discriminating between socially appropriate and inappropriate behaviours from short videos of social interactions compared to younger adults.

Performance on social cognition tests have been shown to be influenced by variables such as personality traits and measures of IQ (e.g., verbal comprehension and perceptual reasoning). Charlton et al. [45] has argued that age-related difficulties in ToM are not independent of measures of intelligence. They found that the association between age and ToM abilities as measured by Happé's Strange Stories test was fully mediated by perceptual reasoning and partially mediated by verbal comprehension. Further studies have found correlations between ToM and verbal abilities [24] and have shown that perceptual reasoning performance accounts for age-related differences, again on Happé's Strange Stories test [28]. These findings suggest that some tests may not be simply assessing our social cognitive abilities and this has important implications for interpretations of age-related differences in performance.

A hallmark characteristic of ASD is pronounced impairments in social cognition [46]. Moreover, research has shown that difficulties in social cognition are responsible for social functioning impairment in ASD [47], suggesting that social cognitive abilities are important contributions to the quality of an individual's social interactions. This finding is relevant for the present study since characteristics typically found in adults with ASD are continuously distributed within the general population [48–50]. Indeed, subclinical autistic-like traits referred to as the Broad Autism Phenotype (BAP) [51] within the general population are related to reductions in social cognitive ability [48]. Individuals who exhibit more BAP traits report experiencing more social and interpersonal problems [50, 52]. Additionally, recent evidence suggests that BAP traits in older adults are associated with lower levels of social support, and increased self-reported levels of depression and anxiety [53]. Given the findings discussed above, it would be of interest to examine the relationship between the ESCoT, measures of intelligence and the BAP, and compare these to the findings of established tests.

To our knowledge, no tests are currently available in the literature that allow clinicians and researchers to examine different aspects of social cognition such as cognitive and affective ToM and understanding of social norms within the same test. Yet, some authors have argued that reliable assessments of a given construct should have multiple measures and these should differ in modality [54]. This could possibly be the reason for contradictory findings in the aging literature [13]. Moreover, while tests like the Movie for the Assessment of Social Cognition (MASC) [55], the Awareness of Social Inference Test (TASIT) [56], the Awkward Moments Test [57] and the Empathic Accuracy Paradigm [58] already exist and are all useful indices of social cognitive functioning, they are not without their limitations. For instance, the TASIT [56] uses excerpts from short interactions so lacks important contextual information, the MASC [55] is dubbed in English, the Awkward Moments Test [57] uses television adverts of exaggerated interactions and the Empathic Accuracy Paradigm [58] uses scenes from hidden filming which limits the range of mental states to be inferred.

We attempted to address these issues using a novel test of social cognition called the Edinburgh Social Cognition Test (ESCoT). We devised the ESCoT to explicitly measure both cognitive and affective ToM in the same test. The ESCoT also provides a much-needed measure of interpersonal and intrapersonal social norm understanding. Few tests measure more than one social cognitive ability in a single test, but the ESCoT provides four distinct and potentially informative insights into social cognitive abilities.

The aims of this study were to investigate the relationship between the ESCoT and a) age, b) measures of intelligence and c) the BAP in comparison to established tests. Additionally, we sought to examine convergent validity between the ESCoT and other measures of social cognition. By closely examining different social cognitive abilities in a systemic manner using the ESCoT, this study sought to shed new light on the consequences of aging on social cognitive abilities in younger, middle-aged and older adults.

Methods
Participants
A total of 91 healthy participants were recruited for this study: 30 aged between 18 and 35 years (15 male, 15 female), 30 aged between 45 and 60 years (15 male, 15 female) and 31 aged between 65 and 85 years (14 male, 17 female). The participants' demographic information is reported in Table 1. None of the participants had any self-reported history of neurological or psychiatric disorders based on the Wechsler Adult Intelligence Scale (WAIS-III) exclusion criteria [59]. Participants were recruited from online advertisement, through a Psychology Department volunteer panel, and were reimbursed for their time. Written informed consent to participate in the study was obtained from each participant. The study was approved by the School of Philosophy, Psychology and Language Sciences (Psychology) Ethics committee at the University of Edinburgh.

Measures
The Wechsler Abbreviated Scale of Intelligence, Second Edition (WASI-II) [60] was administered as a measure of verbal comprehension and perceptual reasoning. Participants completed four subtests: Vocabulary; Similarities; Block Design; and Matrix Reasoning. Scores from each of the four subtests were converted to age-adjusted standardised scores. The Vocabulary and Similarities subsets provided a Verbal Comprehension Index (VCI) and Block Design and Matrix Reasoning provide a Perceptual Reasoning Index (PRI) [60, 61].

The Autism Quotient (AQ) [62] was administered to assess traits related to the autism spectrum. The Empathy Quotient (EQ) [63] was administered to measure the ability to identify and understand the thoughts and feelings of others and to respond to these with appropriate emotions. The Systemizing Quotient assessed the drive to analyse or construct systems such as mechanical systems. All questionnaires were self-report and participants completed them electronically. For the AQ (maximum score = 50), the higher the score, the more autistic-like characteristics the individual possessed. For the EQ (maximum

Table 1 Summary of Demographic Information

	Younger adults N = 30	Middle-aged adults N = 30	Older adults N = 31	Sig*	ηp² (d)
	Age groups				
Age(SD)	26.20 (5.21)	50.60 (5.77)	72.45 (6.05)	-	-
Males:Females	15:15	15:15	14:17	-	-
Years of full-time education	17.03 (2.82)	15.53 (2.88)	14.58 (2.88)	O<Y	.12(.74)

Y= Younger adults; M= Middle-aged adults, O = Older adults.
*Analysis were conducted using one-way ANOVAs, post hoc testing were conducted using Gabriel's procedure for multiple comparisons. All $p < .05$.
https://doi.org/10.1371/journal.pone.0195818.t001

score = 80), higher scores suggested higher levels of empathy. For the SQ (maximum score = 150), higher scores suggested stronger interest systems, for example the drive to construct systems or to understand the underlying rules that govern a system.

The Edinburgh Social Cognition Test (ESCoT)

The Edinburgh Social Cognition Test (ESCoT) measured four social cognitive abilities: cognitive ToM; affective ToM; interpersonal understanding of social norms and intrapersonal understanding of social norms.

The ESCoT consisted of 11 dynamic, cartoon-style social interactions (each approximately 30 seconds long): 1 practice interaction, 5 interactions involved a social norm violation and 5 portrayed everyday interactions that did not involve social norm violations. Each animation had a different context and specific questions relating to that context. The animation was presented in the middle of a computer screen and at the end of each animation, a static storyboard depicting a summarised version of the interaction was presented (see S1 Fig in the supplementary materials). The storyboard remained on the screen for the duration of the trial. Participants were asked to describe what had occurred in the interaction. Then participants were asked one question to assess each of the four subtests of social cognition. To allow participants to give their optimal interpretation of each interaction and capture the quality of their response, they were prompted if they gave a limited response or their response lacked important information from the interaction. They were prompted with the question, 'Can you tell me more about what you mean by that?' or 'Can you explain that in a little bit more detail?'. Each participant was prompted only once for each question.

Each response was scored based on the quality of the answer with maximum points awarded for responses that successfully extracted and integrated the relevant information from the interaction and articulated this response in a contextually specific manner. Importantly, response length was not related to quality; participants could score maximum points with a minimal response. For scoring of the intrapersonal understanding of social norms subtest, responses that considered the social nuances of the interaction were scored more highly than responses that highlighted personal attributes of the participant. Each question was awarded a maximum of 3 points, resulting in a score of 12 points for each social interaction. The total maximum score for the test was 120 points. The ESCoT took appropriately 20–25 minutes to complete and the animations were viewed on VLC media player. Researchers interested in using the ESCoT can contact the corresponding author to obtain the full test with scoring instructions.

Reading the Mind in the Eyes (RME) [18]

The RME was administered to assess affective ToM. Participants were presented with photographs of the ocular region of different human faces and were required to make a force-choice response from four adjectives (one target and three foils) which best described what the individual was thinking or feeling. If participants were unsure or unfamiliar with an adjective, they were provided with a glossary of the adjectives and their definitions to clarify what each word meant. Participants kept this glossary throughout testing and could refer to it when required. Responses were recorded verbally and 1 point was awarded for each correct answer, giving a total score of 36.

Reading the Mind in Films (RMF) [64]

The RMF was administered to assess affective ToM. Participants viewed short scenes from feature films and were instructed to make a forced-choice response from four adjectives (one target and three foils) that best described what the protagonist was thinking or feeling at the end of the scene. Similar to the RME, participants were provided with a glossary of the adjectives for clarification and responded verbally. A correct response was awarded 1 point, giving a total score of 22.

Judgement of Preference (JoP) [65]

The JoP assessed a participant's ability to make affective ToM judgements of a character while inhibiting their own preferences. This version consisted of a pre-experimental condition and two experimental conditions, each comprising of twelve trials each. In the pre-experimental condition, participants were instructed to choose the item that they liked the most out of 4 items. Following this, participants were presented with a small circular face in the middle of a computer screen with 4 objects in the four corners. In the affective condition, participants were told to choose the item the face in the middle of the screen liked. In the physical condition, participants were asked to identify the item that the face was looking at. Participants touched the item in the correct position on the screen of a touch-screen computer. Each participant was instructed to respond as quickly but as accurately as possible. The affective and physical conditions were counterbalanced. A correct response was given 1 point with a maximum score of 12 per condition.

Social Norms Questionnaire (SNQ) [66]

The SNQ examined intrapersonal understanding of social norms. It was originally developed to screen patients for potential behaviour changes and is administered to examine how well participants understand the social standards that govern their behaviour in mainstream culture. Participants were given a list of behaviours (e.g., tell a stranger you don't like their hairstyle?) and asked to indicate whether or not each of the behaviours was socially acceptable to perform in the presence of a stranger or acquaintance, not a close friend or family member. A total score (maximum score = 22) was calculated, with higher scores reflecting better performance.

Procedure

Participants completed all six tasks in a single session, which took approximately two hours to complete. The order of the tasks was kept the same for each participant.

Statistical Analyses

The effects of age, intelligence (verbal comprehension and perceptual reasoning) and the BAP (AQ, EQ and SQ) on the ESCoT and established tests of social cognition were investigated using hierarchical multiple regression analysis. In the first stage, the background predictors (age, gender, years of education, measures of IQ) which showed a correlation with the outcome variables (subtests of the ESCoT, ESCoT total scores and established social cognition tests) at a pre-specified significance level of $p<0.20$ was entered into the analysis [67] using the enter method. While some researchers have suggested that all relevant variables should be included in the regression model regardless of their significance, this approach can result in numerically unstable estimates and large standard errors [68]. We chose a significance level of $p<0.20$ over more traditional levels such as $p<0.05$ because $p<0.05$ can fail in identifying variables known to be important, and simulation studies have shown that a cut-off of $p<0.20$ yields better outcomes than a cut-off of $p<0.05$ [68, 69]. The scores of VCI and PRI were entered into the first stage independently along with the other background predictor variables in separate regression models. In the second stage, AQ, EQ and SQ scores were entered using the stepwise method (entry criterion $p<0.05$, removal criterion

$p>0.10$) to examine their effect on performance. Furthermore, adjusted scores based on the regression analyses were calculated. These age adjustments were calculated using the unstandardized β coefficients from the regression analysis and the mean age of the sample, the calculations for these can be found in the supplementary materials (S2 Fig). To investigate the relationship between the ESCoT and standard tests of social cognition, correlational analyses were conducted to validate the ESCoT against established tests.

Results

Table 2 demonstrates the preliminary correlational analyses between cognitive ToM, affective ToM, inter- and intrapersonal understanding of social norms with VCI scores, PRI scores, age, years of education and gender. Variables with correlations that were significant at the $p<0.20$ level were included in the regression analysis. Table 3 shows a summary of the regression analyses for the subtests of the ESCoT.

ESCoT total scores and IQ scores. The ESCoT total scores correlated with age (r = –0.42, $p<0.20$). Years of education (r = 0.13, $p>0.20$), gender (males = 1, females = 2, r = 0.09, $p>0.20$), VCI scores (r = 0.11, $p>0.20$) and PRI scores (r = 0.09, $p>0.20$) did not correlate with ESCoT total scores at $p<0.20$. Therefore, these variables did not meet criteria for inclusion in the model.

In the regression model, age was the only significant predictor of ESCoT performance ($p<0.001$, R^2 = 0.18). The inclusion of AQ, EQ and SQ scores produced a significant F-change (F-change = 5.44, $p<0.05$, ΔR^2 = 0.05). In the final model, only age ($p<0.001$) and AQ scores ($p<0.05$) were significant predictors of ESCoT performance, with older age and higher AQ scores predicting poorer performance on the ESCoT. EQ and

Table 2 Correlational Analysis Between the Background Predictors and Measures of the ESCoT

Outcome Variable	Age	Years of Education	Gender	VCI	PRI
Cognitive ToM	–0.32*	0.18*	0.01	0.12	0.04
Affective ToM	–0.17*	0.09	0.23*	0.15*	0.18*
Interpersonal Understanding of Social Norms	–0.38*	0.12	0.06	–0.08	–0.09
interpersonal Understanding of Social Norms	–0.16*	-0.09	–0.13	–0.09	–0.11

*P<0.20.

Predictor variables which correlated with the outcome variable at the p<0.20 level met criteria for inclusion in the regression model. Predictor variables with correlations p>0.20 did not meet criteria for inclusion in the regression model. Results of the regression analyses that included the correlated variables can be seen in Table 3. VCI = Verbal Comprehension Index; PRI = Perceptual Reasoning Index.

https://doi.org/10.1371/journal.pone.0195818.t002

Table 3   Regression Analyses for the Subtests of the Escot with VCI and PRI Scores

	Model 1 Summary	Significant Predictors in Model 1	Excluded Predictors in Model 2	F-change & ΔR^2	Significant Predictors in Model 2
Cognitive ToM	$R^2 = 0.11$, $P<0.01$	Age($P<0.01$)	AQ, EQ & SQ	-	-
Interpersonal Understanding of social Norms	$R^2 = 0.14$, $P<0.01$	Age($P<0.0001$)	EQ & SQ	F-change = 10.55, $P<0.01$, $\Delta R^2 = 0.08$	Age ($p<0.001$) & AQ ($P<0.01$)
Interpersonal Understanding of social Norms	$R^2 = 0.03$, $P>0.05$	-	EQ & SQ	F-change = 7.27, $p<0.01$, $\Delta R^2 = 0.08$	AQ ($P<0.01$)
VCI: Affective ToM	$R^2 = 0.03$, $P<0.05$	Age ($P<0.05$) & Gender ($P<0.05$)	AQ,SQ & SQ	-	-
PRI: Affective ToM	$R^2 = 0.12$, $P<0.05$	Age ($P<0.05$) & Gender ($P<0.05$)	AQ,SQ & SQ	-	-

SQ scores were excluded as predictors from the final regression model.

RME and IQ scores. For the RME scores, VCI scores ($r = 0.28$, $p<0.20$) met criteria for inclusion in the first stage of the analysis. Age ($r = -0.10$, $p>0.20$), years of education ($r = -.07$, $p>0.20$) and gender ($r = -0.06$, $p>0.20$) were not included. In the first model, VCI scores ($p<0.05$, $R^2 = 0.06$) predicted performance on the RME. Higher VCI scores predicted better RME performance. AQ, EQ and SQ scores were not retained in the final model.

RMF and IQ scores. Gender ($r = 0.23$, $p<0.20$), VCI scores ($r = 0.38$, $p<0.20$) and PRI scores ($r = 0.27$, $p<0.20$) met the criteria for inclusion in the regression models. Age ($r = .02$, $p>.20$) and years of education ($r = -0.03$, $p>0.20$) did not correlate with RMF scores at $p<0.20$. In the first model, VCI scores ($p<0.01$) and gender ($p<0.05$) were significant predictors of RMF performance ($p<0.001$, $R^2 = 0.18$). Female participants and participants who had higher VCI scores performed better on the RMF. No variables were entered into the model in the second stage as they did not meet criteria for inclusion.

In a regression model with PRI scores, both gender ($p<0.05$) and PRI scores ($p<0.05$) were predictors of RMF scores ($p<0.01$, $R^2 = 0.13$). Female participants and participants with higher PRI scores were associated with better performance on the RMF. AQ, EQ and SQ scores were not retained in the final model.

SNQ and IQ scores. Age ($r = 0.14$, $p<0.20$) and VCI scores ($r = 0.23$, $p<0.20$) met criteria for inclusion. Gender ($r = 0.07$,

$p>0.20$), years of education ($r = -0.12$, $p<0.20$) and PRI scores ($r = 0.06$, $p>0.20$) did not meet criteria for inclusion in the regressions. However, all regression analyses were not significant (all $p>0.10$).

JoP and IQ scores. Age ($r = 0.05$, $p>0.20$), years of education ($r = -0.05$, $p>0.20$) gender ($r = -0.13$, $p>0.20$), VCI scores ($r = -0.06$, $p>0.20$) and PRI scores ($r = -0.09$, $p>0.20$) did not meet criteria for inclusion in the regression models. Moreover, all regression analyses for the JoP were not significant (all $p>0.10$).

Age Adjusted Scores
Cognitive ToM

The regression analysis demonstrated a negative association with age; as age increased, performance on cognitive ToM decreased. Rather than producing separate normative data for each age group, we suggest that raw cognitive ToM scores should be adjusted for age accordingly: 18–22 years old = –1 point, 23–77 years old = no change in raw score and 78 years and older = +1 point.

Affective ToM

The regression analysis revealed that age negatively predicted performance on affective ToM. As participants' ages increased, performance on affective ToM decreased. Therefore, raw affective ToM scores should be adjusted for age: 18–26 years old = –1 point, 27–73 years old = no change in raw score and 74 years and older = +1 point.

Gender predicted performance on affective ToM with being female predicting better performance better than being male. However, the difference between the male and female groups was only 0.36 standard deviations (less than 1 point on the ESCoT). Therefore, it is not necessary to adjust the raw affective ToM scores for gender.

Interpersonal Understanding of Social Norms

Since the regression analysis revealed that age predicted performance on interpersonal understanding of social norms, raw scores should be adjusted as follows: 18–19 years old = –2 points, 20–34 years old = –1 point, 35–65 years old = no change, 66–80 years old = +1 point and 81 years and older = +2 points.

Correlations between the ESCoT and Established Tests

Correlational analyses with the Holm correction for multiple comparisons showed that the ESCoT significantly correlated with the RME ($r = 0.33$, $p<0.01$) and showed a trend towards significance with the SNQ ($r = 0.19$, $p>0.05$). The RME correlated with the RMF ($r = 0.38$, $p<0.001$) and SNQ ($r = 0.34$, $p<0.01$). The RMF also showed a trend towards significance with the SNQ ($r = 0.19$, $p>0.05$). None of the tests significantly correlated with the JoP (all $p>0.10$).

ESCoT Inter-rater Reliability and Internal Consistency

To establish the reliability of the scoring, we calculated inter-rater reliability for the ESCoT using intraclass correlation (ICCs). A second independent rater scored a sample of 5 participants from each age group. The consistency (ICCs) for the 15 ratings was 0.90, indicating high inter-rater reliability.

We assessed internal consistency for the ESCoT by calculating Guttman's Lambda 4 reliability coefficient. This method has been shown to be a better measure of internal consistency than Cronbach's alpha [70]. Guttman's Lambda 4 reliability coefficient for the ESCoT was 0.70 which is acceptable [71].

Discussion

The current study presented a new within subjects' measure of social cognition that assesses cognitive and affective ToM, as well as intra- and interpersonal social norm understanding, within the same test. We examined the effects of age, measures of intelligence and the BAP on the ESCoT and established tests of social cognition. Additionally, we investigated the relationship between the ESCoT and established measures of social cognition. Total ESCoT scores were predicted by the age of participants and their AQ scores, here increasing age and AQ scores resulted in poorer performance. Investigation of the

subcomponents of the ESCoT revealed that performance on cognitive ToM was significantly predicted by age, with increasing age resulting in decreased performance on cognitive ToM. Affective ToM was also predicted by age but also gender; in this instance, better performance was associated with being younger and female. Moreover, performance on interpersonal understanding of social norms was predicted by age and AQ scores–increasing age and AQ scores were predictive of poorer performance. On the subtest of intrapersonal understanding of social norms, higher AQ scores predicted poorer performance.

Notably, the ESCoT total score and sub-test measures were not associated with the two measures of intelligence; verbal comprehension (VCI) and perceptual reasoning (PRI). This contrasts with performance on some of the more standard tests of social cognition. In the present study, we found that participants with higher verbal comprehension scores performed better on the RME, while RMF performance was significantly predicted by measures of verbal comprehension, perceptual reasoning and gender. Here, female participants and those with higher verbal comprehension and perceptual reasoning scores performed better on this measure of affective ToM. The correlation analysis demonstrated that ESCoT total scores significantly correlated with the RME and showed a trend towards significance with the SNQ, indicating convergent validity.

Similar to previous findings in the literature which have demonstrated aged-related difference in cognitive ToM [20, 22, 23, 26, 30, 36–38], age predicted poorer performance in cognitive ToM on the ESCoT. This provides further evidence that, as we get older, we experience difficulties in our ability to infer what another individual is thinking. Moreover, we found that increasing age predicted poorer performance in participants' ability to infer what another is feeling, comparable to some [21, 28, 36, 40], but in contrast to other studies [22, 33, 35]. It could be argued that the findings here are more representative of the population, as we included adults aged 18–85 years while Bottiroli *et al.* [22] only included younger and older adults. Or, as Henry *et al.* [13] have argued, age-related differences can be the consequence of the type of task used. For example, Phillips *et al.* [34] examined how well older adults were able to assess the severity of contextual emotions of individuals in short stories. They found younger and older adults did not significantly differ in this ability. However, forced choice tests offer limited insights in understanding the relationship between age and social cognition. Primarily because there are few real-world social interactions where inferring what another person is feeling is forced-choice in nature. Overall, these results suggest that the process of healthy aging is associated with difficulties in both components of ToM.

To our knowledge, this is the first study to assess the ability to understand social rules in the same test as ToM and explicitly examine interpersonal (did X behave as other people should behave?) and intrapersonal (would you have acted the same as X?) understanding of social norms. Age was found to predict poorer performance on interpersonal understanding of social norms. These findings add to the preliminary findings of Halberstadt *et al.* [44] who showed poorer performance of older adults compared to younger adults on interpersonal understanding of social norms. We provide a novel finding in regards to intrapersonal understanding of social norms; we showed that the age of participants was not a predictive variable of performance. This suggests that age does not impact our own knowledge of how we should behave in social situations, and not all our social cognitive abilities are negatively affected by age. Both of these findings demonstrate that understanding of social norms warrants further investigation.

Although both cognitive and affective ToM were affected negatively by age, we do provide some evidence for a dissociation between the two processes in that performance is predicted by different demographic variables. This is analogous to the findings that cognitive and affective ToM correlate with different cognitive processes [22]. Cognitive ToM performance was negatively predicted by age while affective ToM was significantly predicted by age and gender. Like Duval *et al.* [23], we found that both cognitive and affective ToM show impairments with advancing age in the same study. The advantage in this study was that we were able to measure cognitive and affective ToM within the same test, unlike Duval *et al.* [23] who relied on different tests to measure these abilities and was therefore unable to control for task difficulty. Gender was only found to predict performance on affective ToM; this is similar to research found in the literature which has shown that women are significantly better at inferring what a character is feeling compared to men [18, 72, 73]. These results show that, as well as considering the consequences of aging on our social cognitive abilities, we should consider the gender of the sample population. Furthermore, they highlight the importance of adopting social cognitive tests that assess cognitive and affective ToM separately and suggest composite tests are not appropriate to accurately examine ToM in aging populations. Using within subjects tests are essential if we are to better understand whether aging does indeed affect cognitive and affective ToM in the same way.

The only test of social cognition that was associated with the measures of the BAP was the ESCoT, suggesting that perhaps the ESCoT is more sensitive to difficulties in social abilities of individuals on the BAP compared to established tests. Here, lower scores in inter- and intrapersonal understanding of social norms were associated with higher scores on the AQ. Additionally, we found that the presence of more autistic traits predicted poorer overall performance on the ESCoT. These are novel findings but makes sense in the context of the BAP, as impaired

social cognition is related to the milder social-behavioral phenotype described as part of the BAP [48, 50, 52]. Research on the understanding of social norms in healthy aging is limited but these findings are in line with research that show that adults with ASD perform poorer than controls on tests such as the Faux Pas which implicitly assess social norms understanding [74]. However, the relationship between ASD and intrapersonal understanding of social norms is less clear and requires further investigation For example, Baez *et al.* [7] found that adults with ASD do not significantly differ on this ability compared to controls. Nonetheless, the observed relationship between the ESCoT and the AQ demonstrates that this new test of social cognition may offer new insights into the relationship between the BAP and social cognition in healthy aging populations and may be valuable in ASD research.

An advantage of the ESCoT over other tests of social cognition, is that overall performance was not related to measures of IQ, namely verbal comprehension and perceptual reasoning performance. However, this is not the typical finding with social cognition measures. Charlton *et al.* [45] found that performance on Happé's Strange Stories test (a composite ToM task) was fully mediated by performance IQ, executive function, and information processing speed and was partially mediated by verbal IQ. Moreover, again on Happé's Strange Stories test, Sullivan and Ruffman [28] both found that ToM abilities were related to perceptual reasoning abilities. In both the current study and previous studies in the literature [64, 72, 75], performance on the RME and RMF was found to be predicted by verbal comprehension. In one study, the only significant predictor of performance on the RME test was verbal comprehension which accounted for 11.7% of the variance [76]. This has implications for studies using the RME and RMF to investigate affective ToM as they appear to be tests of verbal comprehension as well as affective ToM.

A limitation of the present study is that we did not examine the relationship between executive functions and the ESCoT. Given that social cognition has been associated with executive abilities in aging [22, 23, 27, 72], future work might explore potential associations between the ESCoT and processes such as inhibition, set-shifting and updating. Finally, it has been suggested that the clinical assessment of social cognition should emulate the way in which individuals process social situations in everyday life [4]. As argued by Henry *et al.* [13], dynamic-visual information such as images depicting a social interaction that lead to a protagonist in a particular mental state is more ecologically valid and information-rich compared to verbal narratives. Consequently, dynamic cartoons were chosen as the mode of presentation in the ESCoT. This allowed perceivers to use many more cues to make inferences [77], similar to real-life. Videos of real individuals interacting would be the ideal stimuli for assessing social cognitive abilities to maximise ecological validity. However, social interactions are highly complex [78] and social information can be difficult to control in real interactions. Therefore, it may be difficult to separate the specific social cognitive process that the test is intending to measure. With animated characters, specific social cognitive abilities can be more easily isolated and individual social differences can be controlled; essentially all of the parameters can be regulated. For these reasons, we chose to use animated interactions for the ESCoT.

This study is the first to assess cognitive ToM and affective ToM, as well as interpersonal and intrapersonal understanding of social norms within the same test in younger, middle-aged and older adults. We have provided further evidence for similar but distinct components of ToM and evidence for social norm understanding. These findings are useful in furthering our understanding of the consequences of aging on our social cognitive abilities. They also demonstrate specific advantages of the ESCoT over other tests of social cognition. The ESCoT is able to assess distinct aspects of social cognition within a single task and using a within subjects design, allowing for systematic comparisons of these abilities. This important feature of the ESCoT allows it to be a useful test for researchers examining age-related changes in social cognition, and perhaps as a test for clinicians in populations such as adults with ASD, traumatic brain injury patients or psychiatric and neurological patients with suspect social cognitive impairments. As a consequence of its design, the ESCoT can provide researchers and clinicians with an objective measurement of four important social cognitive abilities that are needed to interact with others. This is particularly useful in clinical settings since the results can be used to personalise interventions or educate caregivers about the difficulties the patient might be experiencing in processing social information and interacting with others. In conclusion, these findings show that the ESCoT is a valuable measure of social cognition and, unlike established and standard tests of social cognition, performance is not predicted by measures of verbal comprehension and perceptual reasoning. This is particularly valuable in order to get an accurate assessment of the influence of age on our social cognitive abilities.

. . .

References

1. Adolphs R. The social brain: Neural basis of social knowledge. Annual Review of Psychology. 2009;60:693–716. pmid:18771388
2. Baez S, García AM, Ibanez A. The social context network model in psychiatric and neurological diseases. Current Topics in Behavioral Neurosciences. 2016:1–18.
3. Frith CD. Social cognition. Philosophical Transactions of the Royal Society B: Biological Sciences. 2008;363(1499):2033–9.
4. Henry JD, Cowan DG, Lee T, Sachdev PS. Recent trends in testing social cognition. Current Opinion in Psychiatry. 2015;28(2):133–40. pmid:25630050
5. Love MCN, Ruff G, Geldmacher DS. Social sognition in older adults: A review of reuropsychology, neurobiology, and functional connectivity. Medical & Clinical Reviews. 2015.
6. Baez S, Herrera E, Villarin L, Theil D, Gonzalez-Gadea ML, Gomez P, et al. Contextual social cognition impairments in Schizophrenia and Bipolar Disorder. PLoS One. 2013;8(3):e57664. pmid:23520477
7. Baez S, Rattazzi A, Gonzalez-Gadea ML, Torralva T, Vigliecca N, Decety J, et al. Integrating intention and context: Assessing social cognition in adults with Asperger Syndrome. Frontiers in Human Neuroscience. 2012;6:1–21.
8. Scheibe S, Carstensen LL. Emotional aging: Recent findings and future trends. The Journals of Gerontology Series B: Psychological Sciences and Social Sciences. 2010:135–44.
9. Luong G, Charles ST, Fingerman KL. Better with age: Social relationships across adulthood. Journal of Social and Personal Relationships. 2010;28(1):9–23.
10. English T, Carstensen LL. Selective narrowing of social networks across adulthood is associated with improved emotional experience in daily life. International Journal of Behavioral Development. 2014;38(2):195–202. pmid:24910483
11. Blanchard-Fields F. Everyday problem solving and emotion an adult developmental perspective. Current Directions in Psychological Science. 2007;16(1):26–31.
12. Hess TM. Memory and aging in context. Psychological Bulletin. 2005;131(3):383. pmid:15869334
13. Henry JD, Phillips LH, Ruffman T, Bailey PE. A meta-analytic review of age differences in theory of mind. Psychology and Aging. 2013;28(3):826. pmid:23276217
14. Kemp J, Després O, Sellal F, Dufour A. Theory of Mind in normal ageing and neurodegenerative pathologies. Ageing Research Reviews. 2012;11(2):199–219. pmid:22186031
15. Shamay-Tsoory SG, Harari H, Aharon-Peretz J, Levkovitz Y. The role of the orbitofrontal cortex in affective theory of mind deficits in criminal offenders with psychopathic tendencies. Cortex. 2010;46(5):668–77. pmid:19501818
16. Kalbe E, Schlegel M, Sack AT, Nowak DA, Dafotakis M, Bangard C, et al. Dissociating cognitive from affective theory of mind: a TMS study. Cortex. 2010;46(6):769–80. pmid:19709653
17. Sebastian CL, Fontaine NM, Bird G, Blakemore S-J, De Brito SA, McCrory EJ, et al. Neural processing associated with cognitive and affective Theory of Mind in adolescents and adults. Social Cognitive and Affective Neuroscience. 2011:1–11.
18. Baron-Cohen S, Wheelwright S, Hill J, Raste Y, Plumb I. The "Reading the Mind in the Eyes" test revised version: A study with normal adults, and adults with Asperger Syndrome or High Functioning Autism. Journal of Child Psychology and Psychiatry. 2001;42(2):241–51. pmid:11280420
19. Stone VE, Baron-Cohen S, Knight RT. Frontal lobe contributions to theory of mind. Journal of Cognitive Neuroscience. 1998;10(5):640–56. pmid:9802997
20. Bailey PE, Henry JD. Growing less empathic with age: Disinhibition of the self-perspective. The Journals of

Gerontology Series B: Psychological Sciences and Social Sciences. 2008;63(4):P219–P26. pmid:18689763

21. Bailey PE, Henry JD, Von Hippel W. Empathy and social functioning in late adulthood. Aging and Mental Health. 2008;12(4):499–503. pmid:18791898

22. Bottiroli S, Cavallini E, Ceccato I, Vecchi T, Lecce S. Theory of mind in aging: Comparing cognitive and affective components in the faux pas test. Archives of Gerontology and Geriatrics. 2016;62:152–62. pmid:26434925

23. Duval C, Piolino P, Bejanin A, Eustache F, Desgranges B. Age effects on different components of theory of mind. Consciousness and Cognition. 2011;20(3):627–42. pmid:21111637

24. Maylor EA, Moulson JM, Muncer AM, Taylor LA. Does performance on theory of mind tasks decline in old age? British Journal of Psychology. 2002;93(Pt 4):465–85. pmid:12519529

25. McKinnon MC, Moscovitch M. Domain-general contributions to social reasoning: theory of mind and deontic reasoning re-explored. Cognition. 2007;102(2):179–218. pmid:16480974

26. Moran JM, Jolly E, Mitchell JP. Social-cognitive deficits in normal aging. The Journal of Neuroscience. 2012;32(16):5553–61. pmid:22514317

27. Rakoczy H, Harder Kasten A, Sturm L. The decline of theory of mind in old age is (partly) mediated by developmental changes in domain general abilities. British Journal of Psychology. 2012;103(1):58–72. pmid:22229774

28. Sullivan S, Ruffman T. Social understanding: How does it fare with advancing years? British Journal of Psychology. 2004;95(Pt 1):1–18. pmid:15005864

29. Happé FG, Winner E, Brownell H. The getting of wisdom: Theory of mind in old age. Developmental Psychology. 1998;34(2):358. pmid:9541787

30. Castelli I, Baglio F, Blasi V, Alberoni M, Falini A, Liverta-Sempio O, et al. Effects of aging on mindreading ability through the eyes: An fMRI study. Neuropsychologia. 2010;48(9):2586–94. pmid:20457166

31. Keightley ML, Winocur G, Burianova H, Hongwanishkul D, Grady CL. Age effects on social cognition: faces tell a different story. Psychology and Aging. 2006;21(3):558. pmid:16953717

32. Li X, Wang K, Wang F, Tao Q, Xie Y, Cheng Q. Aging of theory of mind: The influence of educational level and cognitive processing. International Journal of Psychology. 2013;48(4):715–27. pmid:22515730

33. MacPherson SE, Phillips LH, Della Sala S. Age, executive function and social decision making: a dorsolateral prefrontal theory of cognitive aging. Psychology and Aging. 2002;17(4):598. pmid:12507357

34. Phillips LH, MacLean RD, Allen R. Age and the understanding of emotions neuropsychological and sociocognitive perspectives. The Journals of Gerontology Series B: Psychological Sciences and Social Sciences. 2002;57(6):P526–P30.

35. Wang Y, Su Y. Theory of mind in old adults: The performance on Happé's stories and faux pas stories. Psychologia. 2006;49(4):228–37.

36. Fischer AL, O'Rourke N, Thornton WL. Age differences in cognitive and affective theory of mind: Concurrent contributions of neurocognitive performance, sex, and pulse pressure. The Journals of Gerontology Series B: Psychological Sciences and Social Sciences. 2016:gbw088.

37. German TP, Hehman JA. Representational and executive selection resources in 'theory of mind': Evidence from compromised belief-desire reasoning in old age. Cognition. 2006;101(1):129–52. pmid:16288734

38. Saltzman J, Strauss E, Hunter M, Archibald S. Theory of mind and executive functions in normal human aging and Parkinson's disease. Journal of the International Neuropsychological Society. 2000;6(07):781–8.

39. Pardini M, Nichelli PF. Age-related decline in mentalizing skills across adult life span. Experimental Aging Research. 2009;35(1):98–106. pmid:19173104

40. Slessor G, Phillips LH, Bull R. Exploring the specificity of age-related differences in theory of mind tasks. Psychology and Aging. 2007;22(3):639–43. pmid:17874961

41. Phillips LH, Bull R, Allen R, Insch P, Burr K, Ogg W. Lifespan aging and belief reasoning: Influences of executive function and social cue decoding. Cognition. 2011;120(2):236–47. pmid:21624567

42. Eddy CM, Beck SR, Mitchell IJ, Praamstra P, Pall HS. Theory of mind deficits in Parkinson's disease: a product of executive dysfunction? Neuropsychology. 2013;27(1):37. pmid:23356595

43. Carr AR, Paholpak P, Daianu M, Fong SS, Mather M, Jimenez EE, et al. An investigation of care-based vs. rule-based morality in Frontotemporal Dementia, Alzheimer's Disease, and healthy controls. Neuropsychologia. 2015;78:73–9. pmid:26432341

44. Halberstadt J, Ruffman T, Murray J, Taumoepeau M, Ryan M. Emotion perception explains age-related differences in the perception of social gaffes. Psychology and Aging. 2011;26(1):133. pmid:21280951

45. Charlton RA, Barrick TR, Markus HS, Morris RG. Theory of mind associations with other cognitive functions and brain imaging in normal aging. Psychology and Aging. 2009;24(2):338–48. pmid:19485652

46. American Psychiatric Association. Diagnostic and statistical manual of mental disorders. 5th ed. Arlington, VA: APA; 2013.

47. Klin A, Jones W, Schultz R, Volkmar F, Cohen D. Visual fixation patterns during viewing of naturalistic social situations as predictors of social competence in individuals with autism. Archives of general psychiatry. 2002;59(9):809–16. pmid:12215080

48. Sasson NJ, Nowlin RB, Pinkham AE. Social cognition, social skill, and the broad autism phenotype. Autism. 2013;17(6):655–67. pmid:22987889

49. Wainer AL, Block N, Donnellan MB, Ingersoll B. The broader autism phenotype and friendships in non-clinical dyads. Journal of autism and developmental disorders. 2013;43(10):2418–25. pmid:23430176

50. Wainer AL, Ingersoll BR, Hopwood CJ. The structure and nature of the broader autism phenotype in a non-clinical sample. Journal of Psychopathology and Behavioral Assessment. 2011;33(4):459.

51. Piven J, Palmer P, Jacobi D, Childress D, Arndt S. Broader autism phenotype: evidence from a family history study of multiple-incidence autism families. American Journal of Psychiatry. 1997;154(2):185–90. pmid:9016266

52. Losh M, Piven J. Social cognition and the broad autism phenotype: identifying genetically meaningful phenotypes. Journal of Child Psychology and Psychiatry. 2007;48(1):105–12. pmid:17244276

53. Wallace GL, Budgett J, Charlton RA. Aging and autism spectrum disorder: Evidence from the broad autism phenotype. Autism Research. 2016;9(12):1294–303. pmid:26970433

54. Devine RT, Hughes C. Silent films and strange stories: theory of mind, gender, and social experiences in middle childhood. Child Development. 2013;84(3):989–1003. pmid:23199139

55. Dziobek I, Fleck S, Kalbe E, Rogers K, Hassenstab J, Brand M, et al. Introducing MASC: a movie for the assessment of social cognition. Journal of autism and developmental disorders. 2006;36(5):623–36. pmid:16755332

56. McDonald S, Flanagan S, Rollins J, Kinch J. TASIT: A new clinical tool for assessing social perception after traumatic brain injury. The Journal of head trauma rehabilitation. 2003;18(3):219–38. pmid:12802165

57. Heavey L, Phillips W, Baron-Cohen S, Rutter M. The Awkward Moments Test: A naturalistic measure of social understanding in autism. Journal of autism and developmental disorders. 2000;30(3):225–36. pmid:11055458

58. Roeyers H, Buysse A, Ponnet K, Pichal B. Advancing advanced mind reading tests: empathic accuracy in adults with a pervasive developmental disorder. Journal of Child Psychology and Psychiatry. 2001;42(2):271–8. pmid:11280423

59. Wechsler D. Wechsler Adult Intelligence Scale: Technical and interpretive manual. 3rd ed. San Antonio, TX: The Psychological Corporation; 1997.

60. Wechsler D. Wechsler Abbreviated Scale of Intelligence–Second Edition (WASI-II). San Antonio, TX: NCS Pearson; 2011.

61. McCrimmon AW, Smith AD. Test Review: Review of the Wechsler Abbreviated Scale of Intelligence, Second Edition (WASI-II). Journal of Psychoeducational Assessment. 2013;31(3):337–41.

62. Baron-Cohen S, Wheelwright S, Skinner R, Martin J, Clubley E. The autism-spectrum quotient (AQ): Evidence from Asperger Syndrome/High-Functioning Autism, males and females, scientists and mathematicians. Journal of Autism and Developmental Disorders. 2001;31(1):5–17. pmid:11439754.

63. Baron-Cohen S, Wheelwright S. The empathy quotient: An investigation of adults with Asperger Syndrome or High Functioning Autism and normal sex differences. Journal of Autism and Developmental Disorders. 2004;34(2):163–75. pmid:15162935.

64. Golan O, Baron-Cohen S, Hill JJ, Golan Y. The "reading the mind in films" task: complex emotion recognition in adults with and without autism spectrum conditions. Social Neuroscience. 2006;1(2):111–23. pmid:18633780

65. Girardi A, MacPherson SE, Abrahams S. Deficits in emotional and social cognition in amyotrophic lateral sclerosis. Neuropsychology. 2011;25(1):53–65. pmid:20919762

66. Rankin KP. Social Norms Questionaire NINDS Domain Specific Tasks of Executive Function. 2008.

67. Altman DG. Practical statistics for medical research. London: Chapman and Hall; 1991.

68. Bursac Z, Gauss CH, Williams DK, Hosmer DW. Purposeful selection of variables in logistic regression. Source code for biology and medicine. 2008;3(1):17.

69. Lee PH. Should we adjust for a confounder if empirical and theoretical criteria yield contradictory results? A simulation study. Scientific reports. 2014;4:6085. pmid:25124526

70. Sijtsma K. On the use, the misuse, and the very limited usefulness of Cronbach's alpha. Psychometrika. 2009;74(1):107. pmid:20037639

71. Nunnally J. Psychometric Theory. 2 ed. New York: McGraw-Hill Book Company; 1978.

72. Ahmed FS, Miller LS. Executive function mechanisms of theory of mind. Journal of Autism and Developmental Disorders. 2011;41(5):667–78. pmid:20811770

73. Baron-Cohen S, Bowen DC, Holt RJ, Allison C, Auyeung B, Lombardo MV, et al. The "Reading the Mind in the Eyes" Test: Complete Absence of Typical Sex Difference in similar to 400 Men and Women with Autism. Plos One. 2015;10(8). doi: ARTN e0136521 PubMed PMID: WOS:000360144000065. pmid:26313946

74. Zalla T, Sav A-M, Stopin A, Ahade S, Leboyer M. Faux pas detection and intentional action in Asperger Syndrome. A replication on a French sample. Journal of Autism and Developmental Disorders. 2009;39(2):373–82. pmid:18726150

75. Peterson E, Miller S. The eyes test as a measure of individual differences: how much of the variance reflects verbal IQ? Frontiers in psychology. 2012;3:220. pmid:22783217

76. Lawrence EJ, Shaw P, Baker D, Baron-Cohen S, David AS. Measuring empathy: reliability and validity of the Empathy Quotient. Psychological medicine. 2004;34(05):911–20.

77. Moran JM. Lifespan development: The effects of typical aging on theory of mind. Behavioural Brain Research. 2013;237:32–40. pmid:23000532

78. Van Overwalle F. Social cognition and the brain: A meta analysis. Human Brain Mapping. 2009;30(3):829–58. pmid:18381770

Critical Thinking

1. Discuss the contradictions among the variety of cognitive tests mentioned in this article.

2. Why is it important to understand Theory of Mind and social norm understanding across the lifespan?

3. How do you think the ESCoT could affect resource acquisition in elementary, middle, high schools and college, as well as in the workforce?

Internet References

American Psychiatric Association
   https://www.psychiatry.org/

Autism Research Institute
   https://www.autism.com/

Neurology MedLink
   http://www.medlink.com/

Baksh RA, Abrahams S, Auyeung B, MacPherson SE (2018) The Edinburgh Social Cognition Test (ESCoT): Examining the effects of age on a new measure of theory of mind and social norm understanding. *PLoS ONE* 13(4): e0195818. https://doi.org/10.1371/journal.pone.0195818

Article   Prepared by: Elaina Osterbur, *Saint Louis University*

Gastric Balance: Heartburn Not Always Caused by Excess Acid

JAMES ENGLISH

Learning Outcomes

After reading this article, you will be able to:

- Discuss the cause and treatment of poor stomach acid production.

- Explain symptoms and chronic conditions associated with poor stomach acid production.

- Explain the importance of healthy digestion across the life span.

The human requirement for vitamins, minerals and other nutrients remains relatively constant throughout adult life. Unfortunately our ability to properly digest food and absorb vital nutrients declines with advancing age. Surprisingly, one of the most common age-related causes of impaired digestive function is the reduction of hydrochloric acid produced by the stomach.

Hydrochloric acid (HCl) is an important gastric secretion that enables the body to break down proteins, activate important enzymes and hormones, and protect against bacterial overgrowth in the gut. *Achlorhydria* (the complete absence of stomach acid) and *hypochlorhydria* (low stomach acid) are common digestive problems. Symptoms of low stomach acid include heartburn, indigestion and bloating, among others (Table 1). Additionally, a number of chronic health conditions are correlated with impaired acid secretion, including allergies, asthma and gallstones (Table 2).

HCl and Digestion

Digestion is a complex body function that starts when food enters the mouth and continues as material is processed and passed on to the stomach, small intestine and large intestine. In the stomach, digestion begins with the release of a number of gastric secretions, including HCl, pepsinogen and a protective mucus coating. Secretion of hydrochloric acid and pepsin is a prerequisite for

Table 1   Symptoms of Poor Stomach Acid Production
(*Alt Med Rev* 1997; 2(2):116-127)

• Stomach Bloating	• Weak, Cracked Fingernails
• Nausea When Taking Supplements	• Dilated Capillaries in Cheeks and Nose (non-alcoholics)
• Burping	• Post-adolescent Acne
• Upset Stomach	• Iron Deficiency
• Burning	• Mineral Deficiencies
• Flatulence	• Chronic Intestinal Infections
• Diarrhea	• Undigested Food in Stool

Table 2   Disorders Associated with Poor Stomach Acid Output (*Alt Med Rev* 1997; 2(2):116-127)

• Addison's Disease	• Lupus
• Asthma	• Osteoporosis
• Celiac Disease	• Pernicious Anemia
• Chronic Autoimmune Disorders	• Psoriasis
• Diabetes	• Acne rosacea
• Eczema	• Thyrotoxicosis
• Food Allergies	• Urticaria
• Gall Bladder Disease	• Vitiligo
• Gastric Cancer	• Colitis (Ulcerative)
• Gastritis	• Hair Loss
• Graves Disease	• Multiple Sclerosis (MS)
• Hepatitis	• Rheumatoid Arthritis

healthy digestion. Normally the stomach contains enough free hydrochloric acid (HCl) to maintain a constant stomach acidity of between pH 1 and 2. The amount of HCl produced increases rapidly following the ingestion of food. HCl has an important role in the digestion and absorption of a number of nutrients, including:

- **Protein:** HCl initiates the digestion of protein in the stomach by converting pepsinogen into the proteolytic enzyme, pepsin. Once formed, pepsin acts to break proteins into smaller peptides that can be absorbed by the small intestine. Without adequate gastric secretions, incompletely digested macromolecules can be absorbed into the systemic circulation.
- **Carbohydrates and Fats:** HCl supports the digestion and absorption of carbohydrates, fats, and vitamins A and E by stimulating the release of pancreatic enzymes and bile into the small intestine.
- **Vitamins and Minerals:** HCl also aids in the absorption and assimilation of vitamins and minerals such as folic acid, ascorbic acid, beta-carotene and iron, by increasing their bioavailability and effecting their release from food. Jonathan Wright, MD, Medical Director of the Tahoma Clinic, reports observing that a number of minerals and micro-trace elements are poorly absorbed in cases of low stomach acid, including calcium, magnesium, zinc, copper, chromium, selenium, manganese, vanadium, molybdenum and cobalt. (1)

Protection from Pathogens

In addition to breaking down and absorbing vital nutrients, HCl also plays an important role in maintaining a sterile environment in the stomach. HCl does this by protecting against orally ingested pathogens and acting as a barrier to prevent bacterial or fungal overgrowth of the small intestine. Researchers have shown that a common pathogen, E. coli (*Escherichia coli*) is inactivated when stomach acidity is high, with a pH ranging between 1.5 and 4.0. (2)

Conversely, low stomach acidity is associated with the rapid invasion of microorganisms from the colon, leading to gastric and intestinal bacterial colonization and overgrowth. (3) And in tests where researchers induced a temporary state of low acid (pH greater than 4.0) all subjects experienced bacterial overgrowth in the proximal small intestine. (4) Conversely, E coli is not found in the gastric contents of patients with achlorhydria following treatment with HCl. (5)

An additional finding of a Japanese team was a strong correlation between low stomach acidity and increased infection by *Helicobacter pylori* (H. pylori), (6) one of the most common chronic bacterial infections of humans and recognized as a major cause of gastritis, gastric ulcer disease, gastric carcinoma and B-cell gastric lymphoma. (7)

Low Stomach Acid and Age

Numerous studies have shown that hydrochloric acid secretion declines with advancing age (Fig. 1). In one study US researchers found that over 30 percent of men and women past the age of 60 suffer from *atrophic gastritis*, a condition marked by little or no acid secretion. (8) A second study found that up to 40% of postmenopausal women have no basal gastric acid secretions. (9)

In a second study involving 3,484 subjects, researchers found that among both males and females, 27% suffered from achlorhydria, with the greatest incidence (39.8%) occurring in females aged 80 to 89 years. (10)

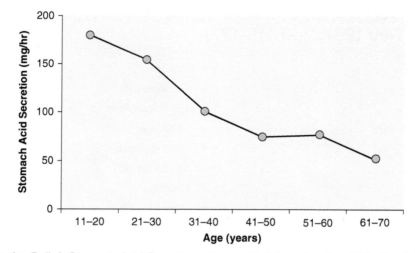

Figure 1   Contrary to Popular Belief, Stomach Acid Secretions Drop with Advancing Age. This Graph Shows Average Decline in Stomach Acid Secretion in Humans Between Age 20 to Age 80. (From *"Why Stomach Acid is Good For You."*)

Researchers in Japan have also measured a similar age-related drop in gastric acidity in elderly Japanese subjects. In 1984 researchers found that 60 percent of Japanese men and women over 50 years age suffered from achlorhydria. New research based on data collected from 1989 to 1999 continued to substantiate a substantial age-related decrease in stomach acid production, though the total percentage of achlorhydric subjects dropped from 60 percent to 40 percent. (7)

Conditions of Low Stomach Acid

Symptoms of low stomach acid frequently occur several hours after eating and can include a desire to eat when not hungry, a sense of fullness after meals, flatulence, constipation and diarrhea. Symptoms that may persist regardless of eating food can include feeling soreness and burning of the mouth. (10)

Heartburn

Heartburn, a burning sensation in the chest caused by the regurgitation of bile through the stomach into the lower esophagus, is a frequent symptom of low gastric acid. The traditional approach of treating heartburn is to suppress gastric acid by taking antacids or alkalizers. This approach is the opposite of what should often be done, and in many cases only worsens the problem by suppressing gastric acidity when it is needed and promoting it (rebound phenomenon) when it is unnecessary.

Jonathan Wright, MD, states, "In 24 years of nutritionally oriented practice, I've worked with thousands of individuals who've found the cause of their heartburn and indigestion to be low stomach acidity. In nearly all of these folks, symptoms

have been relieved and digestion improved when they've taken supplemental hydrochloric acid and pepsin capsules. (Certainly it would be preferable that our stomach production of hydrochloric acid and pepsin be restored on its own, but a reliable way to do this hasn't been found.)" (11)

Supplemental Hydrochloric Acid

Hydrochloric acid was routinely prescribed for many symptoms and clinical conditions for over 100 years. Use of HCl by the medical establishment began to decline in the late 1920s. The decline in HCl replacement therapy, according to Jonathan Wright, was due to poorly designed and misinterpreted research that convinced medical practitioners that HCl and pepsin replacement therapy was not necessary.

> "Encouraged by the legal drug industry, medical students are not taught that hypochlorhydria (inadequate stomach acid production) is treatable only with unpatentable, natural replacement therapies. Instead, their education concentrates on hyperchlorhydria (excess stomach acid production) and its treatment with patentable acid blocker drugs and highly profitable over-the-counter antacids." (11)

Hydrochloric acid has been shown to be effective in relieving symptoms associated with achlorhydria and hypochlorhydria. Substances shown to support healthy acid secretion and digestion include:

- **Betaine hydrochloride** (HCl) is a nutritional supplement that has been used for over 100 years to safely restore normal gastric acidity and to support healthy gut function. Betaine HCl should not be confused with another popular nutritional supplement, anhydrous Betaine, a methyl-donor nutrient taken to control homocysteine levels.

- **Pepsin** has a long history of medicinal use and is considered very safe when administered to assist digestion, typically in conjunction with hydrochloric acid.
- **Peppermint** is used to aid the various processes of digestion due to its antibacterial and gastric-acid-promoting effects. Peppermint also aids digestive function by combating gas, increasing the flow of bile, and healing the stomach and liver. The spasmolytic property of peppermint has been found to decrease the tone of the lower esophagus sphincter so that the escape of air is made easier, which is particularly useful for relieving discomfort caused by spasms in the upper digestive tract. (12)
- **Gentian:** The bitter principles of the dried root of Gentiana lutea have been used in Europe as a digestive aid for centuries, especially in Swedish bitters. Gentian roots were historically used topically to treat skin tumors, and internally to treat fever and diarrhea. (13) Modern research has shown that gentian, which contains two of the most bitter substances known, the glycosides gentiopicrin and amarogentin, acts on taste bud receptors to stimulate the secretion of saliva in the mouth and hydrochloric acid in the stomach. (14)

Summary

Healthy digestion and absorption of nutrients is dependent upon the secretion of gastric acid. When gastric secretions are reduced the result can lead to nutritional deficiencies and a variety of chronic disorders. Low secretion of gastric acid can also allow orally-ingested pathogens to prevail and contribute to their overgrowth in the stomach and small intestine. HCl supplementation is a safe and effective means of restoring normal gastric levels, particularly in cases where age or chronic conditions indicate that nutrients, particularly B vitamins and minerals, are not being properly utilized.

References

1. Wright JV. Treatment of childhood asthma with parenteral vitamin B12, gastric re-acidification, and attention to food allergy, magnesium and pyridoxine. Three case reports with background and an integrated hypothesis. J Nutr Med 1990;1:277-282.
2. Takumi K, de Jonge R, Havelaar A. Modeling inactivation of Escherichia coli by low pH: application to passage through the stomach of young and elderly people. J. Appl Microbiol 2000 Dec;89(6):935-43.
3. Saltzman JR, Kemp JA, Golner BB, et al. Effect of hypochlorhydria due to omeprazole treatment or atrophic gastritis on protein bound vitamin B12 absorption. J Amer Coll Nutr 1994;13:584-591.
4. Tang G, Serfaty-Lacrosniere C, Camilo ME, et al. Gastric acidity influences the blood response to a B-carotene dose in humans. Am J Clin Nutr 1996;64:622-626.
5. Brummer P, Kasanen A. The effect of hydrochloric acid on the indican metabolism in achlorhydria. Acta Medica Scan 1956;155:11-14.
6. Morihara M, Aoyagi N, Kaniwa N, Kojima S, Ogata H.Assessment of gastric acidity of Japanese subjects over the last 15 years. Biol Pharm Bull 2001 Mar;24(3):313-5.
7. Young DG. A stain for demonstrating Helicobacter pylori in gastric biopsies. Biotech Histochem 2001 Jan;76(1):31-4.
8. Krasinski SD, Russell RM, Samloff IM, Jacob RA, Dallal GE, McGandy RB, Hartz SC. Fundic atrophic gastritis in an elderly population. Effect on hemoglobin and several serum nutritional indicators. J Am Geriatr Soc. 1986 Nov;34(11):800-6.
9. Grossman MI, Kirsner JB, Gillespie IE. Basal and histalog-stimulated gastric secretion in control subjects and in patients with peptic ulcer or gastric cancer. Gastroenterology 1963;45:15-26.
10. Sharp GS, Fister HW. The diagnosis and treatment of achlorhydria: ten-year study. J Amer Ger Soc 1967;15:786-791.
11. Jonathan Wright, MD, The Digestive Theory of Aging, Part I, http://www.tahoma-clinic.com/aging.shtml.
12. Schilcher, H,: Deutshe Apotheker Zeitung 124:1433-1443 (1984) (Brundesanzeiger (Cologne, Germany): Nov. 30, 1985; March 13, 1986.
13. Duke JA. CRC Handbook of Medicinal Herbs. Boca Raton, FL: CRC Press, 1985.
14. Bradley PR, ed. British Herbal Compendium (Vol. 1): A handbook of scientific information on widely used plant drugs. Guilford and King's Lynn, Great Britain: Biddles Ltd; 1992:109-111.

Critical Thinking

1. Discuss how poor stomach acid production affects socialization.
2. Discuss risk factors that influences stomach acid production.

Internet References

Livestrong.org
https://www.livestrong.com/
MedlinePlus
https://medlineplus.gov/

Article   Prepared by: Elaina Osterbur, *Saint Louis University*

Caregiving Youth

Today's Caregiver Editorial Staff

Learning Outcomes

After reading this article, you will be able to:

- Explain the role of parents in easing children into caregiving roles.
- Identify the benefits of youth caregiving.

The face of caregivers in the United States today represents every race, ethnicity and religious sect. They can be found in virtually every zip code. And yet, there is still a population of caregivers that often remains invisible. It is estimated that 1.4 million children in the United States participate in the care of a family member or loved one who is either critically or chronically ill. Either living in the same home or nearby the ailing person, these children partake in a wide variety of activities of daily living including everything from bathing to shopping. However, they are often not included in the training or the support structures designed to help caregivers.

But as a parent who is also a caregiver, there are ways to help your child ease into but also successfully maintain a caregiving role.

Often parents want to protect children from the harsh realities of life. But by not giving them the proper information they need about the situation, you can end up doing more harm than good. "Children worry anyhow, even if they are being told everything is okay," explains Laurie Conners, Project Manager of the American Association of Caregiving Youth. Expressing your concerns and fears with your children gives them permission to do the same, preventing them from dealing with it silently. Also by explaining the practicalities of the disease and the treatment, everything from common side effects from certain medications to potential outcomes, prepares the child for what to expect so that nothing is a surprise.

Many times when medical professionals educate and train new caregivers on the different modalities associated with the disease, children aren't involved in learning these necessary techniques. As a parent, find a way to give your children the skills they need to do these jobs as easily as they can. Use the opportunity to teach your children about the disease and caregiving skills as another way to spend time as a family.

A way for you to insure your child talks about what they are going through with the added stress and responsibility of caregiving is to appoint an advocate in the family. This is a person outside of the direct living environment that your child can visit or call on the phone to voice feeling and problems they might encounter. This way, even if your child doesn't feel comfortable talking to you, there is an adult accessible to discuss concerns.

Creating time to be a family outside of caregiving tasks is a great stress reliever for the whole family. Try to remember all the things you used to do as a family. It could be something simple as an hour at your neighborhood park or a night out for pizza just as long as it is time away from the responsibilities of caregiving. If it is not possible for you to get away, plan a game night at home to laugh and enjoy each other's company.

Children in a caregiving role often must neglect outside friends and activities because of the responsibilities at home. Perhaps they need to come home right after school because the parent is still at work and someone needs to take care of the ailing person. Or they may be embarrassed to invite friends over in fear of what they might think. In turn, they become isolated from the rest of the world. However, it is important for kids to maintain relationships with people their own age. Even if it is just one afternoon a week, try to find a way for your child to play with friends or join an activity group.

Just as adult caregivers often must juggle the responsibilities of work and caring for a sick family member, children also play a dual role as student and caregiver. And often children suffer at school because they didn't get a chance to finish their homework the night before because they were helping the ailing person, they had to get up very early to bathe and dress that person or they are simply worried about what is happening at home. As a parent, it is so important to make certain your child is adequately prepared for school each day. And talk to your child's school to let them know the situation at home. If they understand the added constraints, teachers and school administrators can be a valuable asset in your child's wellbeing.

Valuable traits such as independence and confidence often go hand in hand with the responsibility of caring for another person. And children learn valuable life skills that other children may not learn until much later in life. However, what is important is that your child is getting all the support and encouragement they need to be not only a successful caregiver and student, but also have time to be a kid.

Critical Thinking

1. How can medical professionals support youth caregivers?
2. How can communities support youth caregivers?
3. What are the mental health side effects of youth caregiving?

Internet References

American Psychological Association
https://www.apa.org/

National Alliance for Caregivers
https://www.caregiving.org/

Today's Caregiver
https://caregiver.com/

Article Prepared by: Elaina Osterbur, *Saint Louis University*

Caregiver Stress

ALZHEIMER'S ASSOCIATION

Learning Outcomes

After reading this article, you will be able to:

- Identify the 10 symptoms of caregiver stress.
- Discuss the tips to manage stress.

Alzheimer's caregivers frequently report experiencing high levels of stress. It can be overwhelming to take care of a loved one with Alzheimer's or other dementia, but too much stress can be harmful to both of you. Read on to learn symptoms and ways to avoid burnout.

10 Symptoms of Caregiver Stress

1. **Denial** about the disease and its effect on the person who has been diagnosed. I know Mom is going to get better.
2. **Anger** at the person with Alzheimer's or frustration that he or she can't do the things they used to be able to do. He knows how to get dressed — he's just being stubborn.
3. **Social withdrawal** from friends and activities that used to make you feel good. I don't care about visiting with the neighbors anymore.
4. **Anxiety** about the future and facing another day. What happens when he needs more care than I can provide?
5. **Depression** that breaks your spirit and affects your ability to cope. I just don't care anymore.
6. **Exhaustion** that makes it nearly impossible to complete necessary daily tasks. I'm too tired for this.
7. **Sleeplessness** caused by a never-ending list of concerns.
8. What if she wanders out of the house or falls and hurts herself?
9. **Irritability** that leads to moodiness and triggers negative responses and actions. Leave me alone!
10. **Lack of concentration** that makes it difficult to perform familiar tasks. I was so busy, I forgot my appointment.
11. **Health problems** that begin to take a mental and physical toll. I can't remember the last time I felt good.

If you experience any of these signs of stress on a regular basis, make time to talk to your doctor.

Tips to Manage Stress

- **Know what community resources are available.** Adult day programs, in-home assistance, visiting nurses and meal delivery are just some of the services that can help you manage daily tasks. Use our online Community Resource Finder or contact your local Alzheimer's Association® chapter for assistance in finding Alzheimer's care resources in your community. Use Alzheimer's Navigator, our free online tool that helps evaluate your needs, identify action steps and connect with local programs and services.

If you experience signs of stress on a regular basis, consult your doctor. Ignoring symptoms can cause your physical and mental health to decline.

- **Get help and find support.** Our online Care Team Calendar helps you organize friends and family who want to help provide care and support. Our 24/7 Helpline (800.272.3900), ALZConnected online community and local support groups are all good sources for finding comfort and reassurance. If stress becomes overwhelming, seek professional help.
- **Use relaxation techniques.** There are several simple relaxation techniques that can

help relieve stress. Try more than one to find which works best for you. Techniques include:

- Visualization (mentally picturing a place or situation that is peaceful and calm)
- Meditation (which can be as simple as dedicating 15 minutes a day to letting go of all stressful thoughts)
- Breathing exercises (slowing your breathing and focusing on taking deep breaths)
- Progressive muscle relaxation (tightening and then relaxing each muscle group, starting at one end of your body and working your way to the other end) Learn more about relaxation techniques on the Mayo Clinic website.

- **Get moving.**
Physical activity — in any form — can help reduce stress and improve overall wellbeing.
Even 10 minutes of exercise a day can help. Take a walk. Do an activity you love, such as gardening or dancing.

- **Find time for yourself.**
Consider taking advantage of respite care so you can spend time doing something you enjoy. Respite care provides caregivers with a temporary rest from caregiving, while the person with Alzheimer's disease continues to receive care in a safe environment. Learn more about respite care.

- **Become an educated caregiver.**
As the disease progresses, new caregiving skills may be necessary. The Alzheimer's Association offers programs to help you better understand and cope with the behaviors and personality changes that often accompany Alzheimer's. You may also find it helpful to talk to other care partners and caregivers about how they are coping with the challenges of the disease and uncertainty about the future.

- **Take care of yourself.**
Visit your doctor regularly. Try to eat well, exercise and get plenty of rest. Making sure that you are healthy can help you be a better caregiver.

- **Make legal and financial plans.**
Putting legal and financial plans in place after an Alzheimer's diagnosis is important so that the person with the disease can participate. Having future plans in place can provide comfort to the entire family. Many documents can be prepared without the help of an attorney. However, if you are unsure about how to complete legal documents or make financial plans, you may want to seek assistance from an attorney specializing in elder law, a financial advisor who is familiar with elder or long-term care planning, or both. Learn more about planning ahead.

Critical Thinking

1. Discuss how a support group assists caregivers to relieve caregiver stress?
2. Identify community supports that may assist caregivers?

Internet References

American Psychological Association
   https://www.apa.org/
National Alliance for Caregivers
   https://www.caregiving.org/
Today's Caregiver
   https://caregiver.com/

Article   Prepared by: Elaina Osterbur, *Saint Louis University*

Optimism, Pessimism, Coping, and Depression: A Study on Individuals with Parkinson's Disease

Kristen Anzaldi and Kim Shifren

Learning Outcomes

After reading this article, you will be able to:

- Explain types of coping strategies and how they affect health-related quality of life, psychological well-being and stress.

- Discuss how the relationship between problem-focused coping and emotion-focused coping and depressive symptoms depend on high levels of optimism and low levels of pessimism.

Parkinson's disease (PD) is a progressive neurodegenerative disorder with motor dysfunction, affecting more than one million people in the United States and over 10 million people worldwide (Parkinson's Disease Foundation, 2017). Those with PD show tremor, rigidity, postural instability, and bradykinesia as the central motor symptoms of the disease (Guo et al., 2013). Nonmotor symptoms of PD may include neurological impairments, hallucinations, sleep disorders, and depression (Bucks et al., 2011).

Individuals with PD can experience symptoms from their disease that may be associated with increased amounts of stress. Increases in their stress levels may affect individuals with PD by reducing their ability to negotiate their environment and exceeding their personal resources (Eaton & Bradley, 2008). An important protective mechanism against stress is coping. *Coping* is the cognitive and behavioral effort individuals use to manage taxing situations or interactions (Lazarus & Folkman, 1984). Coping strategies are important to investigate

because they are associated with health-related quality of life (Bucks et al., 2011; Whitworth et al., 2013) and mental health (Bucks et al., 2011; Hurt et al., 2011). Understanding which coping strategies are associated with better mental health in those with PD will be helpful in tailoring support and interventions to help those with PD. This study provides an assessment of coping strategies, personality, and depressive symptoms in individuals with PD. The article begins with a discussion of coping strategies, followed by the possible mediating role of personality on the relation between coping and depressive symptoms.

Lazarus and Folkman (1984) discussed three broad dimensions of coping including problem-focused coping, emotion-focused coping, and avoidant coping. *Problem-focused coping* refers to behaviors that manage or change stressors through instrumental actions with the stressor directly analyzed (Lazarus & Folkman, 1984). Problem-focused coping has been associated with higher health-related quality of life, greater psychological well-being, and reduced stress (Bucks et al., 2011; Hurt et al., 2011). Problem-focused coping is the most frequently reported coping style across diverse populations and situations (Hurt et al., 2011). *Emotion-focused coping* involves regulation of emotions felt about stressors. Emotion-focused coping involves effort put toward assigning new meaning in response to a stressor rather than directly changing it (Lazarus & Folkman, 1984; Meléndez, Mayordomo, Sancho, & Tomás, 2012). Emotion-focused coping has been associated with lower health-related quality of life, greater distress, and poorer health (Bucks et al., 2011; Hurt et al., 2011). *Avoidant coping* includes passive behaviors of withdrawal, disengagement, and denial

(Eaton & Bradley, 2008; Meléndez et al., 2012), and avoidant coping is considered the least effective of the three coping dimensions (Meléndez et al., 2012).

Gender may have an influence on an individual's coping strategy. Females use a combination of coping strategies and seek social support when dealing with stress, while males cope with stress by problem-focused or avoidant coping (Eaton & Bradley, 2008). Males tend to suppress or deny their emotions. Society's expectations of masculinity may influence tendencies of denial in males (Eaton & Bradley, 2008). Females appear to use more emotion-focused coping strategies than men (Meléndez et al., 2012). Possible gender differences in coping strategies in those with PD are assessed in this study.

The three coping strategies (problem-focused coping, emotion-focused coping, and avoidant coping) have been examined thoroughly on a variety of samples (Benyamini, 2005; de Ridder, Schreurs, & Bensing, 2000; Eaton & Bradley, 2008; Meléndez et al., 2012). However, to our knowledge, there are few published studies on coping strategies for individuals with PD. Over the past 20 years, there have been about a dozen studies on PD, which include an assessment of coping strategies (e.g., Bucks et al., 2011; da Costa, 2014; Ehmann, Beninger, Gawel, & Riopelle, 1990; Frazier, 2000, 2002; Hurt et al., 2011; Montel, Bonnet, & Bungener, 2009; Whitworth et al., 2013). For example, Frazier (2000) found that PD patients used regulation of emotion as a coping strategy more often than other coping strategies.

The small published literature on coping strategies in individuals with PD is promising, but it lacks the inclusion of personality. Personality may be important to examine in individuals with PD, because personality can affect one's coping preference, perceptions, and response to stress (Connor-Smith & Flachsbart, 2007; Whitworth et al., 2013). One study of note on personality and coping among individuals with PD is Whitworth et al. (2013). In Australia, Whitworth et al. (2013) found that individuals with PD who scored higher on neuroticism reported more use of escape-avoidance coping strategies, while those higher on extraversion reported less of this strategy and more planned problem-solving coping strategies.

A personality orientation of interest in this study is optimism. *Optimism* is the expectation that good outcomes will occur (Scheier & Carver, 1985). Past research has shown that individuals who are more optimistic tend to use more problem-focused coping strategies, while those who are more pessimistic will resort to emotion-based coping strategies such as denial (e.g., Carver, Scheier, & Weintraub, 1989). Optimists spend less time dwelling on negative emotions and more time planning and setting goals for recovery from surgery (Shifren, 1996).

However, optimists are more likely to choose problem-focused coping strategies when they are in situations they can control

(Scheier, Weintraub, & Carver, 1986). Scheier et al. (1986) found that optimists use some emotion-based strategies in situations they cannot control. Carver et al. (1993) found that acceptance, positive reframing, and the use of religion were the most common coping strategies in a sample of breast cancer patients. It is not always possible to control the symptoms of PD (Frazier, 2002). Perhaps optimists use emotion-based strategies such as acceptance when dealing with long-term physical health problems from PD.

There have been a handful of published studies with Parkinson's patients, which include an assessment of individuals' levels of optimism (de Ridder et al., 2000; Gison, Dall'Armi, Donati, Rizza, & Giaquinto, 2014; Gruber-Baldini, Ye, Anderson, & Shulman, 2009; Hurt et al., 2014; Shifren, 1996). To our knowledge, there has been only one prior published study that includes the assessment of both optimism and coping strategies in PD patients (de Ridder et al., 2000). In the United Kingdom, de Ridder et al. (2000) found that a moderate level of optimism was associated with task-oriented coping strategies and avoidant coping strategies in those with PD and multiple sclerosis.

In addition to evaluating coping strategies and optimism in individuals with PD, we assessed their depressive symptoms. Although estimates vary, about 20% of individuals with PD experience mental health issues such as depressive symptoms (de Ridder et al., 2000; Troeung, Gasson, & Egan, 2015). In this study, we assessed the possible mediator role of optimism and pessimism on the relation between coping strategies and depressive symptoms in individuals with PD. Prior research has shown that optimism and pessimism have direct effects on outcomes and are not mediated by coping strategies (e.g., Tomakowsky, Lumley, Markowitz, & Frank, 2001). In fact, there is accumulating evidence that optimism and pessimism may mediate the relationship between coping strategies and outcome variables. Researchers have shown that optimism and pessimism mediated the relationship between coping strategies and distress in a sample of breast cancer patients awaiting biopsy or lumpectomy (David, Montgomery, & Bovbjerg, 2006), and pessimism mediated the relation between coping strategies and well-being in a sample of Norwegian adults (Kvande, Kl€ockner, Moksnes, & Espnes, 2015).

The primary objective of this study is the assessment of a mediator role of optimism and pessimism on the relation between coping strategies and depressive symptoms. There are additional objectives in this study which include the following: (a) examining the data for possible gender differences in personality, coping strategies, and depressive symptoms; (b) determining if individuals with PD report the use of more emotion-focused coping strategies than problem-focused coping strategies as has been reported in prior work on those with PD (Frazier, 2000, 2002); and (c) determining if individuals with PD report more optimism than pessimism.

In this study, we use the Brief Cope (Carver, 1997) to examine coping strategies in those with PD. Carver (1997) created this measure to provide 14 different coping dimensions, and suggested that individuals would need to perform their own factor analysis of the instrument to determine broader coping factors. In this study, we performed an exploratory factor analysis to create coping factors reflective of the coping literature we have discussed in the introduction (problem-focused, emotion-focused, and avoidant coping). The exploratory factor analysis is described in the result section of the article. The coping variables created from the exploratory factor analysis were used for addressing the primary objective of the study, the mediating role of optimism and pessimism on the relationship between coping strategies and depressive symptoms.

Method
Participants
Individuals were recruited for this study from the Michael J. Fox Foundation Parkinson's disease website, with permission to advertise and recruit participants through the Fox Trial Finder. To qualify for this study, individuals needed a diagnosis of PD, and the ability to complete survey questions themselves. The Fox Trial Finder allows for those individuals diagnosed with PD to select studies of interest to them. Eighty-two individuals volunteered and were qualified to participate in this study. Twelve cases were excluded from our study because of incomplete measures or they had a comorbid diagnosis with stroke. We had a total sample of 70 participants diagnosed with PD to include in analyses (35 males and 35 females). Participant's ages ranged from 26 to 79 years, with an average age of 60 years ($SD = 10.11$). The majority of individuals who completed this study were Caucasian American (90.1%). Income level ranged from 15,001—35,000 to over 120,000, with an average income between 60,000 and 120,000. There were 55 who married, 3 who divorced, 2 who separated from their spouse, 4 were single, and 5 cohabitated with another. The amount of time since diagnosis of PD was an average of 5.4 years ($SD = 4.78$), with a range of 1 year to 22 years since diagnosis. Details on characteristics are provided in Table 1.

Measures
Coping. The Brief COPE is an instrument designed to assess and measure a broad range of coping resources, particularly for individuals with chronic illnesses and diseases (Carver, 1997). There are a total of 28 items that provide 14 dimensions consisting of two items each. A sample item is "I've been turning to work or other activities to take my mind off things." Strategies are measured on a 4-point Likert-type scale from *I haven't been doing this at all* (score of 1) to *I've been doing this a lot* (score

Table 1 Demographic Information on Individuals with Parkinson's Disease

Variables	Percentage
Gender	
Male	49.5
Female	49.5
Age at diagnosis	
24–39	8.4
40–49	12.6
50–59	39.3
60–69	35.1
70–74	4.2
Current age	
26–39	4.2
40–49	11.3
50–59	24.3
60–69	45.9
70–79	14.3
Ethnicity	
Caucasian American	90.1
Latin American	2.8
African American	1.4
Asian American	1.4
Religion	
Christian	66.2
Jewish	16.9
Other	5.6
None	9.9
Income	
15,001 to 35,000	4.2
35,001 to 60,000	8.5
60,001 to 99,000	22.5
99,001 to 120,000	18.3
Over 120,000	36.6

Note. N = 70

of 4). The sum of the two items for each dimension indicates the frequency of the dimension. Larger scores indicate a higher use of the resource. No items are reverse scored. Scores ranged from 2 to 8 for each of the 14 dimensions. Coping dimensions consist of active coping ($\alpha = .71$), use of instrumental support ($\alpha = .83$), planning ($\alpha = .77$), acceptance ($\alpha = .69$), use of emotional support ($\alpha = .73$), positive reframing ($\alpha = .76$), humor ($\alpha = .87$), religion ($\alpha = .85$), venting ($\alpha = .49$), self-distraction ($\alpha = .46$), denial ($\alpha = .72$), substance use ($\alpha = .95$), behavioral disengagement ($\alpha = .86$), and self-blame ($\alpha = .81$). All alpha values reported here are those from this study. The 14 dimensions for this instrument were placed in an exploratory factor analysis to create problem-focused, emotion-focused, and avoidant coping factors—three factors discussed in the larger literature on coping strategies. The exploratory factor analysis is in the result section of this article.

Optimism. The Life Orientation Test-Revised (LOT-R) measurement was developed by Scheier, Carver, and Bridges (1994) to assess optimism. The scale has 10 items including four filler items, three items to measure optimism, and three items to measure pessimism. A sample item is "In uncertain times, I usually expect the best". Participants are asked to rate their level of agreement to items on a 5-point Likert-type scale. The responses range from *I disagree a lot* (0) to *I agree a lot* (4). Total scores were computed by adding together the three positively worded items for Optimism and adding together the three negatively worded items for Pessimism. Optimism and pessimism scores have a possible range of 0 to 12, with higher scores indicating more of each construct. The negatively worded items were reversed coded to create the total LOT-R score. LOT-R scores have a possible range of 0 to 24, where higher scores indicate more optimism. Cronbach's α was .88 for the LOT-R, .79 for Optimism and .85 for Pessimism in this study. While providing some information on the total LOT-R in this study, our main focus is primarily on optimism and pessimism as separate factors.

Depressive symptoms. The Center for Epidemiological Studies Depression Scale (CES-D; Radloff, 1977) was used to measure depressive symptomatology. The CES-D is a 20-item self-report measure. A sample item is "In the past week, I was bothered by things that usually don't bother me". Participants are asked to rate each item on a 4-point Likert-type scale. Responses range from *Rarely or none of the time (less than 1 day) (0) to Most of all of the time (5-7 days)* (3). Positive items 4, 8, 12, and 16 are reverse coded. A higher score indicates greater depression, with scores ranging from 0 to 60. The CES-D has been used in much prior research including individuals with PD (Williams et al., 2012). The total CES-D Cronbach's a for this study was .93.

Procedures

Institutional review board approval was received for this study before advertising and data collection began. Participants were obtained by advertising through the Michael J. Fox Foundation for Parkinson's Research (Fox Trial Finder) and data were compiled on SurveyMonkey. Researcher's contact information was included on all advertisements and surveys. Individuals who were interested in participating from the Fox Trial Finder website clicked on the SurveyMonkey link shown in the study description and completed the survey at the secure online website. At no time could participant names or identifying information be linked to their study data.

An individual was required to be over the age of 18 and have Parkinson's for a minimum of 1 year to complete the survey. Before starting, participants have to read a description of the study, its objectives, and the consent form. By checking the box, participants certified that they were over qualifying age, and they consented to participating in the study voluntarily. The questionnaires took no more than 20 minutes to be completed and included the measures for demographics, optimism and pessimism, coping, and depressive symptoms. No monetary compensation was available for participating in this study.

Results

SPSS version 20 was used to perform all statistical analyses. The primary objective of this study is the examination of a mediator effect of optimism and pessimism on the relation between coping strategies and depressive symptoms in those with PD. Before performing analyses that assess this relationship, several other analyses were conducted.

First, demographic characteristics (age, income, religion, and duration of PD) were assessed for possible gender differences among those with PD. An independent sample t test showed there was a gender difference in the age of individuals with PD in this study. Males ($M = 63.06$, $SD = 10.23$) were significantly older than females ($M = 57.00$, $SD = 9.33$), $t(67) = 2.57$, $p = .01$. Independent sample t tests showed no significant gender differences for PD patients on income level ($M = 6.09$, $SD = 1.01$ for males and $M = 5.58$, $SD = 1.32$ for females, respectively), $t(67) = 1.76$, $p = .08$, or duration of PD ($M = 6.23$, $SD = 5.37$ for males and $M = 4.66$, $SD = 4.14$ for females, respectively), $t(67) = 1.37$, $p = .18$. A Chi-square analysis showed no gender difference for PD patients on religion, $x^2(1) = 0.11$, $p = .74$.

Second, to discuss coping variables in relation to the large literature focused on problem-focused, emotion-focused, and avoidant coping strategies, factor analysis was conducted on the Brief COPE. A principal component factor analysis with Varimax rotation on the 14 Brief COPE subscales was used, rather than on the 28 individual items. Researchers have recommended a wide range from 2 participants per item to over 100 participants per item (Costello & Osborne, 2005). While a sample of 70 participants with PD is small, researchers have investigated the use of factor analysis with samples smaller than 50 and found some adequate (deWinter, Dodou, & Wieringa, 2009). This study had five participants per item ($n = 70/14$ sub-scales) by using the 14 subscales.

The subscales were examined for distribution of data. Four of the subscales had a large amount of skew and kurtosis (denial, substance use, behavioral disengagement, and self-blame), and these subscales were not included in the factor analysis. The remaining 10 subscales were kept for the factor analysis. Subscales were retained if they loaded greater than .40 on one factor and less than .40 on any remaining factors. Subscales that did not meet the criteria were removed, and the factor analysis was continued until only those subscales that met the criteria remained. This technique has been used by others for different chronic illness samples involving the Brief COPE (e.g., Willis et al., 2016). We only needed to perform this iterative step once. The initial factor analysis revealed that only two subscales showed factor loadings above .40 on more than one factor (emotional support and religion). In addition, the scree plot was examined to determine the best number of factors (the best number was three factors).

The second factor analysis provided the final solution which included three factors: (a) problem-focused coping (active coping, instrumental support, and planning), (b) emotion-focused coping (humor, positive reframing, and acceptance), and (c) avoidant coping (self-distraction and venting). The factor loadings and Cronbach's alpha for these three coping factors are presented in Table 2. The Kaiser–Meyer–Olkin measure of sampling adequacy was .74, considered above the minimum

of .60. Bartlett's test of sphericity was $x^2(28) = 136.64$, $p \le .001$. The total variance explained by these three factors was 67.77%.

The items for each of the factors were added together into a sum score before conducting any analyses. Problem-focused coping had a sum score that ranged from 10 to 24, emotion-focused coping had a sum score that ranged from 9 to 23, and avoidant coping had a sum score that ranged from 4 to 15.

Next, the data were examined for possible gender differences in the study variables (personality, coping, and depressive symptoms). This was an objective of the study but also helps to determine if gender must be statistically controlled in the mediation analyses. Descriptive information for the study variables (total optimism score, optimism and pessimism subscales, problem-focused coping, emotion-focused coping, avoidant coping, and depressive symptoms) are illustrated in Table 3. And t tests were performed to assess gender differences in the study variables (see Table 3 for these results). There was a significant gender difference in individuals' scores on problem-focused coping, with females reporting more problem-focused coping strategies than males. There were no other gender differences in the study variables.

An additional objective of the study was to determine if more emotion-focused coping strategies were used than problem-focused coping strategies by those with PD. A paired t test showed that there was no significant difference in the amount of these coping strategies reported (mean = 15.72, $SD = 3.78$ for emotion-focused coping and mean = 16.48, $SD = 3.99$ for problem-focused coping, respectively), $t(68) = -1.61$, $p = .111$. Another objective of the study was to determine if individuals reported more optimism than pessimism. A paired t test

Table 2   Exploratory Factor Analysis of the Brief COPE Subscales in Those with Parkinson's Disease

Subscales	Factor 1 Problem-focused Coping	Factor 2 Emotion-focused Coping	Factor 3 Avoidant Coping
Active Coping	.82	.26	−.03
Instrument support	.77	.00	.23
Planning	.72	.40	.08
Humor	.04	.89	.06
Positive reframing	.25	.75	.21
Acceptance	.38	.62	−.12
Self-distraction	.17	−.01	.82
Venting	.01	.12	.78
Total variance (%)	38.68	16.37	12.73
Cronbach's α	.83	.82	.58

Note. The significant factor loadings are in bold.

Table 3   Descriptive Information and t Tests for Gender Differences on Optimism, Pessimism, Coping Factors, and Depressive Symptoms

Variables	Mean(SD)	Males Mean (SD)	Females Mean (SD)	df	t	P
Personality						
Total LOT-R	17.44 (5.30)	16.71 (5.77)	17.97 (4.74)	68	0.99	.32
Optimism	8.75 (2.78)	8.51 (3.16)	8.89 (2.35)	68	0.56	.58
Pessimism	3.31 (2.97)	3.80 (3.05)	2.91 (2.86)	68	−1.25	.21
Coping						
Problem-focused	16.48(3.99)	15.15(3.75)	17.46(3.86)	67	2.52	.01
Emotion-focused	15.72 (3.78)	15.18 (3.85)	16.17 (3.73)	66	1.08	.29
Avoidant	8.16 (2.31)	7.81 (2.26)	8.54 (2.33)	65	1.29	.19
Depressive symptoms						
Total CES-D	12.01 (10.70)	13.77 (11.60)	10.34 (9.75)	68	−1.34	.19

Note. N = 70. Higher scores mean that more of the construct is present. LOT-R = Life Orientation Test- Revised; CES-D = Center for Epidemiological Studies Depression Scale.

showed that individuals did report significantly more optimism (mean = 8.75, SD = 2.78) than pessimism (mean = 3.31, SD = 2.97), $t(68) = 8.64, p \leq .0001$.

Finally, analyses were conducted for the main objective of this study, a possible mediator effect of optimism and pessimism on the relation between coping strategies and depressive symptoms. First, demographic/disease characteristics (current age, income level, and duration of time since diagnosis) were examined for their relation to the study variables. Pearson correlations showed that there were no significant relationships between current age, income level, and duration of time since diagnosis and the study variables (see Table 4 for these results).

Because there were gender differences in age and problem-focused coping, we statistically controlled for both gender and age when examining the relationship between the study variables (optimism, pessimism, problem-focused coping, emotion-focused coping, avoidant coping, and depressive symptoms). The relationships between all of the study variables were analyzed with partial correlations (controlling for both age and gender), and these correlations are presented in Table 5. The correlations showed that optimism was positively related to both emotion-focused and problem-focused coping strategies. Pessimism was negatively related to both of these coping strategies. The LOT-R total score and optimism and pessimism were not related to avoidant coping strategies. Avoidant coping strategies were only related to depressive symptoms, with more avoidant coping linked to more depressive symptoms. Both optimism and pessimism were related to depressive symptoms in predictable ways, with more optimistic individuals reporting less depressive symptoms and more pessimistic individuals reporting more depressive symptoms. Both emotion-focused

and problem-focused coping strategies were negatively related to depressive symptoms. It appears that both types of coping strategies are related to the reporting of less depressive symptoms in individuals with PD.

Both theoretical assumptions from Baron and Kenny (1986) and statistic strategies by Preacher and Hayes (2008) were used to assess the mediator role of optimism and pessimism on the relation between coping strategies and depressive symptoms. Baron and Kenny (1986) argue for a relation between the independent variable, the mediator, and the dependent variable.

Table 4   Pearson Correlations of Demographic Characteristics on Personality, Coping, and Depressive Symptoms in Those With PD

Variables	Age	Income	Duration of PD
Optimism	.17	−.03	−.09
Pessimism	−.18	−.05	−.02
Problem-focused coping	.07	.00	.03
Emotion-focused coping	−.06	−.03	.12
Avoidant coping	−.22	−.05	.19
Total CESD	−.22	.03	.01

Note. df = 67. Missing data were excluded listwise for analyses. None of the above correlations was significant at the .05 level or higher.

Table 5 Pearson Correlations for the Relationship Between Personality, Coping Strategies, and Depressive Symptoms in Individuals with Parkinson's Disease

Variables	1	2	3	4	5	6	7
LOT-R	-	.92**	−.93**	.32**	.42**	−.17	−.62**
Optimism	-	-	−.71**	.27*	.31*	−.15	−.51**
Pessimism	-	-	-	−.31*	−.46**	.17	.63**
Problem-focused coping	-	-	-	-	.54**	.29*	−.28*
Emotion-focused coping	-	-	-	-	-	.14	−.36*
Avoidant coping	-	-	-	-	-	-	.28*
Total CES-D	-	-	-	-	-	-	-

Note. N = 70. The aforementioned correlations are partial correlations controlling for both age and gender. LOTR = Life Orientation Test-Revised; CES-D = Center for Epidemiological Studies Depression Scale. *$p \leq$ .01, **$p \leq$ .001.

Once a mediator is included in the analyses, the relation between the independent variable and the dependent variable should be reduced (partial mediator) or eliminated (full mediator). The statistical approach of Preacher and Hayes (2008) involves bootstrapping, a nonparametric resampling procedure, and is a better approach to determine indirect effects. Bootstrapping, with repeated sampling from a data set, includes the estimate for the indirect effect for each resampled data set. This technique is especially helpful with small samples (MacKinnon, 2008).

For this study, the Hayes (2013) PROCESS program was used to examine direct and indirect effects using bootstrapping and bias-corrected and accelerated confidence intervals to determine the possible significance of a mediator in the model. Avoidant coping was not related to personality, so it was not included in analyses. Analyses were first conducted with problem-focused coping and second with emotion-focused coping as the independent variable. Optimism and pessimism were assessed separately as mediators. There were a total of four analyses run with the PROCESS approach. The Preacher and Hayes (2008) PROCESS approach included coping strategy as the independent variable, personality as the mediator, and depressive symptoms as the dependent variable. Bootstrapping (resampling at 10,000) and bias-corrected and accelerated confidence intervals were performed. In order for personality to be a mediator for the relation between coping strategies and depressive symptoms, the lower and upper bootstrap confidence intervals must not include zero (Hayes, 2009; Hayes & Scharkow, 2013).

According to Figure 1, optimism played a full mediator role on the relation between problem-focused coping and depressive symptoms, with bootstrap confidence intervals indicating a significant mediator (lower CI: −.67 and upper CI: −.25), $F(2, 67) = 15.13$, $p \leq .0001$, $R^2 = .31$. The Preacher and Kelley (2011) kappa-squared was significant (effect = .15, boot $SE = .07$, boot lower CI: .04, and boot upper CI: .32), and the normal theory test for the indirect effect was significant (effect $= −.14$, $SE = .06$, $Z = −2.21$, $p = .03$).

According to Figure 2, pessimism played a full mediator role on the relation between problem-focused coping and depressive symptoms (lower CI: .41 and upper CI: .80), $F(2, 67) = 26.36$, $p \leq .0001$, $R^2 = .44$. The Preacher and Kelley (2011) kappa-squared was significant (effect = .22, boot $SE = .07$, boot lower CI: .08, and boot upper CI: .37), and the normal theory test for the indirect effect was significant (effect $= −.21$, $SE = .08$, $Z = −2.68$, $p = .01$).

According to Figure 3, optimism played a full mediator role on the relation between emotion-focused coping and depressive symptoms (lower CI: −.68 and upper CI: −.25), $F(2, 66) = 14.89$, $p \leq .0001$, $R^2 = .31$. The Preacher and Kelley (2011) kappa-squared was significant (effect = .15, boot $SE = .07$, boot lower CI: .04, and boot upper CI: .33), and the normal theory test for the indirect effect was significant (effect $= −.14$, $SE = .07$, $Z = −2.27$, $p = .02$).

According to Figure 4, pessimism played a full mediator role on the relation between emotion-focused coping and depressive symptoms (lower CI: .43 and upper CI: .84), $F(2, 66) = 25.44$, $p \leq .0001$, $R^2 = .44$. The Preacher and Kelley (2011) kappa-squared was significant (effect = .29, boot $SE = .07$, boot lower CI: .16 and boot upper CI: .44), and the normal theory test for the indirect effect was significant (effect $= −.28$, $SE = .08$, $Z = −3.36$, $p = .001$).

Discussion

There is limited published research available on the relationship between personality, coping strategies, and depressive symptoms among Parkinson's patients. Understanding the relationship between these variables may help researchers and practitioners develop better support and interventions that address individual differences in how people deal with living with PD. This study included the assessment of optimism, pessimism, coping strategies, and depressive symptoms in Parkinson's patients.

The main objective of the study was to assess the possible mediator role of optimism and pessimism on the relation between coping strategies and depressive symptoms in those with PD. The findings of this study supported both optimism and pessimism as full mediators on the relation between coping strategies and depressive symptoms in those with PD. Once optimism and pessimism were included in analyses, the relation between coping strategies (problem-focused coping and emotion-focused coping) and depressive symptoms was no longer significant. The results for our PD sample support those found with other kinds of samples including a sample of breast cancer patients (David et al., 2006) and a sample of Norwegian adults (Kvande et al., 2015).

The finding of this study suggests that optimism and pessimism play equally important roles in understanding the influence of coping strategies on mental health outcomes. The relationship between problem-focused coping and emotion-focused coping and depressive symptoms appears to depend on individuals with PD having high levels of optimism and low levels of pessimism. A similar argument is supported for optimism and pessimism and other coping strategies and well-being in a Norwegian sample of adults (Kvande et al., 2015).

Lazarus and Folkman (1984) and others (de Ridder, Schreurs, & Bensing, 1998; Frazier, 2000; Montel et al., 2009) have suggested that it is not useful to assume that one set of coping strategies is good for everyone, while another set is harmful. There may be times when certain coping strategies are more appropriate given specific situations like living with PD.

For an additional objective of this study, we found no significant difference in the amount of emotion-focused and problem-focused coping strategies in the sample of individuals with PD in this study. While these results contradict those of Frazier (2000, 2002), she did not use the same coping instrument or the same number of items to create her coping factors. The Brief COPE items are considered flexible in application and the use will vary for each researcher's needs (Carver, 1997). We found that individuals with PD in this study reported more optimism than pessimism. The optimism mean was similar to a previous study's findings with PD patients (Gruber-Baldini et al., 2009, mean = 8.04).

Limitations

Parkinson's patients were recruited via Fox Trial Finder and filled out self-report measures. The sample may be biased toward those who want to be of help in finding interventions and treatment options. Volunteer samples may include those with PD who are not experiencing extreme symptoms, and the sample may be positively biased. The cross-sectional design limits the ability to discuss temporal relations. A larger sample size in a future study may be beneficial in increasing generalizability.

Implications for Future Research

Researchers suggest that optimism can be learned through different intervention strategies (Koenig, Pearce, Nelson, & Daher, 2015). An intervention to increase the level of optimism in individuals with PD may help to reduce symptoms of depression. The role of pessimism needs to be explored as well, since pessimism also fully mediated the relation between coping strategies and depressive symptoms (Benyamini, 2005). A longitudinal approach to the assessment of personality and coping strategies would be useful to determine the temporal relation between these variables within Parkinson's patients.

. . .

References

Baron, R. M., & Kenny, D. A. (1986). The moderator-mediator variable distinction in social psychological research: Conceptual, strategic, and statistical considerations. *Journal of Personality and Social Psychology*, 51(6), 1173–1182. doi:10.1037/0022-3514.51.6.1173

Benyamini, Y. (2005). Can high optimism and high pessimism co-exist? Findings from arthritis patients coping with pain. *Personality and Individual Differences*, 38(6), 1463–1473. doi:10.1016/j.paid.2004.09.020

Bucks, R. G., Cruise, K. E., Skinner, T. C., Loftus, A. M., Barker, R. A., & Thomas, M. G. (2011). Coping processes and health-related quality of life in Parkinson's disease. *International Journal of Geriatric Psychiatry*, 26(3), 247–255. doi:10.1002/gps.2520

Carver, C. S. (1997). You want to measure coping but your protocol's too long: Consider the Brief COPE. *International Journal of Behavioral Medicine*, 4(1), 92–100. doi:10.1207/s15327558ijbm0401_6

Carver, C. S., Pozo, C., Harris, S. D., Noriega, V., Scheier, M. F., Robinson, D. S., . . .Clark, K. C. (1993). How coping mediates the effect of optimism on distress: A study of women with early stage breast cancer. *Journal of Personality and Social Psychology*, 65(2), 375–390. doi:10.1037/0022-3514.65.2.375

Carver, C. S., Scheier, M. F., & Weintraub, J. K. (1989). Assessing coping strategies: A theoretically based approach. *Journal of Personality and Social Psychology*, 56(2), 267–283. doi:10.1037/0022-3514.56.2.267

Connor-Smith, J. K., & Flachsbart, C. (2007). Relations between personality and coping: A meta-analysis. *Journal of Personality and Social Psychology*, 93(6), 1080–1107. doi:10.1037/0022-3514.93.6.1080

Costello, A. B., & Osborne, J. W. (2005). Best practices in exploratory factor analysis: Four recommendations for getting the most from your analysis. *Practical Assessment, Research & Evaluation*, 10(7), 1–9. Retrieved from http://pareonline.net/getvn.asp?v=10&n=7

David, D., Montgomery, G. H., & Bovbjerg, D. H. (2006). Relations between coping responses and optimism-pessimism in predicting anticipatory psychological distress in surgical breast cancer patients. *Personality and Individual Differences*, 40(2), 203–213. doi:10.1016/j.paid.2005.05.018

da Costa, F. P. (2014). Communicative aspects and coping strategies in patients with Parkinson's disease. *Arquivos De Neuro-Psiquiatria*, 72(6), 480. doi:10.1590/0004-282X20140041

de Ridder, D. T., Schreurs, K. G., & Bensing, J. M. (1998). Adaptive tasks, coping and quality of life of chronically ill patients. *Journal of Health Psychology*, 3(1), 87–101. doi:10.1177/135910539800300107

de Ridder, D. T., Schreurs, K. G., & Bensing, J. M. (2000). The relative benefits of being optimistic: Optimism as a coping resource in multiple sclerosis and Parkinson's disease. British *Journal of Health Psychology*, 5(2), 141–155. doi:10.1348/135910700168829

deWinter, J. C. F., Dodou, D., & Wieringa, P. A. (2009). Exploratory factor analysis with small sample sizes. *Multivariate Behavioral Research*, 44(2), 147–181. doi:10.1080/00273170902794206

Eaton, R. J., & Bradley, G. (2008). The role of gender and negative affectivity in stressor appraisal and coping selection. *International Journal of Stress Management*, 15(1), 94–115. doi:10.1037/1072-5245.15.1.94

Ehmann, T. S., Beninger, R. J., Gawel, M. J., & Riopelle, R. J. (1990). Coping, social support, and depressive symptoms in Parkinson's disease. *Journal of Geriatric Psychiatry and Neurology*, 3(2), 85–90. doi:10.1177/089198879000300206

Frazier, L. D. (2000). Coping with disease-related stressors in Parkinson's disease. *The Gerontologist*, 40(1), 53–63. doi:10.1093/geront/40.1.53

Frazier, L. D. (2002). Stability and change in patterns of coping with Parkinson's disease. *The International Journal of Aging and Human Development*, 55(3), 207–231. doi:10.2190/ua78-79lb-4gcf-8mjt

Gison, A., Dall'Armi, V., Donati, V., Rizza, F., & Giaquinto, S. (2014). Dispositional optimism, depression, disability and quality of life in Parkinson's disease. *Functional Neurology*, 29(2), 113–119. doi:10.11138/FNeur/2014.29.2.113

Gruber-Baldini, A. L., Ye, J., Anderson, K. E., & Shulman, L. M. (2009). Effects of optimism/pessimism and locus of control on disability and quality of life in Parkinson's disease. *Parkinsonism & Related Disorders*, 15(9), 665–669. doi:10.1016/j.parkreldis.2009.03.005

Guo, X., Song, W., Chen, K., Chen, X., Zheng, Z., Cao, B., . . .Shang, H. (2013). Gender and onset age-related features of non-motor symptoms of patients with Parkinson's disease—A study from Southwest China. *Parkinsonism & Related Disorders*, 19(11), 961–965. doi:10.1016/j.parkreldis.2013.06.009

Hayes, A. F. (2009). Beyond Baron and Kenny: Statistical mediation analysis in the new millennium. *Communication Monographs*, 76(4), 408–420. doi:10.1080/03637750903310360

Hayes, A. F. (2013). *Introduction to mediation, moderation, and conditional process analysis: A regression-based approach.* New York, NY: The Guilford Press.

Hayes, A. F., & Scharkow, M. (2013). The relative trustworthiness of inferential tests of the indirect effect in statistical mediation analysis: Does method really matter? *Psychological Science*, 24(10), 1918–1927. doi:10.1177/0956797613480187

Hurt, C. S., Thomas, B. A., Burn, D. J., Hindle, J. V., Landau, S. S., Samuel, M. M., & Brown, R. G. (2011). Coping in Parkinson's disease: An examination of the coping inventory for stressful situations. *International Journal of Geriatric Psychiatry*, 26(10), 1030–1037. doi:10.1002/gps.2634

Hurt, C. S., Burn, D. J., Hindle, J., Samuel, M., Wilson, K., & Brown, R. G. (2014). Thinking positively about chronic illness: An exploration of optimism, illness perceptions and well-being in patients with Parkinson's disease. *British Journal of Health Psychology*, 19(2), 363–379. doi:10.1111/bjhp.12043

Koenig, H. G., Pearce, M. J., Nelson, B., & Daher, N. (2015). Effects of religious vs. standard cognitive-behavioral therapy on optimism in persons with major depression and chronic medical illness. *Depression and Anxiety*, 32(11), 835–842. doi:10.1002/da.22398

Kvande, M. N., Kl€ockner, C. A., Moksnes, U. K., & Espnes, G. A. (2015). Do optimism and pessimism mediate the relationship between religious coping and existential wellbeing? Examining mechanisms in a Norwegian population sample. *The International Journal for the Psychology of Religion*, 25(2), 130–151. doi:10.1080/10508619.2014.892350

Lazarus, R. S., & Folkman, S. (1984). Stress, appraisal, and coping. New York, NY: Springer Publishing Company.

MacKinnon, D. P. (2008). *Introduction to statistical mediation analysis.* New York, NY: Erlbaum.

Meléndez, J. C., Mayordomo, T., Sancho, P., & Tomás, J. M. (2012). Coping strategies: Gender differences and development throughout life span. *The Spanish Journal of Psychology*, 15(3), 1089–1098. doi:10.5209/rev_sjop.2012.v15.n3.39399

Montel, S., Bonnet, A., & Bungener, C. (2009). Quality of life in relation to mood, coping strategies, and dyskinesia in Parkinson's disease. *Journal of Geriatric Psychiatry and Neurology*, 22(2), 95–102. doi:10.1177/0891988708328219

Parkinson's Disease Foundation (2017). *Statistics.* Retrieved from http://parkinson.org/Understanding-Parkinsons/Causes-and-Statistics/Statistics

Preacher, K. J., & Hayes, A. F. (2008). Asymptotic and resampling strategies for assessing and comparing indirect effects in

Optimism, Pessimism, Coping, and Depression: A Study on Individuals with Parkinson's Disease by Kristen Anzaldi and Kim Shifren

107

multiple mediator models. *Behavior Research Methods*, 40(3), 879–891. doi:10.3758/brm.40.3.879

Preacher, K. J., & Kelley, K. (2011). Effect size measures for mediation models: Quantitative strategies for communicating indirect effects. *Psychological Methods*, 16(2), 93–115. doi:10.1037/a0022658

Radloff, L. S. (1977). The CES-D: A self-report depression scale for research in the general population. *Applied Psychological Measurement*, 1(3), 385–401. doi:10.1177/014662167700100306

Scheier, M. F., & Carver, C. S. (1985). Optimism, coping, and health: Assessment and implications of generalized outcome expectancies. *Health Psychology*, 4(3), 219–247. doi:10.1037//0278-6133.4.3.219

Scheier, M. F., Carver, C. S., & Bridges, M. W. (1994). Distinguishing optimism from neuroticism (and trait anxiety, self-mastery, and self-esteem): A reevaluation of the life orientation test. *Journal of Personality and Social Psychology*, 67(6), 1063–1078. doi:10.1037/0022-3514.67.6.1063

Scheier, M. F., Weintraub, J. K., & Carver, C. S. (1986). Coping with stress: Divergent strategies of optimists and pessimists. *Journal of Personality and Social Psychology*, 51(6), 1257–1264. doi:10.1037/0022-3514.51.6.1257

Shifren, K. (1996). Individual differences in the perception of optimism and disease severity: A study among individuals with Parkinson's disease. *Journal of Behavioral Medicine*, 19(3), 241–271. doi:10.1007/BF01857768

Tomakowsky, J., Lumley, M. A., Markowitz, N., & Frank, C. (2001). Optimistic explanatory style and dispositional optimism in HIV-infected men. *Journal of Psychosomatic Research*, 51(4), 577–587. doi:10.1016/S0022-3999(01)00249-5

Troeung, L., Gasson, N., & Egan, S. J. (2015). Patterns and predictors of mental health service utilization in people with Parkinson's disease. *Journal of Geriatric Psychiatry and Neurology*, 28(1), 12–18. doi:10.1177/0891988714541869

Whitworth, S. R., Loftus, A. M., Skinner, T. C., Gasson, N., Barker, R. A., Bucks, R. S., & Thomas, M. G. (2013). Personality affects aspects of health-related quality of life in Parkinson's disease via psychological coping strategies. *Journal of Parkinson's Disease*, 3(1), 45–53. doi:10.3233/JPD-120149

Williams, J. R., Hirsch, E. S., Anderson, K., Bush, A. L., Goldstein, S. R., Grill, S., . . .Marsh, L. (2012). A comparison of nine scales to detect depression in Parkinson disease: Which scale to use? *Neurology*, 78(13), 998–1006. doi:10.1212/WNL.0b013e31824d587f

Willis, K., Timmons, L., Pruitt, M., Schneider, H. L., Alessandri, M., & Ekas, N. V. (2016). The relationship between optimism, coping, and depressive symptoms in Hispanic mothers and fathers of children with autism spectrum disorder. *Journal of Autism and Developmental Disorders*, 46(7), 2427–2440. doi:10.1007/s10803-016-2776-7

Critical Thinking

1. According to the article optimism can be learned through a variety of interventions, would you support an optimism intervention as part of a Parkinson' patient's medical treatment plan?

2. The Michael J. Fox Foundation provided the subjects for this research article through a recruitment mechanism. Discuss the pros and cons of this type of recruitment for research.

Internet References

American Association of Neurological Surgeons
https://www.aans.org/

Michael J. Fox Foundation
https://www.michaeljfox.org/

Parkinson's Foundation
https://www.parkinson.org/

Unit 5

UNIT

Prepared by: Elaina Osterbur, *Saint Louis University*

Retirement: American Dream or Dilemma?

Since 1900, the number of people in America who are 65 years or more of age has been increasing steadily, but a decreasing proportion of that age group remains in the workforce. In 1900, nearly ⅔ of those over the age of 65 worked outside the home. By 1947, this number had declined to about 48 percent, and in 1975, about 22 percent of men age 65 and over were still in the workforce. The long-range trend indicates that fewer people are employed beyond the age of 65. Some choose to retire at age 65 or earlier; for others, retirement is mandatory. A recent change in the law, however, allows individuals to work as long as they want with no mandatory retirement age.

Gordon Strieb and Clement Schneider (Retirement in American Society, 1971) observed that for retirement to become an institutionalized social pattern in any society, certain conditions must be present. A large group of people must live long enough to retire; the economy must be productive enough to support people who are not in the workforce; and there must be pensions or insurance programs to support retirees. We have reached these goals in American society.

Retirement is a rite of passage. People can consider it either as the culmination of the American Dream or as a serious problem. Those who have ample incomes, interesting things to do, and friends to associate with often find the freedom of time and choice that retirement offers very rewarding. For others, however, retirement brings problems and personal losses. Often, these individuals find their incomes decreased; they miss the status, privilege, and power associated with holding a position in the occupational hierarchy. They may feel socially isolated if they do not find new activities to replace their previous work-related ones. Additionally, they might have to cope with the death of a spouse and/or their own failing health.

Older persons approach retirement with considerable concern about financial and personal problems. Will they have enough retirement income to maintain their current lifestyle? Will their income remain adequate as long as they live? Given their current state of health, how much longer can they continue to work? The articles in this unit deal with retirement and changing labor demands that are encouraging older person to work beyond the age of 65.

Article   Prepared by: Elaina Osterbur, *Saint Louis University*

7 Big Estate Planning Mistakes

BOB CARLSON

Learning Outcomes

After reading this article, you will be able to:

- Discuss the seven estate planning mistakes.

- Identify strategies to avoid mistakes when planning your estate.

Experienced estate planners see a high percentage of clients with these recurring mistakes. They know if you've never seen an estate planner or haven't had a plan revised within the last three years, your plan is likely to have at least one of these costly mistakes. (Remember, even if you haven't seen an estate planner, you have an estate plan, and it's probably not a good one.)

· · ·

Mistake #1: Relying Only On A Will

Of course, a written will is essential to every estate plan. People often are criticized for not having wills. But a will isn't enough.

A complete estate plan includes key documents that might be needed before your passing, such as a power of attorney and advanced medical directive. These documents empower one or more people to make decisions and take actions regarding your assets or medical care when you aren't able to.

Without these documents, many actions are taken only after a court appoints someone to act for you, and it could be some-one you wouldn't have selected. Or doctors take the actions they deem best, even if it's not what you would have decided.

I've often heard people say there's no rush to execute these documents. They say they're in fine shape and "aren't there yet." What I've seen over the years is the need for the docu-ments most often arises in two scenarios. One scenario is the occurrence of a sudden event, such as an accident or a health crisis, such as a stroke. Once that occurs, it's too late to have the documents executed. The other scenario is a steady decline that isn't apparent to the person or the person is in denial. By the time others are ready to intervene, either a lot of damage has been done to the person's estate or the legal capacity to execute the documents no longer is there. The bottom line is you need to execute the documents well before there's a need for them.

Another reason a will isn't enough is that ownership of many assets transfers outside the will and probate process. These assets include annuities, life insurance, retirement accounts (such as 401(k)s and IRAs), jointly-owned property, and more. The beneficiary designations of these assets decide who inher-its them, often without reference to your will.

You need to review periodically the beneficiary designation forms for these assets. Numerous court cases and IRS rulings have concluded that the owner's intent and statements in the will rarely matter. The only thing that matters is what was writ-ten in the latest beneficiary designation form.

Trust, with their many uses and flexibility, are another rea-son a will isn't enough.

Trusts can accomplish many goals that a will can't. With a trust, your assets can avoid probate. Your privacy can be main-tained. A trust can protect assets from creditors of you and your heirs. The right trust can provide security for your heirs while protecting the wealth from them.

Once the province of the very wealthy, trusts provide so many benefits they surpass wills as the key documents in many estate plans. . . .

Mistake #2: Expecting too Much from a Power of Attorney

A power of attorney (POA) is an essential estate planning document. But you (and especially your agents) need to know its limits and how to maximize its benefits.

In a POA, the principal (you) names one or more agents (often an adult child) to act on your behalf. The POA can be general, empowering the agent to take any action on your behalf, or limited, restricting the areas in which the agent can act.

You need a POA, because someone needs to manage your assets, pay bills, and make decisions if you become incapacitated. The alternative is for your loved ones to ask a court to declare you incompetent and appoint someone to act on your behalf, known as guardianship in most states.

Ideally, the agent named in your POA smoothly takes over and seamlessly manages your affairs when you aren't able and continues doing so as long as needed.

Based on anecdotes I've heard and my wife's and my experience as my parents' agents, I can tell you things often don't work that way.

Once your agent is ready to act under the POA, the agent has to convince others, usually financial institutions, to recognize and accept the POA.

A financial institution isn't required to accept a POA. Each institution adopts its own standards for accepting POAs.

Many institutions now won't accept a POA that was executed more than six months earlier. Others want the POA on their own forms. Some require you to reaffirm it in writing from time to time if it hasn't been used. Some institutions require specific language in the POA.

At many institutions, the "front line" people won't be able to act on the POA once they receive it. It will be referred to in-house attorneys or POA specialists who will review it and decide whether it will be accepted.

The standards of one one-of-town mutual fund were especially difficult to work with. The firm said the signature on the POA had to be guaranteed, which usually is done by a bank. But the bank said it only guaranteed signatures on its own forms. It wouldn't guarantee signatures on POAs drafted by my parents' lawyers. After a few weeks of back-and-forth on the phone we finally found someone at the mutual fund firm who offered an alternative and eventually accepted the POA.

Once a firm accepts the POA, the agent still has to prove he's the person named in the POA. Most firms will accept a photocopy of a driver's license, but some require additional verification before letting someone act.

Not many years ago, a telephone call or letter from the estate planning attorney verifying the POA would be enough to move things along. But financial institutions these days don't want to take any risk of being involved in identity theft and elder financial abuse. Your agent always can ask a court to require a financial institution to accept the POA. But that takes time and money, and the institution is likely to win if it has any argument that it acted reasonably. To make matters worse, if you lose the court action you could be required to pay the institution's attorneys' fees.

The bottom line is your work isn't done when you leave the estate planner's office with a signed and executed POA. A little more work is needed to ensure your affairs are handled smoothly and your loved ones don't have to climb multiple obstacles to pay your bills.

Consider these actions:

Be sure your agent has a copy of the POA or knows where to find one. The same goes for details about your financial accounts.

Ask each financial institution you deal with what its requirements are for accepting a POA. Then, try to comply with them. I've recommended that people switch financial institutions when their POA requirements had too many hurdles.

Consolidate your accounts. It will be easier for you to manage your finances as you age, and your agent will have to convince a limited number of firms to accept the POA.

Act early. We were lucky that my parents let us take over their finances while they're still alive and have most of their cognitive abilities. In a pinch, we could always bring my parents to a local office or have them participate in a phone call. The early transfer also let my parents monitor things for a while and develop confidence in how we would handle their finances.

Establish relationships. Conducting financial and investment transactions online and over the telephone can be convenient and save money, but it can make it more difficult for someone with a POA to take over your financial matters. Consider having the bulk of your assets at financial firms with at least one local office. Establish a relationship with one or more account representatives at the firm. Give them your POA and ensure it is accepted. Introduce them to the agent. Let them know that if anything happens to you, this is the person who will contact them and take over management of your accounts.

The key goal of having a POA is to ensure someone can pay bills and otherwise manage your finances if you should become unable to. But nothing can happen until financial services firms accept the POA. They won't even tell the agent anything that's going on in an account until the POA is accepted. For the POA to do its job, you and your agent need to work with the financial firms long before the POA is needed.

Mistake #3: Not Avoiding Probate

When an asset passes to others through a will, it has to go through the probate process. Probate can be both time-consuming and expensive. The details vary from state to state and even among localities in a state.

Many states in recent decades enacted less expensive and more streamlined probate procedures, at least for estates of lesser value. But in other states, the delays and costs of the old probate process remain. In addition to being expensive, probate can be disruptive to the management of your assets and leave beneficiaries uncertain when their inheritances will be received and how much they'll receive. When you own assets in more than one state, your estate might have probate procedures in each of the states.

Probate also is a public process. Anyone can go through the probate court records to determine how much your probate estate was worth, what you owned and owed and how you divided it.

Some assets avoid probate by operation of law, as we discussed in the first installment of this series. These include most retirement accounts, life insurance, annuities, and jointly-owned property. Others avoid probate after being transferred to a trust, such as a revocable living trust. The living trust is perhaps the most common way to avoid probate, and we'll discuss it in detail in a later installment of this series.

Despite its disadvantages, probate isn't always bad.

Some people believe it is an advantage to have everything about the estate and how it is distributed in the public record and reviewed by the court. There's less of a chance for shenanigans by the executor or others. Anyone who disagrees with how things are being handled can file a complaint with the court. The probate process also certifies title to the assets, making it more difficult for someone to challenge ownership.

The question to consider is how much of your estate should avoid probate.

When you spend time in more than one state, especially when you own real estate in two or more states, consider the probate situation in each state. Generally, the bulk of your estate is subject to probate in the state where you were a resident or domiciled. But real estate is probated in the estate where it is located. So, your estate might be subject to probate in more than one state without proper planning.

Whether you want to avoid probate depends largely on your privacy concerns, disability planning, and where you live. If you want privacy, you'll want to avoid probate. But if privacy is not a concern and you live in a state with modern probate processes, you might conclude that taking the steps to avoid probate aren't worth the cost and effort.

Discuss the local probate process with your estate planner so you'll know the potential cost and time delay involved. Also, consider your privacy preferences. Then, determine how much of your estate you want to avoid probate.

Mistake #4: Not Making Full Use of a Living Trust

In the typical living trust, you and your spouse transfer title to most of your assets to the trust and serve as co-trustees. You have full control of the assets and deal with them just as before, except you act as a trustee instead of individual owner.

Living trusts have a lot of potential advantages. The main one is the assets in the trust avoid probate. After you pass away, a successor trustee takes over management of the assets and can begin distributing them to the heirs or taking other actions directed in the trust agreement. The expense and delay of probate are avoided. A living trust also provides privacy. The terms of the trust and the assets owned by it aren't recorded in the public record the way a will is.

A living trust also can be a big advantage should the original owner become disabled. Again, a successor trustee can take over and begin managing the assets after being recognized by custodians of the assets. The transfer might be smoother than when you rely on a power of attorney.

Unfortunately, the advantages of living trusts often are lost or diminished by mistakes and oversights.

Perhaps the most common mistake is to fail to transfer legal title of assets to the trust, known as funding the trust.

People often walk out of their estate planner's office with the living trust agreement, and then they put it on a shelf. The trust doesn't own any assets, so none of the assets avoid probate or are subject to the terms of the trust.

For a living trust to work, you have to do the hard work of transferring legal title of assets to it. That means changing the deeds to real estate and recording them as local law requires. It also means re-registering the title to vehicles with the trust as the new owner.

Most financial accounts can be changed to the trust's ownership simply by filing a form required by the financial services firm. Many firms will want a copy of the certificate of trust or the full trust agreement. At most banks and other financial institutions you don't have to change the names preprinted on your checks. They can have either the trust name or your individual name. But the account statements and the financial institution records need to say the trust is the owner of the account.

When these steps aren't taken, the result is an unfunded trust, of which there are many around the country. Your assets won't avoid probate, and a successor trustee won't be able to manage the assets if you are unable to. Instead, a power of attorney must be relied on to ensure your bills are paid and other actions are taken. And all your assets will go through probate and be governed by your will.

Another mistake is not to bring the successor trustees into the picture early enough.

The successor trustees take over management of the trust after you pass away or are unable to manage the trust. For this transition to be smooth, the successor trustees must know you selected them. They also should have copies of the trust agreement and know where the original is located. You also should make them familiar with the assets they will be managing.

A good move is to be sure the custodians of your financial accounts are familiar with the successor trustees. As with the power of attorney, it is best to get to know one or more individuals at your financial institutions and introduce them to the successor trustees. Otherwise, when it is time for the successor trustees to act, they might have to go through a long process or proving who they are and that they are entitled to manage your assets. That would substantially reduce an advantage of having a revocable living trust.

Mistake #5: Leaving Assets Outright to Adult Children

People understand why minor children and even young adults shouldn't inherit property outright. Someone with more maturity and experience needs to manage the assets and make spending decisions. That's why for minors and young adults, inheritances routinely are left in trusts at least until the youngsters are older.

Too often, however, people overlook the benefits of leaving assets in trust for adult children instead of having them inherit the property outright.

Consider the risks of leaving wealth outright even to grown children and these benefits of using inheritance trusts to hold bequests for them.

Reaching a particular age doesn't mean someone is financially sophisticated. As the value of an inheritance increases, so does the level of financial acumen needed to manage it. When one of your goals is for the wealth to last for years, professional management of the wealth might be essential. The adult child could, of course, hire a money manager or financial advisor to manage wealth inherited outright. But someone who isn't sophisticated enough to manage the money might not make a good choice of a financial advisor.

Make an honest assessment of the ability of each of your children to manage the property, and then decide whether to leave the bequest outright or in trust.

Some people are spendthrifts no matter what their age. When you're concerned an adult child won't focus on the long term, consider a trust. You can set rules for distributions from the trust.

For example, you can limit annual distributions to only investment income or a percentage of the trust's value. At the other extreme, you can consider giving the trustee discretion to determine the distributions based on the needs and best interests of the beneficiary. When you're really concerned about the spending of the child, the trustee can pay the expenses of the child directly to providers of essential living expenses instead of distributing cash or property to the child. The rules for distributions generally are limited only by the imaginations of you and your estate planner.

The trust also can have a sort of on/off switch. You might be worried that an adult child has a problem with substance abuse or gambling. In that case, you can give the trustee the discretion to stop making distributions when it is in the beneficiary's best interests. Distributions can be resumed when the trustee determines it is again in the beneficiary's best interests.

A trust also protects your wealth from the creditors of the children. In most states, creditors can't force distributions from a trust, but they can assert claims against income and principal that are distributed to the children. The money is safe as long as it is in the trust. Review state law with your estate planner if creditor protection is a goal. You might want the trust located in a state with stronger protection.

When you leave an inheritance outright to an adult child, the spouse of your offspring often can claim a share of the assets in a divorce or separation. But when you leave the bequest in a trust, it usually isn't considered part of the marital estate. Part of it won't end up with a former spouse of one of your children.

When an inheritance is given through a trust instead of directly, it doesn't have to stay in the trust forever. You can provide that the principal will be distributed to the beneficiary upon reaching a certain age, or that it will be distributed in stages as the beneficiary reaches different ages. Some trusts have principal distributed as other milestones are reached.

A trust isn't needed or appropriate in every case. You should consider your goals and realistically assess your children, Then, decide if it would be better to let your children inherit the wealth outright or through a trust.

Mistake #6: Losing the Portability of a Spouse's Unused Exemption

Before the law was changed in 2010, a major part of the estate planning process for married couples was to equalize the value of assets in which each had legal title. Back then, each spouse had a separate lifetime estate and gift tax exemption, but the exemptions couldn't be shared. A married couple potentially could avoid estate taxes on a joint estate worth up to two individual exemptions, but they had to jump through some hoops.

The joint exemption wasn't automatic.

Suppose when the individual exemption was $3 million a couple had an estate of $7 million. Of that, $1 million was in the wife's name, and $6 million was in the husband's name. None of it was jointly held. If the wife died first, her lifetime exemption would shelter only $1 million of the joint estate. The widower would be left with a $3 million exemption to shelter a $6 million estate, assuming the wife left her $1 million to the children or a bypass trust.

Because the lifetime exemptions couldn't be shared between the spouses and the estate primarily was in the name of one spouse, about $3 million of this estate was subject to estate taxes.

Since 2010, the portability rule allows any unused lifetime estate and gift tax exemption of a deceased spouse to be transferred to the surviving spouse, ensuring it isn't lost. A married couple has a true joint exemption equal to two individual exemptions, and it doesn't matter how much of the estate is legally owned by each spouse.

After inflation indexing the joint exemption in 2018 is $22.36 million ($11.18 million for each spouse). (The IRS finalized the 2018 levels on March 4. The amount was in doubt, because the Tax Cuts and Jobs Act changed the inflation-indexing method.)

Unfortunately, the portability of the exemption isn't automatic. The transfer of the unused exemption amount to the surviving spouse happens only if it is elected by the executor of the first spouse to pass away. It is elected simply by filing an estate tax return.

Very few estates are required to file returns, because the high exemption amount means few will be taxable. Because few estates are required to file estate tax returns, executors who don't understand the portability rule can inadvertently cause the unused exemption amount not to be transferred to the surviving spouse. Whenever an estate doesn't file an estate tax return, the unused exemptions aren't transferred to the surviving spouse.

Executors and surviving spouses need to know that an estate tax return should be filed, even when not required, to transfer the unused exemption amount to the surviving spouse.

Mistake #7: Leaving a Messy Estate

Perhaps the last and best test of how much you care about your survivors and legacy is the level of organization of your estate.

There are two parts of your estate to consider. The first part is your physical estate. For most people it is the home and personal possessions.

I've talked to many people who've dealt with the physical estates of their parents, and most have stories about how much stuff they had to sort through and dispose of. Many people accumulate stuff over their lifetimes and rarely streamline it. Their possessions compound over the decades. Most of them decide, deliberately or by default, to let their children deal with the accumulation. Unfortunately, the children will be doing this while also grieving.

The survivors will feel obligated to sort through all the stuff, because we've all heard stories of people hiding cash or valuable items. One family told me they found a $20 bill in every coat, jacket, and sweater in their parents' house. It added to a nice amount, but they also had to sort through each item of clothing and always wondered how much they missed.

It's not unusual for the surviving children to spend days, weeks, and even longer dealing with the stuff. One family told me they decided the task was so large they agreed to set aside one weekend a month for a year to meet at their parents' house and clean it up.

Don't save stuff because you think the children or grandchildren might want it someday. They won't. Even family heirlooms don't stir much interest these days. Don't think you're saving it for charity. Most charities now are very selective about the donations they'll take. It's the same way with second-hand stores. They won't take a lot of items, because they can't sell them.

Margareta Magnusson introduced the world to *The Gentle Art Of Swedish Death Cleaning*. In her book, Magnusson says part of Swedish culture is for people over age 50 or so to begin streamlining their possessions. It's done partly as a courtesy to survivors and partly to make your life easier and simpler.

The streamlining process can take a long time. You shouldn't delay, because it will become harder the older you are. If you haven't de-cluttered your life for decades, expect this to be a long-term process, not an event. Set aside a day or weekend per month to work on one small part of your house at a time.

I think you'll feel better throughout the process, and your heirs will be appreciative.

The second part of the estate is your legal and financial estate. It's also a good idea to organize and streamline your financial assets.

Many people opened accounts at different financial firms over the years and have 401(k) accounts or other retirement plans at different employers. It's a good idea to consolidate accounts and assets. Consider selling smaller investments and real estate holdings to streamline the estate. You'll find it easier to manage your assets, and your executor will settle your estate more quickly and at lower cost.

If you don't organize and streamline, assets are likely to be lost or misplaced. If your executor and heirs don't know what you own, they won't look for the paperwork. Even if your heirs locate and claim all your assets, they might have to spend a lot of resources in the effort if you haven't streamlined and cleaned up the estate.

Most financial services firms have accounts whose owners they haven't heard from for years. Often, these accounts are transferred to the state, a process known as escheat. It's easier for you than your heirs to prove ownership, so you should check to see if any of your assets have been escheated to any of the states you lived in.

In addition to streamlining your accounts and investments, have your paperwork organized and easy to find. Leave your executor and heirs a roadmap to your estate. This would include a list of all your assets and liabilities. You should include details for each account, such as the firm that has custody of the account, account number, any online access codes, contact persons, and other information that would be helpful to the executor. One way to organization this information is by using my workbook, *To My Heirs: A Book of Final Wishes and Instructions.*

The organization of your possessions and estate is one factor survivors will remember. Decide if you want to leave a messy burden or a more pleasant legacy.

References

Carlson, B. (2018, Feb 21). 7 big estate planning mistakes: relying only on a will. Retrieved from https://www.forbes.com/sites/bobcarlson/2018/02/21/7-big-estate-planning-mistakes-part-1/#322b3a8d5d06

Carlson, B. (2018, Feb 23). 7 big estate planning mistakes: the power of attorney trap. Retrieved from https://www.forbes.com/sites/bobcarlson/2018/02/23/7-big-estate-planning-mistakes-part-2/#76bc362122b5

Carlson, B. (2018, Feb 26). 7 big estate planning mistakes: not avoiding probate. Retrieved from https://www.forbes.com/sites/bobcarlson/2018/02/26/7-big-estate-planning-mistakes-not-avoiding-probate/#5b1d29834503

Carlson, B. (2018, Feb 28). 7 big estate planning mistakes: not making full use of a living trust. Retrieved from https://www.forbes.com/sites/bobcarlson/2018/02/28/7-big-estate-planning-mistakes-not-making-full-use-of-a-living-trust/#784e054f27e2

Carlson, B. (2018, Mar 6). 7 big estate planning mistakes: leaving assets outright to adult children. Retrieved from https://www.forbes.com/sites/bobcarlson/2018/03/06/7-big-estate-planning-mistakes-leaving-assets-outright-to-adult-children/#2f88996e37e1

Carlson, B. (2018, Mar 9). 7 big estate planning mistakes: losing the portability of a spouses unused exemption. Retrieved from https://www.forbes.com/sites/bobcarlson/2018/03/09/7-big-estate-planning-mistakes-losing-the-portability-of-a-spouses-unused-exemption/#4db10958488d

Carlson, B. (2018, Mar 13). 7 big estate planning mistakes: leaving a messy estate. Retrieved from https://www.forbes.com/sites/bobcarlson/2018/03/13/7-big-estate-planning-mistakes-leaving-a-messy-estate/#60312ac12e61

Critical Thinking

1. What type of problems do you think families experience during probate when a loved one passes away?

2. Of all the mistakes mentioned, which ones could have lasting effects on beneficiaries?

Internet References

American Bar Association
https://www.americanbar.org/

EstatePlanning.com
https://www.estateplanning.com/

FindLaw
https://estate.findlaw.com/

BOB CARLSON is the editor of *Retirement Watch.*

Article   Prepared by: Elaina Osterbur, *Saint Louis University*

Why Baby Boomers Refuse to Retire

Classic Notions of Retirement Are no Longer an Option, and Baby Boomers Are Reimagining What the Last Decades of Work Can Hold

GEORGE LORENZO

Learning Outcomes

After reading this article, you will be able to:

- Identify why baby boomers refuse to retire.
- Identify the pros and cons of retirement.

Five years ago, in 2011, the first wave of the oldest U.S. baby boomers reached the common retirement age of 65. Since then, another 10,000 each day continue to reach this stage in their lives. The U.S. Census Bureau calculates that by 2020, 55.9 million people in the U.S. will be age 65 or older, and by 2030, that number will reach 72.7 million.

How will all these aging boomers thrive in the 21st century? According to many experts on aging, it's increasingly by staying in the workforce, at the very least on a part-time basis. As noted by Gallup in their "Many Baby Boomers Reluctant to Retire" report, "Nearly half of boomers still working say they don't expect to retire until they are 66 or older, including one in 10 who predict they will never retire."

Staying Healthy by Working Longer

Boomers don't consider themselves old until around 72 years of age, claimed a Pew Research Center study. And most long-held culturally and historically embedded notions about how to retire are quickly becoming outdated. Many boomers no longer see themselves playing shuffle board, golfing, fishing and generally relaxing for the remainder of their days. Plus, age-related scientists now posit that a life overly focused on leisure and passive entertainment could actually promote poor health.

A 2014 study conducted by the Rush University Alzheimer's Disease Center in Chicago points to living a life of purpose (identified as having a strong sense of meaning, which frequently comes from essential paid employment and/or volunteer work) as highly conducive to reducing one's susceptibility to stroke, dementia, movement problems, disability, and premature death. In short, full retirement is not a smart or healthy option.

The Growing Unretired Cottage Industry

There is an expansive cottage industry that supports the opting-out-of-retirement boomer explosion. The AARP's Life Reimagined site, for example, features a large variety of services focused on assisting boomers with remaining active in the labor force. Since 2006, the growing Encore.org, an organization known for "advancing second acts for the greater good," has provided numerous services related to aging boomers, including "The Purpose Prize," awarded to more than 500 over-60 innovators who have brought their skills and talents to communities all over the world.

Source: FastCompany, www.fastcompany.com/3056475/the-future-of-work/why-baby-boomers-refuse-to-retire. Retrieved May 19, 2016.

A service in Phoenix called Experience Matters is an example of how third-party business entities are bringing together boomers and nonprofit organizations. As noted on their site, "68 percent to 76 percent of the boomer population is in a position both financially and physically to engage in meaningful volunteer or skilled service opportunities." Job sites that emphasize opportunities specifically for boomers are also a growing part of this promising cottage industry, with names like retirementjobs.com and retiredbrains.com.

Aging Experts Endorse Active Engagement

"There are a lot of organizations all over the country that are coalescing around this working-longer theme and helping people figure it out," says Chris Farrell, author of *Unretirement: How Baby Boomers Are Changing the Way We Think About Work, Community, and the Good Life.* "People are using different phrases such as meaning and money, passion and a paycheck, and this notion of reimagining and rethinking."

"The big thing is that people are living longer," says Nancy Collamer, author of *Second-Act Careers: 50+ Ways to Profit from Your Passions During Semi-Retirement* and owner of an informational site for boomers called mylifestylecareer.com. "So you have a dynamic where people work in their primary careers for as long as 40 years, give or take, and then they could be looking at a retirement that lasts 30 years—that is a lot of years to fill and a lot of years to fund."

Not Without Challenges

Paul Irving, editor of *The Upside of Aging* and chairman of the Milken Institute's Center for the Future of Aging, explained how a variety of challenging circumstances are often the root cause for boomers not retiring. "There are different reasons why retirement is changing," he said. "Many people have dramatically inadequate and in some cases no savings beyond social security. The increasing costs of health care and housing present a remarkable challenge. The opportunity to generate income for a longer period of time is not an elective for fun and interests. It is a need for resources and the opportunity to maintain an acceptable life."

According to a Fidelity Investment retirement health care cost estimate, "A couple, both aged 65 and retiring this year, can now expect to spend an estimated $245,000 on health care throughout retirement, up from $220,000 last year. The figure has increased 29 percent since 2005, when it was $190,000."

Overall, there's plenty to scrutinize and act on, both politically and socially, to ensure that the aging boomer generation gets the support they need to keep working productively. "More people are having conversations about it," Farrell said. "We do not have enough institutionalized offerings like phased retirement programs and flexible work schedules. There are a lot of laws that make it difficult for companies to rehire part-time, former employees. There is a lot of underbrush to be cleaned out so that it becomes much simpler for people to keep working."

"As a general matter, this is one of those great challenges we need to address as a society," Irving said. "Both as individuals and as a broader society, we should be encouraging it, enabling it, celebrating it, and making sure that it is an opportunity for all of those who choose to do it."

Collamer referred to the historical dismantling and decrease in pension funds and other employer-paid retirement funding opportunities. "As more employers start to face the so-called brain drain of losing key talent in institutional knowledge, hopefully we will start to see a rise in employers who will offer their employees some form of retirement benefits," she said. In addition, Collamer described the problem of age discrimination in the workplace as being "real, with a lot of people experiencing difficulties finding good, quality part-time work after they retire from their full-time jobs."

Boomers are starting to tackle such challenges in a 21st century way by going online. "The opportunities for doing things like freelancing and consulting work and establishing products and services that you sell on the web have become real possibilities for boomers," Collamer said. "The amount of money required to start online businesses is far less than if you were to try to establish a brick and mortar business."

In a recent blog post, *Gig Economy: Better for Boomers Than Millennials,* on the PBS Next Avenue site for people over 50, Ferrell wrote that "boomers will increasingly and gladly gear up for the gig economy as they enter their 60s and 70s. Already, Uber says more of its drivers are over 50 than under 30, and that about a quarter of its drivers are 50 and older. Last year, incidentally, Uber and AARP's Life Reimagined teamed up to help Uber find more 50-plus drivers."

The baby boomer generation has lived through decades of radical political and social change, so it should be no surprise that they are also revolutionizing retirement.

Critical Thinking

1. How will older adults working beyond retirement age affect job opportunities for younger people?
2. Beyond the services discussed in the article, are their other services that would be necessary given an older working population?

Internet References

AARP
http://www.aarp.org

National Institute on Aging
http://www.nia.nih.org

Article Prepared by: Elaina Osterbur, *Saint Louis University*

Recordkeeping for Retirement Starts with MySSA

KENN BEAM TACCHINO

Learning Outcomes

After reading this article, you will be able to:

- List the reasons that older adults need to provide documentation of income, as well as a Social Security statement, when planning for retirement.
- Discuss the contents of a retirement file.

Vacation time, when clients look to tackle personal projects that they have put off during the work year, may be a good time to assemble all the documentation needed to plan retirement. Every client should have a retirement file that contains the following:

- The retirement plan itself, as well as the summary plan description provided by his/ her employer.
- Benefit statements from IRAs, 401(k) plans, and other plans that show how his/her funds are invested, as well as the current value of these funds.
- Information about the client's health and long-term care policies.
- The will.
- Any living wills or durable powers of attorney for health care.
- Investment policy statements and withdrawal policy statements.
- Any other relevant investment, tax, or legal documents.

For many, a crucial item that is too often missing from the file is their Social Security statement. Clients might ask: "Didn't I used to receive something in the mail from Social Security every year about three months prior to my birthday?" Yes, but . . . .

What Happened and What Now

It used to be the client could request a Social Security statement in the mail by filing the form SSA-7004. However, this option no longer exists. Then from 1999 to 2011 the Social Security Administration mailed Social Security statements to anyone who was 25 or older. In May of 2012 they stopped these automatic mailings and went online to save money. The online statement is created by your clients at the website of the Social Security Administration, using the tab "MySSA." The automated future we all expected for the new millennium had arrived. However, in response to criticism that only a small percentage of people created their accounts online, (about 6 percent), another change was mandated. Starting in September of 2014, the Social Security Administration will resume mailings of the Social Security statement at 5-year intervals to workers who have not made their own accounts on MySSA. The statement will be sent to workers at ages 25, 30, 35, 40, 45, 50, 55, and 60.

Most experts believe that record-keeping would be best served by creating an online account at MySSA and checking it annually (rather than waiting every 5 years for a mailing). Fortunately, accounts are created in three easy steps. First, clients will need to go to www.socialsecurity.gov/myaccount and select "create an account." Second, they will need to provide some personal information to verify their identity. This information includes Social Security number, mailing address, email address, birth date, phone number, and some pesky security questions (such as the name of a bank where (s)he applied for a home equity loan, or the name of his/her high school). And third, your client will need to choose a username and password. Planners need to know that not everyone is eligible to set up an account. To create an account the client must be at least 18 years old, have a valid e-mail address, have a Social

Security number, and have a U.S. mailing address. Some of your clients may be wondering if they are eligible to receive a statement about an ex-spouse so they can tell how much they might receive based on the ex-spouse's Social Security record. If the former spouse is still living, privacy rules prohibit the Social Security Administration from giving out the ex-spouse's statement. However, a visit or call to Social Security can tell the client what to do and know in order to claim any spousal or survivor benefits to which (s)he is entitled.

How Does MySSA Help Plan for Retirement?

One benefit of the Social Security statement is that it can determine whether your client's earnings are accurately posted. Assessing this is crucial because the client's Social Security benefit is based on the amount (s)he earns each year of his/her career. If there is an error in posting earnings, the amount of benefits (s)he receives may be compromised. The sooner your client finds an error, the more documentation (s)he will have available to verify that the Social Security system has it wrong and (s)he actually earned more than (s)he has been given credit for. If your client uncovers an issue, (s)he can go in to the local Social Security office (it might be best to make an appointment to avoid having to sit and wait) or call the Social Security helpline at 800-772-1213, Monday through Friday from 7 A.M. to 7 P.M. In either case, your client should have his/her documents ready when (s)he speaks to the representative. If your client is going into the Social Security office, (s)he should have two copies of his/her benefit statement and two copies of the evidence that supports his/her claim to the higher income. This way the client can leave a copy with the Social Security representative. One important thing for your client to consider when perusing his/her statement is that Social Security has a taxable wage base (e.g., in 2010 and 2011 it was $106,800; in 2012 it was $110,100; in 2013 it was $113,700; and in 2014 it is $117,000), and earnings above that amount will not be shown in his/her earnings history.

Another thing the statement will tell your clients is their full retirement age. Spoiler alert—for anyone born between 1943 and 1954 the full retirement age is 66. For anyone born in 1960 or later the full retirement age is 67. For those in between, add two months per year (e.g., for those born in 1955 it will be 66 and 2 months, and for those born in 1957 it will be 66 and 6 months).

Another crucial element of the statement is that it contains an estimate of the client's retirement benefits. More specifically, the statement contains an estimate of the monthly retirement benefit that (s)he will receive at age 62, full retirement age, and age 70. The estimated benefits take into account certain assumptions such as the fact that for the current year and the

years up to retirement, the individual will continue to work and make about the same as the latest earnings shown on record. If your client earns more or less than is projected, his/her benefits could be higher or lower accordingly. Another consideration regarding these estimates is that the current year's benefit formula is used in the benefit computations. In future years it is likely that this formula will be changed to reflect inflation, and therefore your clients are looking at an estimate of the current projection of their benefits; not the inflated future value of their benefit. Finally, remember that Social Security benefits are inflated after the client retires so the benefit (s)he receive in the first year of retirement will increase every time Social Security gives an annual cost of living adjustment (although purchasing power will remain the same). For a personalized benefit that allows the client to run alternative scenarios based on different future earnings or different future retirement dates the client can go to www.socialsecurity.gov/estimator.

Since Social Security is not just about retirement your client can find out about any disability benefits that might be coming his/her way. In addition, the statement indicates any survivor benefits to which the client's family may be entitled. Other useful information includes:

- An estimate of the Social Security benefits that your client has paid.
- Information about whether your client qualifies for Medicare and how to sign up for it.
- Information about the windfall elimination and government-pension-offset provisions.
- Links to some useful resources.

How Does MySSA Help after Receiving Social Security or Medicare Benefits?

The MySSA site is also useful if your client is already retired. It provides information about benefits and payments. If (s)he needs proof of receiving Social Security benefits, Supplemental Security Income (SSI), and/or Medicare, the client can request a benefit verification letter online. This letter is sometimes called a "budget letter," a "benefits letter," a "proof of income letter," or a "proof of award letter." This tool is an official letter from Social Security that can be used as proof of:

- Income when (s)he applies for a loan or mortgage.
- Income for assisted housing or other state or local benefits.
- Current Medicare health insurance coverage.
- Retirement status.
- Disability.

Clients can select the information they want to be included, or left out of, their online benefit verification letters.

Your client can also use MySSA if (s)he wants to change address or phone number or if (s)he wants to start or change direct deposits of benefit payments.

Marketing Yourself with Full-Service Planning

The MySSA website, the Social Security statement, and the other documents in the client's retirement file provide a number of opportunities for a planner to market himself or herself with clients and provide full-service planning. Here are a dozen services that planners should consider providing:

1. Review the summary plan description with the client to explain the options under the plan and clarify any issues that cause the client confusion.
2. Analyze benefit statements to assess if the client's asset allocation model is optimal for his/her situation. Remember to include "outside" investments and human capital opportunities in your analysis.
3. Review the long-term care policy and health policies to discern if there are gaps in, or duplication of, coverage.
4. Make sure beneficiary designations are up-to-date.
5. Verify that the client has a living will or a durable power of attorney for health care.
6. Review the investment policy statement and withdrawal policy statements.
7. Coordinate the disability benefits provided by Social Security with the client's long-term disability policy. In other words, make sure (s)he has enough disability insurance outside the Social Security system; however, don't double count the private long-term disability policy and Social Security disability when assessing needs.
8. Coordinate the Social Security survivor's benefits with other life insurance benefits.

9. Help the client to create a Social Security account if (s)he needs your assistance.
10. Make sure the client verifies earnings on the Social Security statement and help him/her to make corrections if earnings are misstated.
11. Point out the full retirement age as illustrated in the Social Security statement and review with the client the proper time to retire. Make sure the client realizes that Social Security claiming and retirement can be two different events. Also use the Social Security statement to focus on the replacement ratio provided at age 70 by Social Security.
12. Use the Social Security Estimator to run alternative projections of Social Security based on "what if" scenarios.

Help with these and other record-keeping tasks can engender trust and help the client to think with better clarity about his/her retirement. This creates a win/win scenario for both you and your client.

Critical Thinking

1. How does the MySSA site assist older adults in their retirement planning process?
2. How does the MySSA site assist older adults who are already retired?

Internet References

my Social Security
http://www.ssa.gov/myaccount/
U.S. Social Security Administration
http://www.ssa.gov/l

KENN BEAM TACCHINO, JD, LLM, RICP, is a professor of taxation and financial planning at Widener University in Chester, PA. Professor Tacchino has won awards for both his teaching and his scholarly writing. Among other consulting activities, he conducts retirement planning seminars for employee groups.

Unit 6

UNIT

Prepared by: Elaina Osterbur, *Saint Louis University*

The Experience of Dying

Modern science has allowed individuals to have some control over many aspects of life including the ability to prolong life. Medical technology can keep people alive, can cause disability, and can cure disease. The ability of technology to prolong life has prompted several growing social issues such as physician-assisted suicide, hospice, and palliative care. Six states (California, Oregon, Vermont, Hawaii, Colorado, and Washington) and Washington DC have passed legislation that legalizes physician-assisted dying. The state of Montana has legal physician-assisted dying in the form of court ruling. The rise of the hospice movement and palliative care is another response to the growing number of both young and old patients who have been diagnosed with a terminal disease who wish to live out the rest of their days in comfort.

The experience of dying affects not only the person who is dying but also caregiver, family members, and friends who are left behind. Grieving is an important response to the loss of a loved one. Much research has been done in this area and suggests that the emotional and psychological response to the loss of a spouse is similar between men and women. The five stages of grief (denial, anger, bargaining, depression, and acceptance) are universal and are experienced by all walks of life. During times of mourning, people grieve not only for the loss of a loved one, but also for themselves and for the finiteness of life.

However, life and death defy scientific explanation or reason.

The fear of death leads people to develop defense mechanisms to insulate themselves psychologically from the reality of their own death. The individual knows that someday he or she must die, but this event is nearly always thought to be likely to occur in the far distant future. The individual does not think of himself or herself as dying tomorrow or the next day but years from now. In this way, people are able to control their anxiety about death.

The readings in this unit addresses end-of-life care, bereavement, hospice, and palliative care.

Article   Prepared by: Elaina Osterbur, *Saint Louis University*

Pain Control at the End of Life

CHRIS WOOLSTON

Learning Outcomes

After reading this article, you will be able to:

- Identify how severe pain affects quality of life at the end of life.

- Identify the goals of hospice.

A Better Understanding of Pain—and How to Treat It— Means a Gentler Death for Many Patients with Terminal Illnesses.

People who are near death have more important things to do than suffer. The final days, weeks, and months should be a time to connect with loved ones and reflect on life, says Kandyce Powell, RN. As the executive director of the Maine Hospice Council, Powell has stood at the side of hundreds of dying patients over the years.

Too often, this precious time is clouded with pain. More than half of patients with terminal cancer, for example, suffer from poorly managed pain, according to a report in the *American Journal of Hospice and Palliative Care*. Severe pain at the end of life is distracting, destructive, and, for the most part, unnecessary. "The real sadness is that we forget that we can do so much to improve a person's quality of life," Powell says.

Thanks to recent advances in pain treatments, roughly 90 to 95 percent of all dying patients should be able to experience substantial relief from pain, says June Dahl, PhD, a professor of pharmacology at the University of Wisconsin at Madison, and a founder of the American Alliance of Cancer Pain Initiatives. "Complete freedom from pain is not a realistic goal," she says. Instead, doctors, family members, and patients should fully expect pain to fade into the background. On a scale of 0 to 10, treatments can almost always bring pain down to a 2 or 3, she says.

Unfortunately, many myths and misconceptions stand in the way of relief, Dahl says. Until everyone involved in a patient's care knows the facts about pain control at the end of life, too many patients will suffer needlessly.

Targeting pain

Pain relief should always be a top priority. If the primary focus is on treating disease, even when the prognosis is poor, it might delay admission to a hospice program that can provide more personal, comfort-oriented care, Powell says.

Helen R. from San Francisco, who lost her husband, Walter, to pancreatic cancer in 2006, says Walter's doctors did it right. Before Walter even needed pain medicine, his doctor gave him prescriptions for pain medications complete with instructions for taking them. She also told him what to expect as the disease progressed. "When Walter's dad was in hospice care with pancreatic cancer, Walter made sure he received enough pain medication," his wife said. "So going into his own illness, he wasn't intimidated about taking what he needed to relieve the pain. For him, it was just part of his day."

Many patients and their families find that hospice programs are especially well-equipped to ease both emotional and physical pain. The goal of hospice is to make your loved one's last days as comfortable as possible and to allow him or her to die with dignity—not to treat a disease or prolong life. All hospice programs may not be perfect—they can have the same staffing and quality of care issues found in other areas of medicine—but they do offer a different kind of care to dying patients. Hospice programs can deliver care in a hospice facility or, more commonly, in one's own home. Often patients feel more relaxed and less anxious in their own bed. Members of the hospice team—including nurses, doctors, chaplains, and therapists— visit the home regularly and teach caregivers how to provide comfort and deliver pain-relieving medications, including narcotics. Hospice workers are also specifically trained to help both the patients and family cope with the psychological and spiritual aspects of death.

For people suffering from severe cancer pain, for example, hospice providers often advise caregivers to give them pain medication at safe, regular intervals to prevent "breakthrough" pain—sudden bouts of relentless, uncontrolled pain. If you wait until the patient asks for pain medication, he or she may already be suffering, and the pain will be harder to get under control. If you're working with several caregivers, make sure they all understand that the medications should be used to prevent breakthrough pain—not just to treat it when it appears. This means an around the clock dosing schedule could be necessary in some cases.

Even when patients are taking painkillers at regular intervals, however, they sometimes need a change in medication to keep the pain under control. For this reason, family members should serve as pain monitors. One of their most important jobs is to ask the patients for frequent pain updates, Dahl says. "At the end of life, pain can become much greater very quickly," she says. "You can't depend on the patient to tell you when they are in pain. You have to ask."

Such check-ins may not always be easy—or welcome. Helen says she frequently asked her husband how he was feeling, but that after a while he got tired of it. "He didn't want people hovering," she says. The expression on his face was, "Can you ask me something else?" After checking in, it's good to switch roles—perhaps read to your loved one from a favorite book, or give a gentle back rub.

If direct questions don't work, there are other ways to tell when a patient is in pain. Dahl says that when patients can't describe their pain (whether because of Alzheimer's disease or other impairments), both family members and medical personnel should watch for other signs of pain, including moaning, weeping, grimacing, tensed muscles, clenched hands, thrashing, inability to sleep, or unusual agitation, she says. If the pain is excruciating, you may need to check with your doctor or a hospice provider about the next step. Hospices provide someone for you to call and talk to 24 hours a day.

Painful Emotions

Everyone involved in a patient's care should understand that emotions can shape and fuel pain. Anxiety—certainly a common emotion near the end of life—can make pain feel especially intense. As reported in the *Journal of the American Osteopathic Association* (JAOA), anxiety and pain often feed each other in a vicious circle. Patients worry that they won't get enough pain relief at the end of life, and their worries make them more sensitive to pain.

Some patients are also anxious about burdening the family they're about to leave behind. Helen says Walter always enjoyed being the family "fixer" and protector. When she would get worried or worked up about something, he was the one to calm her down and tell her everything would be all right. That might be why he didn't want to talk to her about his pain, she says: It was one last thing he could protect her from. "He knew what was going to happen," says Helen. "He was supporting me to the end."

Family conflicts are another major source of pain—both physical and emotional. According to the JAOA report, the presence of unsupportive children or an angry spouse can be just as agonizing as anything that's happening in a dying person's body.

While anxiety fuels pain, peace of mind can bring great relief. Family members, as well as doctors, can assure the patient that pain relief will be a top priority. Family members can also work with staff to make sure the patient is as comfortable as possible. Toward the end of Walter's life, when he was unconscious and on an intravenous morphine drip for pain, Helen was able to press a button to deliver more of the drug when she saw signs he needed it.

Most importantly, friends and family need to put any conflicts aside during a person's last days of life. Reassurance and forgiveness are some of the most powerful pain relievers ever utilized.

Doctors can also prescribe antianxiety medications such as Valium (diazepam) to calm nerves, or antidepressants such as Prozac (fluoxetine) to lift spirits, if needed. Ambien (zolpidem) can help patients rest through the night, a hard thing to do when nurses are checking vital signs around the clock. Doctors have recently recognized that anxiety can be a symptom of a treatable physical problem such as low blood sugar or thyroid trouble. In many cases, simply treating these problems will greatly relieve a patient's anxiety.

Multiple Options

Whether a patient is in a hospital, a nursing facility, or the family home, there are many options for pain relief. Drugs are only one part of the picture, Dahl says. Ice, massages, music, relaxation techniques, and guided imagery can all help relieve pain and reduce the need for medications. It's worth noting that even the venerable MD Anderson Cancer Center in Houston offers massage and acupuncture for pain relief.

The World Health Organization recommends a three-step "ladder" for pain relief in people suffering from cancer. The first step is to use relatively mild painkillers such as aspirin. When this isn't strong enough to control pain, the organization recommends moving on to codeine—a mild opioid (narcotic). But when pain gets tough, doctors need to move to the third step on the ladder and prescribe the most effective drugs in their arsenal. That means opioid drugs such as morphine. "Opioids are really essential," Dahl says, especially for patients with cancer pain. Opioids can also be effective for treating the pain from damaged nerves—doctors call it "neuropathic" pain—that's often associated with diabetes or other diseases that attack the nervous system, she says.

Opioids do more than relieve pain. As reported by the Hospice Foundation of America, morphine can "provide a sense of comfort. It makes breathing easier. It lets the patients relax and sleep." In short, pain treatments help patients make the most of their final days. When pain no longer dominates their lives, they can truly focus on the time they have left.

However, opioids can cause side effects that detract from the comfort. The most common side effects include constipation, nausea, itchiness, and mild sedation. Doctors often compensate for these problems by prescribing extra medications, like stool softeners and gentle bowel motility agents to ease constipation, for example. As reported in the *Journal of the American Osteopathic Association*, some side effects usually fade after a few days. Constipation is the one side effect that doesn't usually fade, which is why bowel medications are especially important for people taking opioids regularly.

The first attempt at relief—often morphine pills—isn't always successful. According to a report in *Anesthesiology Clinics of North America*, the drug may fail to control pain or it could cause too many side effects. Even if the first or the second or third try doesn't work, relief may still be in sight. Doctors can try different drugs such as methadone, a drug that has a slightly different mode of action than morphine and may work better for some people, or fentanyl, a fast-acting drug that can bring quick relief. Doctors can also try different methods of delivery. If pills aren't working, liquid morphine can be administered through a dropper, and an IV might also be worth a try. Fentanyl can be delivered through a patch, although safety issues should be discussed with your doctor. Fentanyl can also be prescribed in a lozenge or "lollipop" for quick relief of breakthrough pain, while morphine can be injected near the spine—a procedure that doctors call an epidural injection.

In cases of breakthrough pain during hospice, family members taking care of a loved one are not alone. Ideally, hospice nurses will be on call and can make an emergency visit at any time of the day or night, to give an injection of powerful pain medication, if needed, and discuss how to make the dying person more comfortable.

Putting Fears to Rest

Patients and their families often have fears about opioid treatments. While these fears are completely understandable and are often based on the best intentions, they are also largely unfounded, Powell says. For one thing, there's no danger that a person taking morphine for pain relief will become addicted to the drug, she says. Addiction is a psychological problem that causes people to crave and seek out drugs that they don't need medically and which they have evidence could be harmful to them. A person receiving morphine for chronic pain near the end of life just doesn't fit the picture.

There is a difference between addiction and physical dependence. People will become physically dependent on these drugs if they take them around the clock—that means they will have withdrawal symptoms if they abruptly stop taking the drug. But this is also not something to worry about in the case of a dying patient needing pain relief.

Patients can become tolerant of opioids or their pain may get worse, which means they may need increasing amounts of medication to get the same amount of relief. As a result, patients and their family members often worry that using strong medications now will make it harder to get relief down the road. But when a person is in severe pain, there's no reason to withhold powerful painkillers. As reported in the JAOA, doctors can always adjust the dose to meet a patient's needs.

Sometimes people think that taking morphine or other opioids is akin to giving up or admitting defeat. However, the primary aim should be to make the patient's final days as pain free as possible. This isn't giving up—it's giving comfort.

If every attempt to relieve pain fails, a doctor may suggest palliative sedation. A large dose of drugs will put the patient to sleep, with the goal of helping death to come painlessly. This procedure is rare, and it's never done without full permission of the family and, if possible, the patient. Palliative sedation is not euthanasia, and it is not intended to cause death. It is designed to make the patient unaware and unconscious as the disease follows its natural progression to death. The decision to allow palliative sedation is never easy, even when, as Dahl says, "the alternative is unacceptable suffering."

Some patients decide that they'd rather stay alert as long as possible, pain and all. Unfortunately, many patients don't even know that relief is even an option. "People aren't told what their choices are," Powell says.

When more patients and their families understand their options, and when more doctors make pain relief a priority, more people can spend the last part of their lives in comfort. Dying shouldn't have to hurt.

References

Interview with Kandyce Powell, RN, the executive director of the Maine Hospice Council.

Interview with June Dahl, PhD, a professor of pharmacology at the University of Wisconsin at Madison, and a founder of the American Alliance of Cancer Pain Initiatives.

Interview with Helen R.

Leleszi JP and JG Lewandowski. Pain management in end-of-life care. Journal of the American Osteopathic Association. 105(3): S6–S11.

De Pinto M et al. Pain management. Anesthesiology Clinics of North America. 24: 19–37.

Owens MR et al. A longitudinal study of pain in hospice and pre-hospice patients. American Journal of Hospice and Palliative Care.

Hospice Foundation of America. Common myths about pain. http://www.hospicefoundation.org/endOfLifeInfo/myths_pain.asp

M.D. Anderson Cancer Center. Acupuncture and massage services. http://www.mdanderson.org/departments/wellness/dIndex.cfm?pn=56AEE1F1-60D7-42E6-9E7D04AA35976F7D

American Cancer Society. What is hospice care? http://www.cancer.org/docroot/ETO/content/ETO_2_5X_What_Is_Hospice_Care.asp?sitearea=ETO

Baylor University Medical Care Proceedings. Depression, anxiety, and delirium in the terminally ill patient. 2001. http://www.pubmedcentral.nih.gov/articlerender.fcgi?artid=1291326

National Coalition for Cancer Survivorship. Pain at the end of life. http://www.canceradvocacy.org/resources/essential/pain/end.aspx

American Cancer Society. Pain control: a guide for people with cancer and their families. http://www.cancer.org/docroot/MIT/content/MIT_7_2x_Pain_Control_A_Guide_for_People_with_Cancer_and_Their_Families.asp

The 2nd Joint Clinical Conference and Exposition on Hospice and Palliative Care, Orlando, Florida. Conference report: innovations in hospice and palliative care. http://www.medscape.com/viewarticle/408607_7

Miller KE, et al. Antidepressant medication use in palliative care. American Journal of Hospice and Palliative Medicine. 23(2).

National Cancer Institute, National Institutes of Health. Anxiety Disorder (PDQ) Health Professional Version. http://www.cancer.gov/cancertopics/pdq/supportivecare/anxiety/HealthProfessional/page2

American Pain Society. Definitions related to the use of opioids for the treatment of pain. 2001. http://www.ampainsoc.org/advocacy/opioids2.htm.

Brender E., et al. Palliative Sedation. JAMA;294(14):1850.

WHO's Pain Ladder. World Health Organization. http://www.who.int/cancer/palliative/painladder/en/.

Critical Thinking

1. Discuss the benefits of hospice to both patient and caregiver.
2. Discuss the moral issues that may arise in the process of pain management at end of life.

Internet References

American Academy of Pain Management
http://www.painmed.org/
Hospice Association of America
http://www.nahc.org/haa/

Article   Prepared by: Elaina Osterbur, *Saint Louis University*

Rehabilitation Counselor Ethical Considerations for End-of-Life Care

Jan C. Case, Terry L. Blackwell, and Matthew E. Sprong

Learning Outcomes

After reading this article, you will be able to:

- Define end of life.
- Identify the rehabilitation standards and guidelines that address end-of-life care.

Among the changes in the 2010 revised *Code of Professional Ethics for Rehabilitation Counselors* (Commission on Rehabilitation Certification [CRCC], 2010) are standards and guidelines addressing end-of-life care for clients who are terminally ill. The CRCC standards provide guidance in three key areas: (1) counselor competency for working with end-of-life clients (A.9.a); (2) counselor scope of practice regarding end-of-life clients (A.9.b); and (3) counselor choices pertaining to confidentiality in cases where terminally ill clients are considering hastening their own deaths (A.9.c, A.l.a, A.2.a, A.4.a., B.l.b., B.l.c., B.l.d., B.2.a., I.l.b). With these new guidelines, rehabilitation counselors must now anticipate and consider potential dilemmas that may arise when applying CRCC (2010) Standard A.9 in conjunction with other ethical standards and seek resources to resolve such dilemmas. This article seeks to (1) explore some considerations and implications that Standard A.9 may present for the rehabilitation counseling practitioner, (2) to familiarize rehabilitation counselors with other portions of the Code that will assist their ethical implementation of A.9, and (3) to provide initial best practice considerations.

End-of-Life Issues

Consider the following case scenario:

You prepared yourself for the inevitable phone call from a client, but it still jolted you when it did finally come:

"I knew it was really only a matter of time, and now my doctors think it's probably going to be only a few months until I pass on. I have enjoyed my job so much, and the last few months they have even let me do most of my work out of my parents' home. But now I feel like I am becoming a drag on everyone, and maybe it's time I just gave up trying. My options are limited. Maybe it's time I did something to move my death along. Have you had any experience with this type of thing? I need your advice. I have always admired your wisdom, so I wanted to get together with you about this."

The term "end of life" is understood to mean the developmental period in a person's life when approaching death colors the content of many of their decisions and actions (Papalia & Martorell, 2014). This period of time may differ widely from person to person, and could consist of days, weeks, or months. A person who enjoys good health will be unable to live forever, and by their 70s or 80s, end of life becomes a part of almost everyone's thought process. People in good health often complete living wills or personal care directives, and for those with severe medical issues or with a terminal diagnosis, being able to assure themselves that existential, spiritual, familial, and emotional aspects of their care are also going to be addressed are often cited among the most important concerns of patients (Greisinger, Lorimor, Aday, Winn, & Baile, 1997). Those whose health is less steady or who have progressive disabilities and received terminal diagnoses are even more apt to be preoccupied with end-of-life concerns (Smart, 2012). End of life is not limited to the medical aspect of death; it may include areas such as financial and legacy decisions, creating memorials, attaining a comfortable spiritual acquiescence, and saying goodbye to family and friends. End-of-life concerns impact each theater of a person's life including work roles, educational roles, family roles, and community roles.

Not everyone who is seen by a rehabilitation counselor will need nor seek counseling at end of life. Many may find their needs met by pastoral, rabbinical, or monastic counseling; others will confide in, and receive guidance from, their health-care professionals, including physicians, nurses, or hospice staff. People with disabilities however, especially those with severe disabilities, may also benefit from specialized expertise from a rehabilitation and/or mental health counselor who has knowledge and skills to serve people who are approaching death. Wadsworth, Harley, Smith, and Kampfe (2008) asserted that rehabilitation counselors may be the initial point of contact for employees from diverse cultural backgrounds or employees with a disability who face barriers to accessing hospice and other end-of-life resources. Additionally, clients who have difficulty with end-of-life issues may experience changes in productivity and interpersonal conflicts with coworker and supervisor relationships. In addition, rehabilitation counselors may find themselves involved with end-of-life issues through participation in case management, ethics, research, and administrative committees in which decisions regarding end-of-life practices can occur.

Rehabilitation Counseling Scope of Practice

The Scope of Practice for Rehabilitation Counseling identifies assumptions, underlying values, and specific rehabilitation counseling modalities that are extremely pertinent to clients in end-of-life times. As the Scope of Practice states: "Rehabilitation counseling is a systematic process which assists persons with physical, mental, developmental, cognitive, and emotional disabilities to achieve their personal, career, and independent living goals in the most integrated setting possible through the application of the counseling process" (CRCC, 2010, p. 1). This same systematic process of service can bring important services to the person who is facing end-of-life decisions. Furthermore, the Scope of Practice reminds counselors that their underlying values as rehabilitation practitioners include:

> Facilitation of independence, integration, and inclusion; the belief in the dignity and worth of all persons; commitment to equal justice; and emphasis on the holistic nature of human function; recognition of the importance of focusing on the assets of a person; and commitment to models of service delivery that emphasize integrated, comprehensive services. (p. 1)

These underlying values are also pertinent to the content and the delivery of services to persons in end-of-life times. Finally, the Scope of Practice reiterates the differentiation between a professional scope of rehabilitation counseling practice and an individual scope of practice. While these may overlap, an individual's scope of practice is more specialized and is based on one's own knowledge of the abilities and skills that have been gained through a program of education and professional experience. This insight underscores the importance of continuing education, and suggests that many fellow rehabilitation practitioners may have developed specific expertise in working with clients regarding end-of-life issues. These rehabilitation practitioners have abilities and skills that can assist other rehabilitation practitioners in the effective delivery of their own respective services to clients who face end-of-life transitions and decisions.

Standard A.9

Although there are a variety of informative articles published on specific counseling techniques and considerations in working with end-of-life clients (e.g., Werth & Crow, 2009), much of the literature concerning end-of-life counseling, although valuable and perceptive, does not specifically address the unique roles of rehabilitation counselors and the unique challenges rehabilitation counselors face in formulating and implementing best practice. The challenges in dealing with end-of-life issues are varied and can be quite complex. This fact is made all the more evident in the enumeration of a specific standard in the *Code of Professional Ethics for Rehabilitation Counselors* (CRCC, 2010) that calls attention to this precise issue.

Section A.9: Quality of Care

> Counselors take measures that enable clients to: 1) obtain high quality end-of-life care for their physical, emotional, social, and spiritual needs; 2) exercise the highest degree of self-determination possible; 3) be given every opportunity possible to engage in informed decision-making regarding their end-of-life care; and, 4) receive complete and adequate assessment regarding their ability to make competent rational decisions on their own behalf from mental health professionals who are experienced in end-of-life care practice. (CRCC A.9.a)

The "Quality of Care" standard of the *Code* (A.9.a.1) is poignant and impactful, because while traditionally the goal of rehabilitation counseling has been the optimization and promotion of the lives of those served, Standard A.9.a.2 extends to those wishing to enhance the experience of death. This standard spells out briefly what quality care for an end-of-life client would look like. First, it states that such care addresses physical and emotional health as well as social and spiritual needs. Addressing a client's biological, psychosocial, and spiritual needs is a tall order of business for a single counselor and suggests a team approach (Kaut, 2006; Smart, 2012). This team might include health care and mental health professionals, family, friends, or other support system members, and spiritual advisors. The rehabilitation counselor being guided by the *Code* might do well to take a case-management approach and become the one pulling together all the various components of the client's needs. For example, Olkin (1999) suggested that persons who are older and have disabilities "may have less education, more unemployment, lower income, higher levels of poverty, . . . , increased need for support from family or service agencies, higher medical costs, and more costs associated with assistive devices and modifying the environment to increase accessibility" (p. 154). Moreover, Olkin stated that a decrease in functioning may occur sooner for persons with disabilities and result in being more susceptible to injury, and a quicker onset of fatigue, while cognitive abilities will also begin to diminish (Smart, 2012). For example, the ability to process and retrieve information decreases, working memory deteriorates in speed and function, and speech is slowed and disorganized due to a decline in word retrieval.

Next, standard A.9.a.3 states that clients should be helped to "exercise the highest level of self-determination possible". Self-determination is not easily defined either across cultures or within a single culture; every individual effectively has a sense of what self-determination means to him or her. For persons whose major identification is with the European American dominant culture, self-determination is usually equated with a high level of individual autonomy (Werth & Crow, 2009). Examined across cultures, Standard A.9.a.3. brings up several possible ethical dilemmas which will be discussed later in this paper, but it appears the main thrust of this standard is to attempt to insure that a client will not be influenced in life-and-death decisions by ill-considered or intrusive expressions of values on the part of caregivers or family members (Botsford & King, 2005; Longmore, 2005; Werth, 2005). This is a particularly cogent issue in caring for clients with cognitive disability who might often be easily swayed by the values of those around them (Botsford & King, 2005). Rehabilitation counselors need to be mindful of this and must be careful not to impose their values on the client. However, the ability to recognize that true autonomy or self-determination probably does not exist is beneficial as often times people who need to make these end-of-life decisions probably consult others (e.g., family members, friends) to seek guidance on their values and feelings.

When speaking of self-determination, the *Code* seems to be addressing such things as potential abuse of physicians' or others' authority in influencing persons with disabilities toward a value judgment that life with a severe disability is not worth living (Wachsler, 2007). For example, as discussed by Wachsler, "physicians often urge family members to sign Do Not Resuscitate orders (DNRs) when a child is born with a disability or a parent becomes disabled" (p. 9). Additionally, since self-determination for persons with disabilities cannot be taken for granted but must necessarily be advocated by rehabilitation counselors, facilitating decision making in the end-of-life stage for persons with disabilities is also important. This issue also touches on counselor competency because, while it might be possible to ensure self-determination for clients who clearly can make decisions for themselves, it is not easy to do so at those times when the self-determination of an individual may be challenged by other individuals, as well-intentioned as those individuals may be. Given the complexities of beliefs, traditions and customs associated with death and dying, rehabilitation counselors must be willing to align themselves with other professionals or seek additional educational resources or professional supervision in an effort to function more competently as an advocate for dying clients (Blevins & Papadatou, 2005). In CRCC 2010 Ethical Standard A.9.a.2. deciding what is meant by "self-determination" and what it might look like in different social and cultural contexts is difficult because not every culture believes that the individual is the last resort in decision-making or that the individual's needs and desires should always trump those of family or society. For example, the Chinese culture believes that a dying person should not be given an exact prognosis because it may add additional stress (National Hospice and Palliative Care Organization, 2009). Muller (1992) reported the case of a dominant-culture White American physician who, in the interest of autonomy, seriously harmed the emotional well-being of a terminal patient's family by insisting against their wishes by having a discussion related to having a DNR order. Similarly, the Navajo culture believes that speaking of a person's death is bad luck and doing so will result in a self-fulfilling prophecy (Daitz, 2011).

Third, informed decision making, always a part of ethical counseling, is especially important with end-of-life clients whose decisions often leave no chance for reconsideration. Each person's decision-making is influenced by several issues, such as the presence of physical pain, coexisting psychological conditions, cognitive abilities, fear of loss and abandonment, values, and perceived quality of life. (American Psychological Association [APA], 2001). In addition, a client's capacity to make decisions may vacillate over time as a function of medical treatments or emotional distress that may impair cognitive abilities (Wadsworth et al., 2008). Informed decision making on the part of the client requires that rehabilitation practitioners attend to essential components such as knowledge, competence, and voluntariness on the part of the client (Blackwell & Patterson, 2003). Furthermore, empowering a client for such decision making necessitates the need for the client to consider utilizing a variety of resources in reaching informed decisions, and that these resources include those from both "outside" of the client (e.g., legal counsel, medical counsel, psychological counsel, family counsel, spiritual counsel) and those from "inside" the client (e.g., the client's own preferred method of making decisions, the perceived adequacy of such processes in helping to reach decisions in end-of-life matters).

Ensuring a truly informed decision process for a client exposed to moral values and information sources from widely varying points of view among family, friends, cultural leaders, and health care professionals, can be a difficult task for a rehabilitation counselor. At end of life, family members can become affected by grief to the extent that they may no longer be able to offer cogent advice, and it is the counselor's job to aid those so affected as well as the client; this is all a part of creating a climate in which the client can engage in true informed decision making. Here, as in the entire process, the rehabilitation counselor must carefully refrain from allowing the information presented to be affected by her or his own values and attitudes about death and the meaning of life. End of life informed decision-making is vastly more complex than, for example, a clinical intake for vocational rehabilitation. Throughout history, much of human culture—literature, art, music, philosophy, and theology—has been concerned with the meaning of life and of death. The end-of-life counselor can use a vast array of information sources culturally and personally appropriate to the client with a disability to help access information for the client's personal decision process.

Finally, assessment for competency is a thorny tangle of competing medical, legal, and ethical areas. Traditionally, any individual who has considered ending their life has been viewed as incompetent (Olkin, 1999). Additionally, an array of services are in place to prevent suicide of persons without disabilities, but when a person with a disability requests assistance to commit suicide, services are available to assist in this request (Smart, 2009; as cited in Smart, 2014). However, people with disabilities still encounter health care and other professionals who may assume that any person with a visible disability is, in fact, "incompetent." Within the medical model of disability, the disability itself is often regarded as "pathological." Under this model of disability, even a person with a mild cognitive impairment would be viewed as being unable to handle discussions of "serious" matters such as death (Smart, 2012). Much harm has occurred due to supposedly "experienced" mental health professionals hiding deaths from people with intellectual disability because the thought that extreme disorientation caused by a parent or family member "going on a long trip" is somehow less harmful than an open discussion of death (Botsford & King, 2005). Clearly this is a case where the professional's inability to come to terms with their values and existential dilemmas, yet in many such cases the assessment of client competence by such professionals would pass muster by the *Code* because the professional is considered "experienced in end-of-life care practice." Whether they are aware of it or not, even experienced professionals may allow the assessment process to be swayed by their own ethicospiritual values. Although

Standard A.9.a. implies that clients have a right to be assessed by "mental health professionals who are experienced in end-of-life care practice", experience per se might not be enough to ensure high-quality care, self-determination, or informed decision-making. The standard states that it is the duty of the rehabilitation counselor to seek out and offer access to such professionals, but we take the position that this is not enough, that it is also the rehabilitation counselor's duty to advocate for the client's competency whenever possible and to attempt to create a well-balanced "climate of information" around a client who, because he or she is close to death, must take on the task of making decisions relating to their own end of life.

Rehabilitation Counselor Competence, Choice, and Referral

Rehabilitation counselors may choose to work or not work with terminally ill clients who wish to explore their end-of-life options. Rehabilitation counselors provide appropriate referral information if they are not competent to address such concerns. (CRCC [2010] Code of Ethics A.9.b)

Vital to providing adequate and appropriate services to clients who are terminally ill, rehabilitation counselors must self-assess their desire and ability to provide counseling services. This choice however, is indicated in conjunction with guidelines regarding competency and referral. Basic competency about death and dying should be a primary consideration for rehabilitation counselors choosing to provide services (Allen & Jaet, 1982; Allen & Miller, 1988; Hunt & Rosenthal, 2006). Standard A.9.b deals with scope-of-practice for rehabilitation counselors and alludes to the idea of physician assisted suicide or hastening death. This standard may assist a rehabilitation counselor who feels inexperienced or has moral compunctions about working with clients who are making end-of-life decisions the option of choosing " . . . to work or not work with terminally ill clients who wish to explore their end-of-life options" (p. 6). This sentence gives rehabilitation counselors considerable freedom to opt out if their own value system cannot support a client choosing to end life. When a rehabilitation counselor feels unable to work effectively with such a client, it is stated: " . . . counselors provide appropriate referral information if they are not competent to address such concerns" (p. 6). Appropriate referral is a part of ethical practice in any area which a rehabilitation counselor feels is outside her or his scope of experience and practice. Yet, as many have noted (e.g., Cates, Gunderson, & Keim, 2012; Werth, Hastings, & Riding-Malon, 2010), referral, although the ethically correct thing to do, is not always possible in the modern world of managed care, especially in rural areas with few counseling resources, or for purposes of assuring continuity of care. Even though rehabilitation counselors are trained to regularly conduct self-assessment to determine if their values are being imposed on the clients they serve, death is one in which even competent counseling professionals may allow their strongly held spiritual, philosophical, or religious values to interfere with a self-judgment of lack of end-of-life competence. Referral thus becomes problematic for two reasons: (1) because the automatic response of a rehabilitation counselor who fears to tread in the end-of-life arena; and (2) because a rehabilitation counselor may feel altogether too much confidence and competence in this area due to preconceived moral values.

Confidentiality

> Rehabilitation counselors who provide services to terminally ill individuals who are considering hastening their own deaths have the option of breaking or not breaking confidentiality on this matter, depending on applicable laws and the specific circumstances of the situation and after seeking consultation or supervision from appropriate professional and legal parties. (CRCC [2010])

Standard A.9.c. takes up confidentiality in relation to end-of-life options. Here an attempt is made to chart a neutral course between conflicting state laws, values, and other ethical codes, but the standard is asserting that a client who considers hastening their own death does not necessarily constitute "serious and foreseeable harm" and therefore is not subject to mandatory reporting (Kocet, 2006). Because Standard A.9.c gives the rehabilitation counselor the option of keeping or breaking confidentiality, in effect the decision rests with the rehabilitation counselor who will have to apply his or her own ethical decision making process here which would include legal and professional consultation. This section of the *Code* may not appear to offer much guidance to a rehabilitation counselor faced with an ethical dilemma about a terminal client contemplating suicide, but it does at least state that the rehabilitation counselor has a choice; the end result is to encourage and validate further investigation of the client's unique circumstances.

Rehabilitation counselors examining and applying the end-of-life care standards will recognize the ongoing significance of *principle* ethics (autonomy, beneficence, nonmaleficence, justice, fidelity, veracity), and may struggle making decisions when conflict arises between these fundamental ethical principles. In addition, rehabilitation counselors will recognize the ongoing significance of *virtue* ethics (e.g., recognizing one's own values, recognizing one's own emotions, considering one's own culture, weighing the client's familial and community context), and may struggle in their application of these fundamentals as they serve in end-of-life situations. Dilemmas involving client autonomy, welfare, personal values, and professional

competency in the area of death and dying are conceivable. Given the recent emergence of these new standards, it is likely many rehabilitation counselors have not been formally educated about death and dying or sound ethical end-of-life decision making (Wadsworth et al., 2008). Similarly, professional public and private rehabilitation services entities may have not yet adopted and accommodated for the standards to provide additional ethical guidance for counselors who encounter clients with disability seeking end-of-life counsel. Furthermore, as literature specific to rehabilitation counseling and ethical and effective end-of-life issues is seriously lacking (Zanskas & Coduti, 2006), it becomes even more imperative that the profession examine the applications and implications of section A.9.

The standards relating to end-of-life are a big step in the direction of ethical clarity. However, there are several places where problems could result if not approached with sensitivity, creativity, objectivity, and an awareness of possible discrimination against persons with disabilities. Rehabilitation counselors who have chosen to work with clients who are terminally ill need to be knowledgeable of the legal guidelines surrounding patients' rights to die within their state as well as the policies of employing organizations and agencies. Similarly, rehabilitation counselors choosing to work with terminally ill clients should accommodate for such guidelines within an informed consent addressing the end-of-life services provided and subsequent exceptions or stipulations.

End of Life and Client's Choice: Practice Implications for Rehabilitation Counselors

As previously discussed, the end-of-life care standards underscore the freedom of rehabilitation counselors to work or not work with clients who face end-of-life issues, particularly if the client chooses to explore their end-of-life options. At the same time, these standards reiterate the important role that the respective values of both clients and rehabilitation counselors play in making such decisions, and urge that such choices be made with knowledge, competence (capacity), and voluntariness—on the part of both the client and rehabilitation counselor.

The need for both client and rehabilitation counselor to possess adequate *knowledge* in making this choice raises such questions as: Do the client and rehabilitation counselor possess adequate knowledge regarding the specific illness (or illnesses), the course of the illness, possible treatments for the illness? Do the client and the rehabilitation counselor possess adequate self-knowledge (e.g., awareness of one's values, one's mental health)? Do the client and the rehabilitation counselor possess adequate knowledge regarding other resources that could be utilized to help make such decisions (e.g., community agencies, health-care providers, spiritual consultants)? Do the client and the rehabilitation counselor possess adequate knowledge of pertinent laws? Does the rehabilitation counselor possess adequate knowledge of the Code of Ethics and opinions from their professional organization regarding these matters? Does the rehabilitation counselor possess a best practice framework to utilize in these matters, including adequate decision making models?

The need for both client and rehabilitation counselor to possess *competence (capacity)* in making this choice raises such questions as: Is the client or the rehabilitation counselor incapacitated by previous life experiences (e.g., personal and familial experiences with this issue, unresolved struggles with their grief) that may prevent them from making good decisions? An assessment of such factors as the robustness of family, community, and professional support networks is an essential component in the assessment process (Robinson, Phipps, Purtilo, Tsoumas, & Hamel-Nardozzi, 2006). Are rehabilitation counselors aware of their own values, but at the same time able to prevent their values from diminishing their competency to serve clients facing end-of-life decisions? Do rehabilitation counselors possess adequate time and flexibility in their schedules that may be required to competently serve? Have rehabilitation counselors adequately developed self-care networks, an awareness of the medical and cultural meanings of death, the ability to communicate about death, and appropriate outcome expectations (Wadsworth et al., 2008)?

The need for both client and rehabilitation counselor to possess *voluntariness* in making this choice raises such questions as: Are the client and the rehabilitation counselor "free" to make such a decision, or are they burdened with a sense of guilt in making such a decision? Are they pressured in any way to make expedient decisions rather than good decisions? Are they overly concerned about what others may think of their decision, and, therefore, feel a need to compromise their choice in this matter? "Choice" necessitates that *both* the client and rehabilitation counselor fully examine these issues for themselves, and come to decisions that are, indeed, informed, made with adequate competence, and voluntary.

Competency

Because of the somewhat general nature of the *Code* and the large grey areas that remain even after the promulgation of the end-of-life standards, we believe it is imperative to outline some of the key rehabilitation counselor competencies in end-of-life work. A list of competencies might include: Experience in end-of-life care and/or personal experience of death and loss. The emotions and stages of grief resulting from a sudden loss or death can be set down, analyzed, and discussed, but there is no substitute for a rehabilitation counselor's having personally

experienced death. In order for the counselor to avoid imposing his or her values on a client, the practitioner must assess how these values are related to end-of-life decision making. Without personal experience of loss, a rehabilitation counselor may hold "book values" that he or she thinks would apply in an end-of-life situation (Wadsworth et al., 2008). Dying will cause grieving, both in the client and family. Family members distracted by grief can make the end-of-life stage more difficult for clients (Werth & Crow, 2009).

A major rehabilitation counseling responsibility is to work for beneficence of the client by maximizing the adjustment of the surrounding family members (Millington & Marini, 2015). This should encompass competence in working with families as noted above, but also demands a thoroughgoing knowledge of the grieving process and appropriate interventions when grieving becomes dysfunctional. Olkin (1999) stated there are certain questions that arise for rehabilitation counselors related to physician-assisted suicide (P-AS), including "What are the counselor's beliefs regarding this issue? Can the rehabilitation counselor opt out of participation if she or he works in a setting in which P-AS becomes available? If the counselor opts out, can the counselor still take referrals of elderly or seriously ill clients who may choose P-AS? What are the appropriate interventions with families facing loss of a member through P-AS? How should the issue of remaining minor children be handled? How are "voluntariness" and "capacity" best assessed, and by whom? How does the rehabilitation counselor assess for underlying treatable depression when many symptoms of serious or terminal illness overlap with those of depression?" (p. 267).

Knowledge of Family Systems Theory

Families must be taken into account in end-of-life situations (Lang & Quill, 2004). The client might not be in a conscious state, and to ignore the interplay of family systems and family decision making processes surrounding the client would amount to professional incompetence. No particular theoretical stance is being suggested here, merely that the rehabilitation counselor should acknowledge in his or her approach to counseling that family and support group cannot be ignored when considering a therapy approach or counseling interventions (Millington & Marini, 2014).

Familiarity with Medical Issues

A rehabilitation counselor is required to be familiar with the medical side of disability, but end-of-life medical situations can be even more complex, often involving pain management and use of drugs that in other situations would be lethally addictive. Pharmaceutical knowledge, a good comprehension of the course of treatment for terminal diseases, and an ability to understand the physician's medical and ethical decision making process are all required. Additionally, a competent counselor must often become an advocate for her or his client with the client's health care providers (Smart, 2012). By being seen by the medical providers as competent to discuss the medical situation of a client, the rehabilitation counselor will increase his or her effectiveness in advocating for the client's right to self-determination and informed decision-making.

Client-centered Skills

In keeping with the ethic of maximizing self-determination, it is especially necessary for the counselor to demonstrate objectivity. An essential component of helping clients is to create a non-judgmental and safe environment for the client to interact and speak freely (Ivey, Ivey, & Zalaquett, 2013). This is essential when the client's medical condition may preclude an easy expression of wishes and needs. The emotional turmoil that usually accompanies proximity of death will often make an easy expression of feelings, needs, and thoughts difficult for a client. The ability to always be listening, always be trying to understand the client's experience, is a valuable strength in an end-of-life rehabilitation counselor.

Knowledge of Applicable Laws

This is a highly desirable competency to help a rehabilitation counselor navigate the legal and moral morass of P-AS and mandatory disclosure laws. Every state has enacted their own laws governing disclosure of self-harm and several states have now legalized P-AS. Yet, as most physicians will acknowledge, de facto P-AS occurs everywhere (Barroso, 2012), has probably always occurred, whether it involves a patient demanding withdrawal of medical interventions or terminal sedation. Also, as Olkin (1999) has noted, there are complex laws governing end-of-life and DNR directives. For example, in 1997 there were two cases in which the U.S. Supreme Court rule that "P-AS is not a protected liberty interest under the constitution" . . . "A person is guilty of promoting a suicide attempt when he knowingly causes or aids another person to attempt suicide" (U.S. Legal, 2010, para. 2). These court rulings resulted in the "failure to affirm a right to assisted suicide" (Olkin, p. 267). However, specific states have passed legislation (i.e., Oregon [1997], Washington [2009], and Vermont [2013]), that allows P-AS (Barone, 2014). Furthermore, Barone (2014) stated that in 2009, the state of Montana passed legislation establishing that doctors are protected if they prescribe lethal-medication at the request of a patient who is terminally ill, and the State of New Mexico passed legislation in 2014 that allowed people who are terminally ill to obtain aid in dying. California became the 5th state to pass legislation (October 5, 2015) that legalized P-AS (Pedroncelli, 2015).

Comfort with Spiritual Topics

Spiritual topics are an essential component of end-of-life care; discussion of death and existential concerns for most people cannot occur without reference to spiritual matters at some level (Manis & Bodenhom, 2006). A rehabilitation counselor need not share a client's spiritual or religious values, but a competent rehabilitation counselor must remain respectful of the client's beliefs (CRCC, Standard(s) A.2.a, A.3.c, D.2.a, D.2.b; ACA [2014], Standard A.4.b.). This should include at least a passing acquaintance with many different spiritual belief systems, but more important is the ability to listen respectfully and support the client's application of his or her own beliefs to the process of dying. Naturally, if the client is actively seeking such a contact, a referral to a spiritual adviser might be appropriate and a competent rehabilitation counselor will be open to this kind of action despite his or her personal belief system.

Referral Contacts for Assessment of Client Decision-making Competency

Mental health professionals who are experienced, sensitive, caring, and competent to assess persons with disabilities are not easily found (Caldwell & Freeman, 2009). For example, Caldwell and Freeman pointedly note: Before educating others, rehabilitation counselors must first become more interdisciplinary and collaborative. A rehabilitation counselor should strive to develop such referral sources. Because, as noted above, the assessment process can be subject to imposition of values even by the most well-meaning professionals, the competent counselor must continually be assessing the assessors; matching the assessment professional to the particulars of the client's biopsychosocial situation may be necessary (Anastasi, 1982).

Well-developed and Sensitive Counseling Skills with People of Diverse Backgrounds

End of life is an area where it is especially easy to encounter client-counselor spiritual value clashes and these may often be related to culture because every culture has widely varying ways of dealing with death. Therefore, multicultural counseling skills are required in end-of-life settings (Braun, Pietsch, & Blanchette, 2000) as spirituality may differ from the rehabilitation counselor's own beliefs. However, even if culturally based spiritual differences do not necessarily exist, there are often differences at the sub-cultural or even family level about the appropriateness of speaking about death and dying, disclosing prognosis to the dying person, or even speaking of the dying person and a competent rehabilitation counselor must become sensitive and open to all of this information.

Exploration of a Rehabilitation Counselor's Own Values Relating to the Meaning of Death and Toward Purposeful Ending of One's Own Life

Without such self-reflection, a rehabilitation counselor is in danger of unknowingly imposing his or her own value system on a client and may not be able to recognize when values clash or when a referral might be the ethical thing to do. Many rehabilitation counselors have experience working with suicidal clients (Rogers, Gueulette, Abbey-Hines, Carney, & Werth, 2001). Rehabilitation counselors are trained to value life, to protect the clients against self-harm, and yet this experience may paradoxically prevent them from coming to an unbiased moral stance toward an end-of-life client contemplating hastening their own death. Only by exploring their own conception of death, when it should be avoided and when it should be welcomed, can a rehabilitation counselor maintain a balanced stance when a client needs support at end-of-life. Even apart from the hastening of death, a rehabilitation counselor with his or her own unresolved issues toward death may not be able to offer effective counseling to a person in the end-of-life stage.

A Comprehensive Grasp of the Code of Ethics

Although the implementation of Standard A.9 of the Code may pose many challenges to rehabilitation counselors, other sections of the Code provide important guidance to rehabilitation practitioners that enhance their understanding of Standard A.9 and its efficient implementation. The Preamble of the *Code* reiterates this essential point when it states, "Each Enforceable Standard is not meant to be interpreted in isolation. Instead, it is important for rehabilitation counselors to interpret standards in conjunction with other related standards in various sections of the Code" (p. 2). It is, therefore, incumbent upon rehabilitation counselors to possess a comprehensive understanding of the *Code*. In studying the requirements and the application of A.9 consider significant *Code* sections such as these:

CRCC Code of Professional Ethics for Rehabilitation

- A.4   Avoiding Harm and Avoiding Value Imposition
- E.2   Consultation
- A.8   Termination and Referral
- E.3.b.   Interdisciplinary Team work
- A.7   Group-work (screening, protecting clients)
- A.6   Multiple clients
- Section J   Technology and Distance Counseling
- A.5.d.   Nonprofessional Interactions or Relationships other than Sexual or Romantic Interactions or Relationships
- H.6.   Responsibilities of Rehabilitation Counselor Educators
- L.2.c.   Conflicts between Ethics and Laws
- L.2.d.   Knowledge of Related Code of Ethics
- L.2.f.   Organization Conflicts

Counselors

It is also essential that rehabilitation counselors attend to CRCC Standard L.2.a. (Decision-Making Models and Skills) as they practice A.9. The Preamble of the *Code* also notes the importance of developing decision-making models for the enhanced application of A.9 and all other standards of the *Code*: "While there is no specific ethical decision-making model that is most effective, rehabilitation counselors are expected to be familiar with and apply a credible model of decision-making that can bear public scrutiny."

Tarvydas's (1998) Integrative Model for ethical decision making provides a nice, systematic framework for addressing dilemmas a rehabilitation counselor may encounter when providing end-of-life care. Application of this model first requires the counselor attend to four themes. These themes consist of: (1) Maintaining an attitude of reflection, (2) Addressing the balance between issues and parties to the ethical dilemma, (3) Paying close attention to the context(s) of the situation, and (4) Utilizing a process of collaboration with all rightful parties to the situation. The next step in the Integration Model requires the counselor to systematically review the situation in four stages. The stages are outlined as follows:

Stage I. Interpreting the Situation through Awareness

a. Enhance sensitivity and awareness.
b. Reflect, to determine whether dilemma or issue is involved.
c. Determine the major stakeholders and their ethical claims in the situation.
d. Engage in the fact-finding process.

Stage II. Formulating an Ethical Decision

a. Review the problem or dilemma.
b. Determine what ethical codes, laws, ethical principles, and institutional policies and procedures exist that apply to the dilemma.
c. Generate possible and probable courses of action.

d. Consider potential positive and negative consequences of each course of action.

e. Select the best ethical course of action.

Stage III. Selecting an Action by Evaluating Competing, Nonmoral Values

a. Engage in reflective recognition and analysis of personal competing values.

b. Consider contextual influences on values selection at the collegial, team, institutional, and societal levels.

c. Select preferred course of action.

Stage IV. Planning and Executing the Selected Course of Action

a. Figure out a reasonable sequence of concrete actions to be taken.

b. Anticipate and work out personal and contextual barriers to effective execution of the plan of action, and effective countermeasures for them,

c. Carry out and evaluate the course of action as planned.

The utilization of this particular decision-making framework in the application of A.9 (perhaps in conjunction with other appropriate decision-making frameworks) could facilitate rehabilitation counselors in the identification of potential ethical dilemmas, the identification of pertinent resources in reaching ethical decisions, and the effective implementation of these decisions.

Other pertinent decision-making models are presented in the CRCC Desk Reference (2010). In addition to a comprehensive grasp of the *Code* and the implementation of effective ethical decision-making models, the aspiration to best practice (the best a counselor could be expected to do) in the implementation of A.9 suggests that the rehabilitation practitioner also consult with the CRCC and pertinent opinions that have been rendered by the CRCC with regard to A.9 or other pertinent Standards of the *Code*.

Best practice could also include a variety of continuing education endeavors regarding end-of-life issues, including volunteer experiences (perhaps with a hospital or a hospice program) in order to gain further awareness, knowledge, and skills regarding end-of life issues, resources, and practices. Continuing education experiences could also assist rehabilitation counselors become acquainted with other professionals and agencies in their communities who serve in end-of-life transitions. An enhanced knowledge of such individuals and agencies could also help rehabilitation counselors identify service opportunities for themselves through which they could enhance their knowledge and skills as they simultaneously contribute their own expertise as rehabilitation counselors.

End-of-Life Scenario

Consider the case scenario that was introduced at the beginning of this article. After reading the scenario, identify several pertinent issues that the scenario suggests. Formulate your preliminary responses to the scenario, and then consider the "Discussion Points" and "Sample of Related Standards" that are provided for your further consideration. What further "Discussion Points" would you raise? What other "Related Standards" of the *Code* come to mind?

Case Scenario

You prepared yourself for the inevitable phone call from a client, but it still jolted you when it did finally come: "I knew it was really only a matter of time, and now my doctors think it's probably going to be only a few months until I pass on. I have enjoyed my job so much, and the last few months they have even let me do most of my work out of my parents' home. But now I feel like I am becoming a drag on everyone, and maybe it's time I just gave up trying. My options are limited. Maybe it's time I did something to move my death along. Have you had any experience with this type of thing? I need your advice. I have always admired your wisdom, so I wanted to get together with you about this."

Discussion Points

- What do you think the client meant when saying, "something to move my death along"? How would you explore this further with the client?
- How would you begin to explore the legal options that are available to the client?
- What are cultural considerations need to be evaluated?
- How would you engage the client in such an exploration?
- Would you attempt to include the client's family in this matter? Why? Why not? If you did so, how would you proceed to do so?
- What role does the ethical principle of "beneficence" play in this scenario?
- What role does the ethical principle of "veracity" play in this scenario?
- To what extent would your values play a role in your consultation with this client?

Sample of Related Standards
CRCC
- Preamble
- A.6 Multiple Clients

- B.7 Consultation
- A.4 Avoiding Harm and Avoiding Value Imposition
- B.l.b. Respect for Privacy
- L.2.c. Conflicts between Ethics and Laws

Decision-making Thoughts

Although each theme and each stage of the Integrative Model of Decision Making will likely be important in processing this scenario, consider the significance of these considerations of the Model:

1. Pay close attention to the context(s) of the situation. For example, the client appears to have been aware of this situation for a period of time and has likely been working in collaboration with a variety of specialists. Available treatment options have likely been explored, and have not been effective.

2. Enhance sensitivity and awareness. For example, you are described as being "jolted" by this news? As you strive to remain aware of the client's emotional reactions to this news, it may be equally important for you to remain aware of your own emotional reactions at this time.

3. Determine what ethical codes, laws, ethical principles, and institutional policies and procedures exist that apply to the dilemma. For example, are you aware of those state laws that govern "hastening one's death"?

4. Generate possible and probable courses of action. For example, what options are available to you now and in the days ahead? With whom could you consult further in order to more effectively weigh the implications and consequences of each option?

5. Engage in reflective recognition and analysis of personal competing values. For example, is the "hastening of one's death" compatible with your values? If not, would referral of your client be more in keeping with beneficence? With fidelity?

6. Anticipate and work out personal and contextual barriers to effective execution of the plan of action, and effective countermeasures for them. For example, in implementing your decision what supportive resources would you gather for yourself? What supportive resources could benefit your client as their decision is implemented?

Future Research

Future research in the area of rehabilitation counselors assisting clients in end-of-life decision-making should focus on identifying if rehabilitation counselors are imposing their values in the decision-making process, whether counselor values are impacting how materials are presented to clients who are making end-of-life decisions, and how to increase competencies and comfortableness of rehabilitation counselors in assisting clients who have to make these decisions. Rehabilitation counselors may not feel comfortable assisting this population because they perceive themselves as not having the necessary knowledge needed to be an asset to the client.

Conclusion

Standard A.9 of the revised the *Code of Professional Ethics for Rehabilitation* Counselors (CRCC, 2010) provides an important framework for rehabilitation counselors working with clients who are terminally ill or their families. While the CRCC 2010) *Code* does not solve all of the problems inherent in such work, it provides some standardization of response and some much-needed clarification. Rehabilitation counselors involved in such work would do well to expand their competencies and gain experience with death and dying, grief and loss, and different spiritual value systems. It is also incumbent upon the counselor to develop a best practice framework in the application of Standard A.9. In aspiring to best practice the rehabilitation counselor will possess a comprehensive grasp of the entire *Code* and also be skilled in the application of pertinent ethical decision-making models. Finally, in the small number of potential cases where client wishes for P-AS are encountered, rehabilitation counselors should engage in exploration of their own values and then seek legal and ethical consultation before proceeding.

Two additional issues also help frame an initial appreciation for the complexities of end-of-life counseling. First, persons with disability have a right to live independently; they have as strong a right to die independently. Yet the health-care system with its "medical model" of disability can fail such people. For example, the "medical model" of disability emphasizes two dimensions, "normal" and pathological (Smart, 2012). Disability is generally viewed as being pathological, and people without disabilities are viewed as normal. The stigma attached to disability can result in the belief that there is "no point to live because I can never be normal." This may naturally lead to the presumption that P-AS is a better alternative than attempting to focus on strengths and abilities, and not what a person is "unable" to do when someone acquires a disability.

Second, a wide-ranging philosophical and moral debate continues on the topic of P-AS. Doctors are divided between those who see it as their duty to preserve life at all costs and those who see a doctor's primary function as working for the beneficence of the patient where beneficence includes happiness even over life (Smart, 2012). Furthermore, the public is divided on the issue as well, often forming lines highly correlated with religious preference or moral stance. The present article is not primarily concerned with this subject; to the extent that it is taken up, it is treated as simply another facet of the end-of-life decision-making process.

Finally, rehabilitation counselors must continuously self-assess themselves to determine what their values are related to end-of-life decisions, and P-AS and disability. As working with in any context related to rehabilitation counseling, the values of the rehabilitation counselor may not be consistent with the values of the client. The rehabilitation counselor should note that they are not making the decision that the client should end their life but rather guiding him or her throughout the decision-making process.

References

Allen, H. A. & Miller, D. M. (1988). Client death: A national survey of the experiences of certified rehabilitation counselors. *Rehabilitation Counseling Bulletin, 32,* 58-64.

Allen, H. A. & Jaet, D. N. (1982). The rehabilitation counselor's experience of client death. *Journal of Applied Rehabilitation Counseling 13(2),* 17-21.

Anastasi, A. (1982). Psychological testing (5th ed.). New York, NY: Macmillan.

Barone, E. (2014, November 3). See which states allow assisted suicide. *Time Magazine.* Retrieved from http://time.com/3551560/brittany-maynard-right-to-dielaws/

Blevins, D. & Papadatou, D. (2005). Effects of culture on end-of-life situations. In Werth, J. L. & Blevins, D. (APA), *Psychosocial issues near the end of life: A resource for professional care providers* (1st ed., pp. 27-55). Washington DC: American Psychological Association.

Blackwell, T. L., & Patterson, J. B. (2003). Ethical and legal implications of informed consent in rehabilitation counseling. *Journal of Applied Rehabilitation Counseling, 34(1),* 3-9.

Barroso, L. R. (2012). Here, there, and everywhere: Human dignity in contemporary law and in the translational discourse. *Boston College International and Comparative Law Review, 35(2),* 331-393.

Botsford, A. L. & King, A. (2005). End-of-life care policies for people with an intellectual disability. *Journal of Disability Policy Studies, 16(1),* 22-30.

Braun, K. L., Pietsch, J. H., & Blanchette, P. L. (2000). An introduction to cuture and its influence on end-of-life decision making. In K. L. Braun, J. H. Pietsch, & P. L. Blanchette (Eds.). *Cultural issues in end of life decision making* (pp. 1-11). Thousand Oaks, California: Sage.

Caldwell, C. D. & Freeman, S. J. (2009). End-of-life decision making: A slippery slope. *Journal of Professional Counseling Practice, Theory, and Research, 37,* 21-33.

Cates, K. A., Gunderson, C., & Keim, M. A. (2012). The ethical frontier: Ethical considerations for frontier counselors. *The Professional Counselor, 2(1),* 22-32.

Commission on Rehabilitation Counselor Certification. (2010). *Code of professional ethics for rehabilitation counselors.* Schaumburg, IL: Author.

CRCC Desk Reference. (2010). The CRCC desk reference on professional ethics: A guide of rehabilitation counselors. Athens, GA: Elliot & Fitzpatrick.

Daitz, B. (2011, January 24). With poem, broaching the topic of death. *The New York Times.* Retrieved from http://www.nytimes.com/2011/01/25/health/25navajo.html?pagewanted=all&_r=0

Greisinger, A. J., Lorimor, R. J., Aday, L. A., Winn, R. J., & Baile, W. F. (1997). Terminally ill cancer patients. Their most important concerns. *Cancer Practice, 5(3),* 147-154.

Hunt, B. & Rosenthal, D. A. (2000). Rehabilitation counselors' experience with client death and death anxiety. *Journal of Rehabilitation, 66(4),* 44-50.

Kaut, K. P. (2006). End-of-Life assessment within a holistic bio-psycho-social-spiritual framework. In Werth, J. L. & Blevins, D. (APA), *Psychosocial issues near the end of life: A resource for professional care providers* (1st ed., pp. 111-132). Washington DC: American Psychological Association.

Kocet, M. M. (2006). Ethical Challenges in a Complex World: Highlights of the 2005 ACA Code of Ethics. *Journal of Counseling & Development, 84(2),* 228-234.

Lang, F. & Quill, T. (2004). Making decisions with families at the end of life. *American Family Physician, 70(4),* 719-723.

Longmore, P. K. (2005). Policy, prejudice, and reality: Two case studies of physician assisted suicide. *Journal of Disability Policy Study, 16(1),* 3 8-45.

Manis, A. A., & Bodenhorn, N. (2006). Preparation for counseling adults with terminal illness: Personal and professional parallels. *Counseling and Values, 60,* 197-207.

Millington, M. J., & Marini, I. (2014). *Families in rehabilitation counseling: A community-based rehabilitation approach.* New York, NY: Springer Publishing Company.

Muller, J. H., & Desmond, B. (1992). Ethical dilemmas in a cross-cultural context. A Chinese example. *Western Journal of Medicine, 157(3),* 323-327.

National Hospice and Palliative Care Organization. (2009). Chinese-American outreach guide. Retrieved from http://www.nhpco.org/sites/default/files/public/Access/Chinese_American_Outreach_Guide.pdf

Olkin, R. (1999). What psychotherapists should know about disability? New York, NY: The Guilford Press.

Papalia, D. E., & Martorell, G. (2014). Experience human development. Columbus, OH: McGraw-Hill.

Robinson, E. M., Phipps, M., Purtilo, R. B., Tsoumas, A., & Hamel-Nardozzi, M. (2006). Complexities in decision making for persons with disabilities nearing end of life. *Topics in Stroke Rehabilitation, 13,* 54-67.

Rogers, J. R., Gueulette, C. M., Abbey-Hines, J., Carney, J. V., & Werth, J. L., Jr. (2011). Rational suicide: An empirical investigation of counselor attitudes. *Journal of Counseling & Development, 79(3),* 365-372. doi: 10.1002/j.1556-6676.2001.tb01982.x

Smart, J. F. (2009). The power of models of disability. *Journal of Rehabilitation, 75,* 3-11.

Smart, J. (2012). Disability across the developmental life span: For the rehabilitation counselor. New York, NY: Spring Publishing Company.

Tarvydas, V. M. (1998). Ethical decision making processes. In R. R. Cottone & V. M. Tarvydas (Eds.), Ethical and professional issues in counseling (pp. 144-158). Upper Saddle River, NJ: Prentice-Hall.

Wadsworth, J., Harley, D., Smith, S. M., & Kampfe, C. (2008). Infusing end-of-life issues into the rehabilitation counselor education curriculum. *Rehabilitation Education, 22,* 113-124.

Werth, J. L., Jr., Hastings, S. L., & Riding-Malon, R. (2010). Ethical challenges of practicing in rural areas. Journal of Clinical Psychology, *66,* 537-548.

Werth, J. L., Jr., & Rogers, J. R. (2005). Assessing for impaired judgment as a means of meeting the "duty to protect" when a client is a potential harm-to-self: Implications for clients making end-of-life decisions. *Mortality, 70,* 7-21.

Werth, J. L. & Crow, L. (2009). End-of-life care: An overview for professional counselors. *Journal of Counseling & Development,* 87(2), 194-203.

Critical Thinking

1. Discuss self-determination and it's importance at end of life.

2. The article suggests further research should be conducted in identifying whether rehabilitation counselors expose their own values when their clients make end-of-life decisions. How does this happen and why?

Internet References

American Rehabilitation Counseling Association
http://www.arcaweb.org//

National Center for Ethics in Health Care
http://www.ethics.va.gov/

Article Prepared by: Elaina Osterbur, *Saint Louis University*

Coping with the Death of Your Pet

How to take care of yourself, your family, and other pets when you've had to say goodbye

THE HUMANE SOCIETY OF THE UNITED STATES

Learning Outcomes

After reading this article, you will be able to:

- Discuss the coping strategies of children and older adults.
- Explain the recommendations for getting another pet.

. . .

When a person you love dies, it's natural to feel sorrow, express grief, and expect friends and family to provide understanding and comfort.

Unfortunately, you don't always get that understanding when a pet dies. Some people still don't understand how central animals can be in people's lives, and a few may not get why you're grieving over "just a pet."

Members of the Family

We know how much pets mean to most people. People love their pets and consider them members of their family. Caregivers often celebrate their pets' birthdays, confide in their animals and carry pictures of them in their wallets. So when a beloved pet dies, it's not unusual to feel overwhelmed by the intensity of your sorrow.

Animals provide companionship, acceptance, emotional support, and unconditional love. If you understand and accept this bond between humans and animals, you've already taken the first step toward coping with pet loss: knowing that it is okay to grieve when your pet dies.

Finding ways to cope with your loss can bring you closer to the day when memories bring smiles instead of tears.

. . .

The Grief Process

The grief process is as individual as the person, lasting days for one person, years for another. The process typically begins with denial, which offers protection until individuals can realize their loss.

Some caregivers may try bargaining with a higher power, themselves, or even their pet to restore life. Some feel anger, which may be directed at anyone involved with the pet, including family, friends, and veterinarians. Caregivers may also feel guilt about what they did or did not do; they may feel that it is inappropriate for them to be so upset.

After these feelings subside, caregivers may experience true sadness or grief. They may become withdrawn or depressed. Acceptance occurs when they accept the reality of their loss and remember their animal companion with decreasing sadness.

Coping with Grief

While grief is a personal experience, you need not face your loss alone. Many forms of support are available, including pet-bereavement counseling services, pet-loss support hotlines, local or online pet-bereavement groups, books, videos, and magazine articles.

Here are a few suggestions to help you cope:

Acknowledge your grief and give yourself permission to express it.

Don't hesitate to reach out to others who can lend a sympathetic ear. Do a little research online and you'll find hundreds of resources and support groups that may be helpful to you.

Write about your feelings, either in a journal or a poem, essay, or short story.

Call your veterinarian or local humane society to see whether they offer a pet-loss support group or hotline, or can refer you to one.

Prepare a memorial for your pet.

Children

The loss of a pet may be a child's first experience with death. The child may blame themself, their parents, or the veterinarian for not saving the pet. And they may feel guilty, depressed, and frightened that others they love may be taken from them.

Trying to protect your child by saying the pet ran away could cause your child to expect the pet's return and feel betrayed after discovering the truth. Expressing your own grief may reassure your child that sadness is ok and help them work through their feelings.

Seniors

Coping with the loss of a pet can be particularly hard for seniors. Those who live alone may feel a loss of purpose and an immense emptiness. A pet's death may also trigger painful memories of other losses and remind caregivers of their own mortality. What's more, the decision to get another pet is complicated by the possibility that the pet may outlive the caregiver and that the decision to get another pet hinges on the person's physical and financial ability to care for a new pet.

For all these reasons, it's critical that senior pet owners take immediate steps to cope with their loss and regain a sense of purpose.

If you are a senior, try interacting with friends and family, calling a pet-loss support hotline, even volunteering at a local humane society.

Other Pets

Surviving pets may whimper, refuse to eat or drink, and suffer lethargy, especially if they had a close bond with the deceased pet. Even if they were not the best of friends, the changing circumstances and your emotional state may distress them. (However, if your remaining pets continue to act out of sorts, there could actually be a medical problem that requires your veterinarian's attention.)

Give surviving pets lots of TLC and try to maintain a normal routine. It's good for them and for you.

Getting Another Pet

Rushing into this decision isn't fair to you or your new pet. Each animal has their own unique personality and a new animal cannot replace the one you lost. You'll know when the time is right to adopt a new pet after giving yourself time to grieve, considering whether you're ready, and paying close attention to your feelings.

When you're ready, remember that your local animal shelter or rescue is a great place to find your next special friend.

Critical Thinking

1. Discuss your experience if you have ever lost a family pet.
2. Discuss the similarities between the grief process of losing a loved human versus losing a loved pet.

Internet References

American Veterinary Medical Association
https://www.avma.org/
HealGrief.org
https://healgrief.org/
Human Society of the United States
http://www.humanesociety.org/

Article   Prepared by: Elaina Osterbur, *Saint Louis University*

Death with Dignity Acts

DEATH WITH DIGNITY

Learning Outcomes

After reading this article, you will be able to:

- Identify states with Death with Dignity laws.

- Discuss the Acts requirements for eligibility for physician-assisted dying options.

Death with dignity laws, also known as physician-assisted dying or aid-in-dying laws, stem from the basic idea that it is the terminally ill people, not government and its interference, politicians and their ideology, or religious leaders and their dogma, who should make their end-of-life decisions and determine how much pain and suffering they should endure.

Death with dignity statutes allow mentally competent adult state residents who have a terminal illness with a confirmed prognosis of having 6 or fewer months to live to voluntarily request and receive a prescription medication to hasten their inevitable, imminent death. By adding a voluntary option to the continuum of end-of-life care, these laws give patients dignity, control, and peace of mind during their final days with family and loved ones. The protections in the Act ensure that patients remain the driving force in end-of-life care discussions.

Existing physician-assisted dying laws mirror Oregon's Death with Dignity Act, which is widely acclaimed as successful and which independent studies prove has safeguards to protect patients and prevents misuse. The Death with dignity process is robust: Two physicians must confirm the patient's residency, diagnosis, prognosis, mental competence, and voluntariness of the request. Two waiting periods, the first between the oral requests, the second between receiving and filling the prescription, are required.

Current Death with Dignity Laws

Five states and Washington, D.C., have death with dignity statutes:

- California (End of Life Option Act; approved in 2015, in effect from 2016)
- Colorado (End of Life Options Act; 2016)
- District of Columbia (D.C. Death with Dignity Act; 2016/2017)
- Hawaii (Our Care, Our Choice Act; 2018/2019)
- Oregon (Oregon Death with Dignity Act; 1994/1997)
- Vermont (Patient Choice and Control at the End of Life Act; 2013)
- Washington (Washington Death with Dignity Act; 2008)

Montana does *not* currently have a statute safeguarding physician-assisted death. In 2009, Montana's Supreme Court ruled nothing in the state law prohibited a physician from honoring a terminally ill, mentally competent patient's request by prescribing medication to hasten the patient's death. Since the ruling, several bills have been introduced to codify or ban the practice, none of which have passed.

Critical Thinking

1. Discuss the ethical issues relative to physician-assisted dying.

2. Do you think that the state requirements for eligibility are comprehensive?

Internet References

Death with Dignity
   http://www.deathwithdignity.org/
Ethical Rights
   https://www.ethicalrights.com/

Article   Prepared by: Elaina Osterbur, *Saint Louis University*

Palliative Care: Impact on Quality and Cost

JESSICA D. SQUAZZO

Learning Outcomes

After reading this article, you will be able to:

- Discuss the definition of palliative care.

- Identify the role of family in the discussion of palliative care.

- Discuss the professional's role in the management of palliative care options for patients and families.

Palliative care is an emerging piece of the healthcare system that many predict will have a profound ability to improve quality of care, communication and coordination for seriously ill patients and their families and, through this process, reduce reliance on emergency departments and hospitals. Different in name and function than hospice and end-of-life care, palliative care is a unique, team-oriented approach to caring for the sickest of patients who are also, without doubt, the costliest.

Though not a new concept, it is perhaps one of the least understood service lines. It is, however, showing signs of growth, with the number of U.S. hospitals offering palliative care rising rapidly, according to the Center to Advance Palliative Care. Data from the Center and the American Hospital Association reveal that the number of programs in U.S. hospitals with 50 or more beds increased from 658 (24.5 percent) to 1,635 (66 percent) from 2000 to 2010—a 145.8 percent increase.

One person on the front lines of the emergence of palliative care programs in the U.S. healthcare system is Diane E. Meier, MD, FACP, director of the New York-based Center to Advance Palliative Care. "My mission is to improve access to palliative care across all settings," Meier told the audience at the ACHE program "Palliative Care: Impact on Quality and Cost." The program, funded in part by the Foundation of ACHE's Fund for Innovation in Healthcare Leadership, was held Sept. 11, 2012, in conjunction with ACHE's Atlanta Cluster Program.

During her keynote address, Meier, who is also vice chair of public policy and professor of geriatrics and palliative medicine and Catherine Gaisman Professor of Medical Ethics at Mount Sinai School of Medicine in New York City, made the case for why palliative care is so important to healthcare today and how organizations can begin to develop such programs.

According to Meier, it isn't difficult to make the business case for establishing palliative care programs, especially at a time when, she said, the largest cause of bankruptcy in the U.S. is healthcare bills, and a very large portion of our population is underinsured.

"It is the costliest, very small proportion of patients that drive the vast majority of spending," she said. "Healthcare spending is highly concentrated on the sickest and most vulnerable 5 percent of patients. Palliative care models have been shown to improve quality of life for these patients and families, to prolong life in a number of studies and, as a result, to enable patients to avoid the preventable crises and emergencies that land them in the hospital. The costliest patients are palliative care patients. That's why palliative care is so critical to improving quality and reducing costs."

Defining Palliative Care

Meier said one key way to help organizations think about palliative care and distinguish it from other service lines is to remember that, "Palliative care is not what we do when there's nothing else to do." Palliative care is delivered *at the same time* as appropriate disease-related therapies, she said. "You don't move to hospice until disease-directed therapies are no longer working or their burdens begin to outweigh their benefits."

Palliative care differs from hospice or end-of-life care because the patients benefiting from palliative care programs aren't necessarily dying. Often they are patients who are very sick but have a good prognosis and are expected to live. Most people with serious and complex chronic illness in the United States are not dying, but living with significant burden of illness for many years. Meier said the fact that there are pediatric palliative care programs operating at some organizations highlights the importance of not linking palliative care to end-of-life care. In Meier's program at Mount Sinai, they are very accustomed to taking care of patients who are likely to be cured, such as bone marrow transplant patients, she said.

Meier shared the Center to Advance Palliative Care's definition of palliative care with the audience. The definition was crafted using language that was most highly rated among the public, according to a public opinion survey conducted by the Center, so as to use language that is meaningful and important to patients and families:

"Palliative care is specialized medical care for people with serious illnesses. This type of care is focused on providing patients with relief from the symptoms, pain and stress of a serious illness—whatever the diagnosis. The goal is to improve quality of life for both the patient and the family. Palliative care is provided by a team of doctors, nurses and other specialists who work with a patient's other doctors to provide an extra layer of support. Palliative care is appropriate at any age and at any stage in a serious illness, and can be provided together with curative treatment."

As described in the above definition, palliative care is delivered by a care "team." The team consists of key players such as physicians, nurses and advance practice nurses, social workers, chaplains or spiritual advisors, pain management specialists and others. The emphasis is on treating the patient's medical condition but also helping him or her through the difficult practical challenges and emotional and spiritual distress that accompany a serious illness.

Patients' family members and other loved ones also play a key part in palliative care. In a successful palliative care program, they are part of the conversation at the moment treatment begins. Palliative care programs also provide the proper counseling and support, including bereavement programs, if necessary, to patients' loved ones.

Meier said the impact of serious illness on patients' family members—including increased mortality and morbidity and post-traumatic stress disorder—cannot be ignored. "The cost to society from this is incalculable . . . [resulting in] people who can't function as mothers, who can't go to work, who can't

return to their role in society," she said. "That is a fault in the system we don't think about much."

Palliative care addresses three domains, said Meier. By addressing these domains, quality of care is improved and because patients feel better and remain in control, costs are reduced:

- Physical, emotional and spiritual distress
- Patient-family-professional communication about achievable goals for care and the decision making that follows
- Coordinated, communicated continuity of care and support for practical needs of both patients and families across settings

Evidence showcasing these and other benefits of palliative care programs is mounting, with hundreds of studies showing how palliative care can improve care quality, Meier said. A Harvard Medical School/Massachusetts General Hospital study published by the *New England Journal of Medicine* in 2010 found that in a randomized trial of patients receiving standard cancer care with palliative care co-management from the time of diagnosis versus a control group receiving standard cancer care only, the group receiving palliative care co-management experienced improved quality of life, reduced major depression, reduced "aggressiveness" in treatment (e.g., less chemotherapy before death, less likely to be hospitalized during the last month of care, etc.), *and improved survival rates* (11.6 months versus 8.9 months). Other studies have pointed to cost savings including reductions in use of costly imaging and pharmaceuticals and reductions in ED visits and time spent in the ICU.

Making Palliative Care Work

Meier provided attendees with an overview of what it takes in a healthcare organization to make palliative care succeed. At the top of the list is medical staff engagement. "If you don't have respectful and strong relationships with front-line medical staff working with the patients and families, it won't work," Meier said. "A social worker alone can't do it. Palliative care teams without a doctor are not going to work well." Meier says having medical staff on the palliative care team provides added credibility to the information presented to patients and their families.

Other strategies for convincing physicians and others in the organization to get on board with palliative care include identifying opinion leaders in the organization and getting their interest and investment to help you sell the idea to others; interviewing others in the organization about what problems/issues they perceive and how they feel they should be addressed (this aids in relationship building); gathering quality data; focusing on quality; and, finally, seeking senior leadership's support for a universal, systemwide palliative care screening checklist. "Palliative care should be part of the admission process," said Meier. "They should be screening for unmanaged illness just as they screen for pressure ulcer or fall risk."

Palliative care is sure to gain more ground in the future, as it is already on the radar of several national healthcare groups such as the National Quality Forum, which has listed it as one of six of its National Priorities for action; The Joint Commission, which in September 2011 released its Palliative Care Advanced Certification Program; MedPAC; and the Institute for Healthcare Improvement.

"Palliative care is key to survival under a capitated, global budget," said Meier. "When fee-for-service goes away and you're not managing the sickest 5 percent in the best way possible, they will bankrupt your budget."

After her keynote address, Meier introduced the program's three panelists, who each discussed their organization's experiences with palliative care.

Advance Care Planning

Bernard "Bud" Hammes, PhD, director, medical humanities, and director, Respecting Choices, at Gunderson Lutheran Health System in La Crosse, Wis., discussed advance care planning (ACP) as a complement to palliative care. He said the health system, which serves approximately 560,000 people in 19 counties in western Wisconsin, has invested heavily in the quality of the planning process—the process of knowing and honoring a patient's informed plans.

Hammes outlined the three key desired outcomes of advance care planning:

- Creating an effective plan, including selecting a well-prepared healthcare agent or proxy when possible and creating specific instructions that reflect informed decisions geared toward a person's state of health
- Having advance care plans available to the treating physician
- Incorporating the plans into medical decisions when and wherever needed

"Planning isn't enough," said Hammes. "We have to make sure these plans are available to the treating physicians, and they incorporate them correctly into decisions."

Hammes discussed the relationship of ACP to advance directives. According to Hammes, the successful implementation of an advance directive is directly tied to the quality of the planning process or advance care planning. "If the process of planning has a poor quality to it, the plan will not work," said Hammes. "Quality of communication with the patient and the family predicts the quality of the outcome."

There are four key elements in designing an effective ACP program, according to Hammes. They are:

1. **Systems design**—build an infrastructure that assists in hardwiring excellence, including effective, standardized documentation, reliable medical records storage and retrieval, and an ACP team and referral mechanism. According to Hammes, advance care planning must be made routine among staff members and a part of the care process. "It has to be hardwired into how we relate to our patients," he said. "No matter where patients are being treated, the written care plan must be available to the treating physicians."

2. **Advance care plan facilitation skills training**—build confidence among staff and create an effective ACP team. Hammes said Gunderson Lutheran Health has experienced success with teams featuring "facilitators" who on behalf of doctors talk with patients about their values and goals in order to develop their care plans. Facilitators help take some of the burden off already-busy physicians.

   Once the team is in place, staff training and use of a standardized curriculum are paramount. This ensures delivery of a consistent, reliable ACP service, according to Hammes.

3. **Community education and engagement**—reach out to communities with consistent messages about advance care planning. Because care in the La Crosse region involves two integrated health systems, all ACP-related materials distributed throughout the community have the names of both systems on them so patients know they can contact both systems related to their advance care plans, according to Hammes. This makes it possible to work effectively with all community groups and institutions.

4. **Continuous quality improvement**—measure and improve. Hammes noted the importance of continuously measuring your organization's ACP program—and constantly looking for ways to improve it.

"We didn't create a successful system because we were smart—we created a successful system because we were persistent," said Hammes. "We redesigned it and redesigned it until it worked."

Making the Case for Palliative Care

Stacie T. Pinderhughes, MD, director of palliative medicine at Banner Good Samaritan Medical Center in Phoenix, told the audience about her experience with setting up a palliative care program at the system, which comprises 23 acute-care hospitals, when she began her job at the organization in 2010. She shared several important lessons learned.

One key lesson was to know your organization s culture before you jump in. For Pinderhughes, she was fortunate to be at a hospital where "the doctors were very receptive and open to the whole concept of palliative care," she said.

That buy-in from physicians is critical to the success of a palliative care program, according to Pinderhughes. But there was some education of physicians that had to be done, especially among the specialty groups such as hospitalists, primary care doctors and the hospital's two large intensivist groups.

She recalled how it was helpful at Good Samaritan to have physicians round with the palliative care team to gain a better understanding of how a palliative care program works and see the variety of services it offers. According to Pinderhughes, it also helped clinicians understand that palliative care is different from hospice care. "We made a deliberate decision at Banner Health System to debrand palliative care from hospice," she said.

During year one of the palliative care program, the team consisted of Pinderhughes, a nurse practitioner and one social worker. Pinderhughes said bringing a social worker on board helped make connections in the community, an important aspect of palliative care.

Another key lesson Pinderhughes and her colleagues learned was the importance of getting C-suite buy-in. Showing senior leaders the cost benefit of a palliative care program is key.

"We found significant cost avoidance among these patients, which got the attention of the C-suite early," recalled Pinderhughes. In the first year of its program, Good Samaritan's palliative care team had seen approximately 500 patients. Since the program's start, Pinderhughes said, the total cost avoidance attributed to Good Samaritan's palliative care program is approximately $1.5 million.

At the end of the program's first year, a Palliative Care System Developmental Initiative was convened and charged with developing a stable platform for the delivery of palliative care across the healthcare continuum. This group called together stakeholders across the system, including providers, risk management staff and administrators. The group began the process of defining palliative care for the system and developed a business plan, a plan for educating others about the program and an IT infrastructure for documentation. The palliative care team also defined the program's mission and vision (and alignment with Banner Health's overall mission and vision) and defined its patient population.

Pinderhughes recalled how crucial it was to have the CFO's support with developing the business plan. Good Samaritan's CFO was involved from the beginning, even accompanying the palliative care team on walk rounds. "Now he is an effective ally in the C-suite," said Pinderhughes.

Pinderhughes said the team created tools to ensure palliative care at Good Samaritan was standardized. The team created an information card, which they distributed to physicians, residents, nurses, social workers and case managers. The organization's EHR now includes a Palliative Care Rounding Tool in which palliative care team members document information. Palliative care information is also captured on the Palliative Medicine H&P (history and physical) Template the team developed.

Banner Health is now looking at developing palliative care programs in several of its hospitals and plans to work with its ACO to develop palliative care further across other settings. "We've laid the infrastructure, now we're moving to the design phase," Pinderhughes said.

Buy-In from the C-Suite

When John M. Haupert, FACHE, became CEO of Grady Health System in Atlanta in 2011, one of his priorities was improving the way the system was managing the significant number of patients in need of hospice and palliative care. At least one-third of those patients were being improperly placed in the ICU.

As a safety net provider for Atlanta and one of the nation's largest public hospitals with 625 acute-care beds, Grady's payor mix is 30-30-20-20 (charity, Medicaid, Medicare, commercial). "To make this work economically takes a lot of work," Haupert told the audience.

The development of Grady's palliative care program is one major solution developed to help more efficiently and economically manage the most vulnerable among Grady's patient population. Haupert and his staff established a vision statement for palliative care at the system, which "has become our calling card for everything we do, every action we take and every action we put our energy behind," he said. The vision is: "The program assists patients and their families by providing relief from the symptoms, pain, and stress of a serious illness with the goal of improving their quality of life. The program affirms life and recognizes death as a normal process; helps people live as actively as possible and, in the event of terminal illness, neither postpones nor hastens death but helps them experience the end of their life with dignity and comfort."

Haupert said the vision is inclusive and looks at the full continuum of palliative and hospice services. "We wanted to avoid a model consisting of just life-prolonging care," Haupert said. An ideal model, he said, is a palliative care team working *with* hospice care staff and supportive services including after-care support.

The palliative care program at Grady is constantly evolving and improving as the organization learns what works best to serve its patient population. The focus is always on doing what's best for patients and their families in difficult times. "We have a lot of work to do to treat people with the dignity they deserve," Haupert said.

Grady's palliative care program has been developed in three levels. The organization is currently working to get from level two to level three, and Haupert says they have identified the following factors that must be in place to make that happen:

- **Enhanced leadership**—including identifying clinical leaders
- **Established operational infrastructure**—including implementation of a palliative care service scorecard and deployment of resources to meet demand for services
- **Enhanced system integration**—including clinical partnerships with other service lines such as oncology and internal medicine

Haupert knows firsthand the importance of having C-suite buy-in for a palliative care initiative. "With my commitment, we will get there and make this happen," he said.

Attendee Tammie Quest, MD, associate professor of emergency medicine and director, Emory Center for Palliative Care, which has a close working relationship with Grady

Health, emphasized Haupert's sentiment. It makes a difference in the success of a palliative care program when you work with senior leaders who are "incredibly motivated and enthusiastic," she said.

"When you don't have that from the C-suite, it's really hard to take these programs to the next level."

Critical Thinking

1. What are the considerations that need to be discussed between professionals and patients in order to ensure that patients are making informed decisions?

2. What is the role of advance directives in the palliative care treatment option?

Internet References

National Hospice and Palliative Care Organization
www.nhpco.org
Open Society Foundations: Health: Palliative Care
www.opensocietyfoundations.org/topics/palliative-care

JESSICA D. SQUAZZO is senior writer with *Healthcare Executive*.

Squazzo, Jessica D. From *Healthcare Executive Magazine*, January/February 2013, pp. 27–28, 30, 32, 34, 36, 38. Copyright ©2013 by American College of Healthcare Executives—ACHE. Used with permission.

Unit 7

Prepared by: Elaina Osterbur, *Saint Louis University*

UNIT

Living Environment in Later Life

Old age is often a period of shrinking life space. This concept is crucial to an understanding of the living environments of older Americans. When older people retire, they may find that they travel less frequently and over shorter distances because they no longer work. As the retirement years roll by, older people may feel less in control of their environment due to a decline in their hearing and vision as well as other health problems. As the aging process continues, elderly people are likely to restrict their mobility to the areas where they feel most secure. This usually means that an increasing amount of time is spent at home. Estimates show that individuals aged 65 years and above spend 80–90 percent of their lives in their home environments. The house, neighborhood, and community environments are, therefore, more crucial to elderly individuals than to any other adult age group. The interaction with others that they experience within their homes and neighborhoods can either be stimulating or foreboding, pleasant, or threatening. Across the country, older Americans live in a variety of circumstances, ranging from desirable to undesirable.

According to the Administration on Aging, A Profile of Older Americans, 2017, 59 percent of older adults (noninstitutionalized) live with their spouse (including partner), and 28 percent of older adults live alone. Some older adults live with their grown children, and a relatively small number of older adults live in institutional settings such as nursing homes. Since 2015, the percent of older adults living with spouse or partner has increased 3 percent, and the percent of older adults living alone has declined by 1 percent.

The readings in this section include the top senior housing trends, creating community, information regarding Ombudsman programs, and planning for Alzheimer's Disease.

Article   Prepared by: Elaina Osterbur, *Saint Louis University*

Creating Communities That Support Healthy Aging

NANCY LEAMOND

Learning Outcomes

After reading this article, you will be able to:

- Identify key components of the adaptations necessary to create a community that supports healthy aging.

- Explain why communities need to consider an aging population.

The dramatic aging of our population will be one of America's greatest challenges of the 21st century. For some of us *Policy & Practice* readers, the aging of America already is part of our everyday world of thought and planning, and has been for some time. For others, it may have, so far, played only an incidental, or peripheral, role in your daily responsibilities.

But—please believe me—the aging of our population is a phenomenon that will profoundly affect all sectors of our society. Everyone who is privileged to be in a position to make a difference will be tasked with an important role in dealing with it. And when historians years from now look back at our time and at what we did, one of their primary points of measurement will be how we met this great challenge.

A key component of meeting the challenge will be our nation's communities successfully adapting to accommodate their aging residents by making changes in infrastructure and services that will benefit all age groups. If community leaders have a range of information, tools, successful strategies, and best practices available to assist them at the outset, the task will be easier and less costly. AARP is committed to being a primary go-to resource. Here are some key points everyone needs to know.

Point 1: There is no escape! The aging of America is happening everywhere

By 2030, just 17 years from now, when the last of the baby boomers turns 65, the 65 and older population will have doubled from what it is today—to more than 70 million. Today, the nation's "oldest" city is Scottsdale, Arizona, where one of every five residents is 65 or older. In 2030, one of every five residents of the entire United States will be 65 or older.

All 50 states will see a rapid acceleration in the growth of their 65 and older populations. By 2030, 10 states will actually have more 65 and older residents than school-age children. That's never happened before in our nation's history—in even one state. Utah is projected to be our "youngest" state in 2030, yet their 65 and older population will still have nearly doubled.

Point 2: Too many of our communities are just not prepared for their aging populations

A report several years ago by the International City/County Management Association documented that less than half of our country's jurisdictions were prepared for the aging of their residents. Clearly, there have been pockets of encouraging innovation and experimentation. The approach to date in too many communities and states has been one of "let's wait and see." We just can't afford any longer to play the "wait and see" game.

Point 3: Forget about the old myths concerning aging in America

Supporting "wait and see" has been a pervasive string of myths. Let's start with the myth that suggests the cherished dream of most Americans nearing retirement is to pack up and retire in Florida, or Arizona, or some other place with palm trees. The fact is, this may be true for some, but not for the vast majority.

Since 1990, roughly 90 percent of older Americans have stayed in the same county they've lived in during their working years—most in the very same home. And we expect this to continue. AARP's research on the topic has found repeatedly that more than eight of every 10 boomers want to remain in their current home or community during retirement. The number one reason is the desire to stay close to their families.

Another myth suggests that preparing a community to retain older residents will make it less attractive to younger residents. Not true! I can't stress this enough: This isn't an "old versus young" issue. Livable communities benefit residents of *all* ages and we must consider *all* ages at every stage in the planning process.

Residents of all ages benefit from safer, barrier-free buildings and streets; as well as from better access to local businesses and more green spaces. A curb-cut designed for a wheelchair user also benefits a parent pushing a baby stroller. A crosswalk safe for a senior is a crosswalk safe for a child. A community that is friendly for an 80 year old can be friendly for an 8 year old—and everyone else in between.

Then, there's the myth that creating livable communities will cost too much and will never yield a decent return on the investment. Cost too much? Well, certainly there is cost, but creating livable communities doesn't mean tearing down our communities and starting over. It means, primarily, adapting and building upon existing programs, services, and infrastructure to make them accessible and safe for residents with varying needs and capacities.

How about the cost of not making our communities livable? The cost to our communities and our families—and to our nation—of not having age-friendly housing, streets and sidewalks is enormous—well into the tens of billions of dollars.

Here's a prime example. The biggest cause of hospitalization for Americans 65 and older today isn't cancer, or heart-related episodes. It is falls. Each year, one of every three Americans 65 and older falls, and a third of those require medical treatment. The Centers for Disease Control and Prevention project that annual direct treatment costs from older Americans falling will escalate from just under $20 billion today to nearly $44 billion by 2020. That's more than the current annual budget of the federal Department of Homeland Security.

Point 4: People want solutions, and creativity is the key to finding them

We can't just look to the federal government for solutions anymore. It will require working across unique coalitions involving nonprofits, state and local governments, foundations, businesses, and engaged citizens. Finding the best ways to create successful communities for all ages will require input from just about everyone. Some solutions will emerge naturally. Others will be developed through plans of action, driven by robust research and focused commitment.

Finding the best ways to create successful communities for all ages will require input from just about everyone. Some solutions will emerge naturally. Others will be developed through plans of action, driven by robust research and focused commitment.

Communities and state and local public service administrators need to be thinking of livable communities in terms of the enormous potential for more efficient and less costly delivery of health and other human services. This will require those responsible for transportation planning, human services, and care coordination to work across department and agency lines to solve the challenges related to ensuring that seniors get access to the care they need.

Here are a couple of already successful models for building on existing community structures.

Programs in "*Naturally Occurring Retirement Communities,*" known as NORCs, are now being developed across the nation. NORCs are geographic areas or building developments that feature multigenerational populations, but which already include a significant number of residents that are 60 and older.

Eldercare agencies are creating community-based interventions that build on these "natural" concentrations of elders called NORC-Supportive Service Programs. They connect elders to a variety of health care and home care services that allow them to remain healthy and independent. By serving relatively large numbers of elders in small areas, this model benefits from economies of scale in the organization and delivery of services, and creates related cost savings. We know of more than 100 of these programs moving forward nationwide.

Preserving existing affordable housing near accessible transit is essential, especially for lower-income older adults who desire to age in their homes. Mixed-use neighborhoods with safer, denser, walkable streets engender more physical activity. Public transit users are more likely than nontransit users to meet federally recommended physical activity goals by walking. Nationally, 29 percent of those who use transit are physically active for 30 minutes or more each day, solely by walking to and from public transit stops.

AARP is playing a proactive role, as well through the work of our state offices located in the 53 states and territories. We're excited about the AARP Network of Age-Friendly Communities we launched last year in affiliation with the World Health Organization's *Age-Friendly Cities and Communities Program.* To be selected for the network, a city or community must commit to undertake a 3-year process of continually assessing and improving its age-friendliness, and involve its older residents in a meaningful way. The AARP Age-Friendly Communities Network launched with eight pilot programs in the District of Columbia, and in Georgia, Iowa, Kansas, Michigan, New York, Oregon, and Pennsylvania.

Another example is the AARP HomeFit workshops that have been held by AARP State Offices. The workshop teaches people about inexpensive modifications they can make to their homes so they can stay in their own homes and communities and remain independent as long as possible.

And, with all of the innovation underway in the states to reform their Medicaid long-term care system, human service administrators should use this opportunity to shift resources away from costly institutional nursing home care to less expensive more desirable quality home-and community-based services and supports.

Communities and state and local administrators should also recognize the contribution of caregivers who provide an estimated $450 billion dollars a year in uncompensated support to family members that allows them to remain in their homes. Caregivers can be supported by increasing access to information; connecting them to community-based respite services, and protecting them from losing their jobs because of time spent caring for loved ones.

The late author, Peter Drucker, used to say, "The best way to predict the future is to create it."

I believe strongly that we have an obligation to work together, to identify and share solutions, and to celebrate the opportunities and challenges of Americans living longer and healthier lives, and communities opening their arms to all generations.

I encourage *Policy & Practice* readers to visit our new AARP Livable Communities: Great Places for All Ages web site (*www.aarp.org/livable*). This new site is a go-to resource for the latest information, best practices, research, policy analysis, advocacy resources, including model acts that address both complete streets and universal design, and funding sources that support livable communities. It is the first time that resources from a wide-range of sources have been compiled in one place and organized with the needs of local officials in mind.

Creating Livable Communities for all ages will be a key component in creating brighter and economically stronger futures for our nation's communities. The challenges are formidable, to be sure. But for those communities that succeed, the rewards will be much greater.

Critical Thinking

1. Do you think that aging myths will cloud the views of community leaders when making change to accomodate this population?
2. Discuss current programs, innovations, and accommodations that are being made by communities and agencies.

Internet References

AARP: Livable Communities
   http://www.aarp.org/livable-communities
American Public Human Services Association
   http://www.aphsa.org/content/APHSA/en/home.html

Article   Prepared by: Elaina Osterbur, *Saint Louis University*

Long-Term Care Ombudsman Program

ADMINISTRATION FOR COMMUNITY LIVING

Learning Outcomes

After reading this article, you will be able to:

* Define long-term care, as defined by the program.

* Define ombudsman and the services provided through the program.

What Is the Long-Term Care Ombudsman Program?

Long-term care ombudsmen are advocates for residents of nursing homes, board and care homes, assisted living facilities, and similar adult care facilities. They work to resolve problems of individual residents and to bring about changes at the local, state, and national levels to improve care. While many residents receive good care in long-term care facilities, others are neglected, and other unfortunate incidents of psychological, physical, and other kinds of abuse do occur. Thus, thousands of trained staff and volunteer ombudsmen regularly visit long-term care facilities, monitor conditions and care, and provide a voice for those unable to speak for themselves.

The Swedish word "ombudsman" means "a public official appointed to investigate citizens' complaints against local or national government agencies that may be infringing on the rights of individuals." This concept has been applied in many U.S. settings to include complaints against nongovernmental organizations and advocacy for individuals and groups of individuals, as with the Long-Term Care Ombudsman Program.

History

Begun in 1972 as a demonstration program, today the Long-Term Care Ombudsman Program is established in all States under the Older Americans Act which is administered by the Administration on Aging (AoA). Local ombudsmen work with and on behalf of residents in hundreds of communities throughout the country.

Results

In federal fiscal year 2012, over 11,000 volunteers, 8,712 of whom were certified to investigate complaints, and 1,180 staff served in Long-Term Care Ombudsman Programs in 573 localities nationwide. Ombudsmen investigated and worked to resolve 193,650 complaints made by 126,398 individuals. In addition, ombudsmen provided information on rights, care, and related services 405,589 times.

Residents' Rights

Ombudsmen help residents and their families and friends understand and exercise rights guaranteed by law, both at the Federal level for nursing homes and for States that provide rights and protections in board and care, assisted living, and similar homes. Residents have the right to:

* Be treated with respect and dignity
* Be free from chemical and physical restraints
* Manage their own finances
* Voice grievances without fear of retaliation
* Associate and communicate privately with any person of their choice
* Send and receive personal mail
* Have personal and medical records kept confidential
* Apply for State and Federal assistance without discrimination
* Be fully informed prior to admission of their rights, services available, and all charges
* Be given advance notice of transfer or discharge

Ombudsman Responsibilities

Ombudsman responsibilities outlined in Title VII of the Older Americans Act include:

* Identify, investigate, and resolve complaints made by or on behalf of residents

- Identify, investigate, and resolve complaints made by or on behalf of residents
- Provide information to residents about long-term care services
- Represent the interests of residents before governmental agencies
- Seek administrative, legal, and other remedies to protect residents
- Analyze, comment on, and recommend changes in laws and regulations pertaining to the health, safety, welfare, and rights of residents
- Educate and inform consumers and the general public regarding issues and concerns related to long-term care and facilitate public comment on laws, regulations, policies, and actions
- Promote the development of citizen organizations to participate in the program
- Provide technical support for the development of resident and family councils to protect the well-being and rights of residents
- Advocate for changes to improve residents' quality of life and care

Resources

The National Long-Term Care Ombudsman Resource Center supported with AoA funding and operated by the National Consumer Voice for Quality Long-Term Care, provides technical assistance and intensive training to assist ombudsmen in their demanding work.

Critical Thinking

1. What kind of training do you think would be beneficial for an Ombudsman?
2. What do you think the attitude will be toward Ombudsman in the future?

Internet References

The National Consumer Voice for Quality Long-Term Care
http://theconsumervoice.org/
The National Long-Term Care Ombudsman Resource Center
http://ltcombudsman.org/

Administration for Community Living. "Long-Term Care Ombudsman Program", U.S. Department of Health and Human Services, 2016.

Article   Prepared by: Elaina Osterbur, *Saint Louis University*

Planning for Alzheimer's

Nothing Will Erase the Emotional Toll This Disease Takes on Families. But You Can Take Steps to Stem the Financial Bleeding.

KIMBERLY LANKFORD

Learning Outcomes

After reading this article, you will be able to:

- Identify measures to prepare for long-term care, protecting finances and finding resources when a family member has been diagnosed with Alzheimer's disease.

- Define the stages of Alzheimer's disease.

Rebecca Barnard of St. Louis spent her career as a software developer, but her passion was fine-art photography. She was detail-oriented in both her job and her hobby, says her husband, Richard Rubin. So he was surprised when he began noticing small missteps: She'd park her car at an odd angle and forget to close the car door, and she started to get lost. They had a major scare when she took the wrong train to visit family in New York and didn't know where she was.

"There was a point at which it became apparent that something awful was going on," says Rubin. Seven years ago, he took Barnard to a memory clinic for tests and discovered she had Alzheimer's disease. She was just 53 years old.

A diagnosis of Alzheimer's before age 65 is rare. But one in eight people age 65 and older start showing signs of the disease, and 45 percent of people age 85 and older have it, according to the Alzheimer's Association. All told, more than five million Americans have Alzheimer's. The cost of medical and long-term care for Alzheimer's patients was $200 billion in 2012—not counting the estimated $17 billion hours of unpaid care by family members and friends.

Part of the tragedy of the disease is that it often strikes healthy, vigorous individuals, who then go through a series of stages that rob them of their memory, their awareness of their surroundings and, eventually, their ability to do even the most basic tasks. They typically live nearly a decade after the diagnosis and usually need full-time care, initially at home but ultimately in a nursing home (see "What to Expect," on page 67). "Costs associated with Alzheimer's disease cripple families at a time when they are also coping with the huge practical, social and emotional toll of this chronic brain disorder," says Carol Steinberg, executive vice president of the Alzheimer's Foundation of America.

Scrambling for Care

At first, Rubin, a software developer, worked at home and was able to take care of Barnard. "During the first year, most people couldn't tell that anything was wrong," says Rubin, now 65. But Barnard started getting lost in the house, and eventually even doing her morning routine became difficult. Rubin quit his job at age 60 to care for his wife full-time.

"Alzheimer's sneaks up on you," he says. "You think you can live with it and say you'll manage, but then it changes again." For some people, the middle stage can last five to seven years. But the middle stage for Barnard lasted just a few months.

After a long and complicated application process, Barnard qualified for Social Security Disability Insurance benefits of $1,700 per month and received retroactive payments back to her diagnosis in 2006. Qualifying for benefits has become simpler—early-onset Alzheimer's disease is now on the government's "compassionate allowance" list of conditions subject to fast-track benefits approval (see www.socialsecurity.gov/disability).

Rubin hired a caregiver to give him some relief a couple of times a week. Then Barnard had a sharp decline and started to need about 12 hours of care per day. The caregivers charged about $20 per hour—totaling $240 per day. Barnard's Social Security payments barely put a dent in her monthly care bill of $7,000, and the couple continued to drain their savings to make up the difference.

Qualifying for Social Security disability also made Barnard eligible for Medicare two years after her diagnosis, even though she was younger than 65. Medicare covered most of her medical expenses but not what Alzheimer's patients need most: custodial care, or the nonmedical care associated with the tasks of daily living, such as help with bathing, dressing and eating. Medicare covers that care for only a short time when skilled care is also needed, such as when an Alzheimer's patient treated by a nurse for a broken hip needs help bathing.

Rubin eventually found an assisted-living group home with just nine residents. Barnard moved out of the couple's home in December 2008. "Being together all the time was over, and it was the hardest thing I did in my life," says Rubin.

The assisted-living facility cost $6,000 per month, which they paid from Barnard's Social Security and the couple's savings. "Basically, we had to start liquidating IRAs, and that was at the bottom of the market," says Rubin. They spent about $160,000 for Barnard's care during her two years there—more than their house had cost.

In fewer than four years from the time she started needing care, half of the couple's retirement savings was gone. "I had always been frugal," says Rubin. "I bought used cars and wasn't a big spender. But with $6,000 going out the door every month, that's serious money."

The Medicaid Option

Rubin met with an elder-law attorney to start planning for Medicaid to pay for Barnard's care. But qualifying for Medicaid was tricky because Rubin was so young and had to spend down so much of his retirement kitty. The spouse who lives at home (called the *community spouse*) can keep all of his own income and, in Missouri, $115,920 in countable assets (such as savings). The spouse who needs care must have very little income and assets; those amounts also vary from state to state, but in Missouri, the spouse who lives in the nursing home can't have more than $999 in assets.

If you're the community spouse, you're allowed to keep your home, car and assets in certain kinds of trusts. Giving away money to anyone other than your spouse within five years of applying for Medicaid can delay your eligibility.

(See www.medicaid.gov for state eligibility rules and www.naela.org to find an elder-law attorney in your area.)

Because Rubin was in his early sixties, the $115,920 asset allowance would be way too little to cover the 20 or 30 years he might live in retirement. So he did some "financial acrobatics" to shift money around and keep more for his own future. He sold some stocks to buy a special Medicaid annuity, which converted that money from countable assets to noncountable income (see www.elderlawanswers.com). He also used some money to pay down his mortgage because the value of his primary residence wasn't included in the calculation.

But even after Barnard qualified for Medicaid, the couple faced another problem: Medicaid generally doesn't cover home care or assisted-living facilities (some states have voucher programs that let people in assisted living or home care use Medicaid). Rubin worked with the Missouri Department of Health and Senior Services' long-term-care ombudsman and finally found a nearby nursing home that had a Medicaid bed open. "The new place is just ten minutes away and has a beautiful view of the Mississippi River," he says. "Beck and I watch the boats on our sad, low river," which has been affected by drought.

Even if you find a Medicaid-eligible nursing home, the facility may not be equipped for the special needs of active Alzheimer's patients. Julie Dobson's mother, Elizabeth Dobson, 80, started showing signs of Alzheimer's about ten years ago. Elizabeth's husband, Charles, took care of her in their rural New Hampshire home for several years, but eventually he needed more help. When Charles had knee surgery near Julie's home in the Washington, D.C., area last year, he and Julie moved Elizabeth into a nursing home nearby. The facility cost $9,300 per month, which they planned to pay themselves until Elizabeth qualified for Medicaid.

The nursing home accepted Medicaid, but it wasn't equipped to deal with physically active Alzheimer's patients. "My mother is 80 years old, but she looks 60 and is as healthy as an ox," says Julie. "People don't understand that Alzheimer's patients can be very active—they walk and walk." But the nursing home told Julie that she'd need to hire someone to watch her mother in the nursing home—at an extra $17 per hour.

Instead, she found a memory-care facility near her home in Potomac, Md. "The people are much more like my mother," says Julie. "The facility keeps them active—they sing and dance." The new facility costs $7,500 per month, but it doesn't take Medicaid. Charles is paying the bills from his savings, and Julie, 56, plans to cover the cost as long as she can after her father spends all his money. But she is also saving for retirement and for college for her two teenagers.

"You think you've saved enough, and it's overwhelming," says Julie. "My father felt financially comfortable. You can have a couple hundred thousand dollars in the bank, and it can all go in just a year or two."

The Insurance Option

Neither Elizabeth Dobson nor Rebecca Barnard has long-term-care insurance. That's the only way to get broad coverage for custodial care in a variety of locations: your home, an assisted-living facility or a nursing home.

For the policy to pay benefits, you generally must need help with at least two out of six activities of daily living (such as bathing and dressing) or provide evidence of cognitive impairment. Most policies have a waiting period—generally 60 or 90 days—before benefits kick in.

Contact the insurance company immediately after discovering your family member has Alzheimer's. Many policies have a care-coordinator service that can help you find caregivers or facilities before the benefits kick in, says Marilee Driscoll, author of *The Complete Idiot's Guide to Long-Term Care Planning*. Some newer policies from Genworth, the largest long-term-care insurer, offer its CareScout service to policyholders who are searching for care for their parents—even if their parents don't have long-term-care insurance themselves. The program recommends caregivers and facilities and negotiates discounts.

Some policies pay for any caregiver who is not a family member, and others pay only for licensed caregivers who work for an agency. Hiring an eligible caregiver upfront helps you avoid having to find a new caregiver after the waiting period is over.

Find out how the benefits are calculated. You can't use more than your daily benefit per day, but you can usually stretch your benefit over longer periods if you use less than the allotted amount. For example, if you choose a three-year benefit period at $200 a day but spend only $100 a day for caregivers, you may be able to stretch your coverage to six years. Or if your care costs more than your daily benefit, you might hire a licensed caregiver to provide care up to the benefit limit, then get less-expensive care from adult day care or help with basic tasks from unlicensed providers.

Seven Stages
What to Expect

Individuals with Alzheimer's disease tend to live eight to ten years, on average, from the time of diagnosis. Alzheimer's sufferers go through a series of stages (the Alzheimer's Association identifies seven), but the speed of progression varies, and not everyone goes through each stage separately.

At first, people diagnosed with Alzheimer's may have trouble coming up with the right words or lose track of everyday objects. Then they start to have more trouble remembering words and names, more difficulty performing social or work tasks, and more difficulty with I planning or organizing. In the middle stages, they may forget their address or phone number, get confused about what day it is and need help with simple decisions—such as how to dress for the season. But usually they don't yet need help with most personal care.

By the next stage, they start to lose awareness of their surroundings, have trouble remembering their own personal history, need help dressing and using the bathroom, may exhibit personality changes and tend to wander. At the final stage, they are unable to have a conversation or control movement and need help with most of their personal care.

Critical Thinking

1. Discuss the emotional toll of both family and patient after a diagnosis with Alzheimer's disease.

2. Can you think of more solutions to protecting your family should you be diagnosed with Alzheimer's disease?

Internet References

Alzheimer's Association
   http://www.alz.org/

Kiplinger
   http://www.kiplinger.com/

Article   Prepared by: Elaina Osterbur, *Saint Louis University*

The Top 10 Senior Housing Trends for 2016

Janet Marshall

Learning Outcomes

After reading this article, you will be able to:

- Discuss the 2016 senior housing trends.

- Identify statistics relative to long-term care desires of older adults.

- Define person-centered care and it's importance to the older adult.

The shape of senior living communities across the world has changed drastically over the past several years. Baby boomers have their own unique ideas of what their retirement years are going to look like, and the industry must change in order to fit the shape of their unique preferences. 2016's anticipated trends don't look like your grandmother's retirement!

1. Technology

Changes in technology make it possible for seniors to adapt to many of the challenges that come with the aging process. From wearable devices that automatically alert caregivers or emergency assistance of a fall to large-screen phones, remotes, and other important devices, seniors have more high-quality care options than ever before. There are even geofencing options available that can help keep individuals with Alzheimer's and dementia inside safe spaces.

2. Home Care

Aging in place has become increasingly attractive to many seniors. They want to be able to remain in their own homes for as long as possible. Affordable in-home care and changes in technology have helped to make home care a more viable option for many individuals. Senior Planning Services, a tristate area Medicaid planning firm, cites a recent AARP study which estimates that early 90 percent of people over age 65 want to stay in their home for as long as possible.

3. Senior Living Partnerships

Senior living providers are rapidly becoming major power players in the health-care scene. Physicians, hospitals, insurers, and other organizations within the United States health-care system are coming together to create more comprehensive care that provides exactly what many seniors need. As the baby boomer generation hits their senior years, their increased numbers give senior providers increased impact.

4. Person-Centered Care

Everyone deserves to age with dignity and to be cared for as a whole person. Person-centered care isn't a new trend, but it is one that is rapidly gaining ground. When aging individuals receive person-centered care from nursing homes, doctors, and other health care organizations, they are assured that they will be treated as an individual, rather than being treated based only on the capabilities that they no longer have.

5. Life Plan Community

Instead of "Continuing Care Retirement Communities," many aging individuals prefer the image created by a "life plan community." Life plan communities are dedicated to helping seniors make the most out of every moment, from living a full and active life to maintaining their health for as long as possible.

These communities are based on living in the moment now, as younger seniors, not just on the need for continuing care past a certain age or health level.

6. Memory Care

More and more memory care units are embracing the theory behind reminiscence therapy and extending it. They're stimulating all the senses—not just sight and sound, but even smell and touch—and creating communities that are reminiscent of the world in which seniors grew up. This helps give many seniors a firmer foundation for retrieving long-term memories of the past.

7. Senior Cohousing

Senior cohousing offers all the convenience of a single-family dwelling while simultaneously reducing costs and providing a sense of companionship. They have shared responsibilities and access to communal caregivers to assist with daily tasks. It's the perfect balance between institutionalized living and remaining at home, especially for those seniors who might not have a solid support system in place if they continue to live on their own.

8. Going Green

Many assisted living facilities are embracing the green movement. The goal isn't just to entice earth-conscious baby boomers. Going green also helps cut heating and cooling costs, improve water conservation efforts, and meet Energy Star standards across many of the devices used in the facility.

9. Location

One of the most critical changes to senior housing trends is the changes made to appropriate locations. Many facilities are considering the area's appeal to younger seniors. What makes it a great retirement destination? What amenities are readily available throughout the area? Many senior living communities are learning that the smart thing is no longer to build next to a mall or urban center with lots of shopping. Instead, they're looking for new opportunities for engaging, senior-friendly activities for those early retirement years.

10. Independent Living, Not Assisted Living

More facilities now are being designed to appeal to the under-80 crowd. Baby boomers know that they can expect to live comfortably on their own, experiencing reasonable health, for a long time. The senior housing market is gradually adapting to that need by providing independent living facilities that celebrate independence.

Developers and providers will need to enhance seniors' living environments in ways they might never have considered before in order to compete with the rapidly shifting market. The current goal is to create environments based around the baby boomer mindset: to create a place where they will want to live, not just a place where they need to live. Today's seniors won't settle for less!

Critical Thinking

1. Discuss how the needs of the current older generation translates to the next generation?
2. What kind of long-term housing expectations will your generation consider?

Internet References

AARP
   https://www.aarp.org/
National Council on Aging
   https://www.ncoa.org/

Article   Prepared by: Elaina Osterbur, *Saint Louis University*

The Culture Change Movement in Long-term Care: Is Person-Centered Care a Possibility for the Looming Age Wave?

Laci Cornelison

Learning Outcomes

After reading this article, you will be able to:

- Explain the culture change movement in long-term care.

- Discuss the reasons that some nursing homes directors have not adopted culture change.

I. Introduction

In a time when our population is aging at the fastest rate in history, a movement is under way to change the culture of long-term care.[1] This is timely given that nursing homes are often cited as places to be feared,[2] which is reinforced by media reports of poor care and abuse in them. In a 1997 *Journal of the American Geriatrics Society* article, the authors found that more than half of hospitalized adults reported that they were unwilling to live permanently in a nursing home or that they preferred death over living permanently in a nursing home.[3] Despite this reluctance, each year more than 1.4 million people spend time living in the nation's 16,000 nursing homes[4] and nine out of 10 children can expect one of their parents or their spouse's parents to spend time living in a nursing home.[5]

Traditional nursing homes align with what Erving Goffman described as "a place of residence and work where a large number of like-situated individuals, cut off from the wider society for an appreciable period of time, together lead an enclosed, formally administered round of life."[6]

Within Goffman's framework, nursing homes are a place where elders live a rigid, cutoff life with limited autonomy until death. This may be why Bill Thomas, MD, well-known leader of the culture change movement in long-term care, calls himself an "abolitionist" of the traditional nursing home.[7] His goal is to replace traditional nursing homes with more humanized care approaches such as his Green House model, a quintessential iteration of the culture change philosophy.[8] Given the doom and gloom expressed in the aforementioned paragraphs, it seems wise to widely adopt culture change in long-term care; however, there is more to the story. The purpose of this article is to clarify the issues surrounding the culture change movement and its future.

This article will further educate readers about culture change and person-centered care in long-term care facilities, a key practice used within the movement. It will provide information about how widespread the movement is in the United States. The article will also discuss some of the challenges of the movement raised in *The Gerontologist* in 2014,[9] along with suggested possibilities for overcoming these challenges. Finally, the article will discuss the role of government and policy in advancing the movement, including value-based purchasing practices that states have implemented to provide financial incentives for the adoption of person-centered care.

II. Background

The need to provide care for frail elders is longstanding. Most of this care was traditionally provided through the family or informal networks; however, even in the 20th century, abandoned elders were provided for in poor houses and later almshouses, which were essentially rudimentary precursors to today's nursing homes.[10] In 1935, more funds became available through the enactment of Social Security, which provided money that elders could use to pay for their own care. With more money available to pay for care, public criticism arose about the quality of care in available care settings.[11] Social Security pensions were not allowed to be used for government housing such as the poor houses or almshouses, which contributed to the rise in other types of care models. The 1960s marked the next substantial reform movement as Medicare and Medicaid programs began funding care to providers that opted to become licensed. Regulations, licensing specifications, building code standards, and financial reimbursement structures followed to ensure quality of care. Thus, the number of nursing homes rose dramatically during the 1960s and 1970s.[12]

In the 1980s, consumers, lawsuits, and state and federal reports criticized nursing homes for poor quality.[13] In 1987 Congress passed the Omnibus Budget Reconciliation Act (OBRA '87), with a goal of ensuring that nursing homes strive for high standards of well-being for residents.[14] The reform placed resident's rights and quality of life as equal priorities with quality of care.[15] In addition, the Act brought in enforcement agencies to monitor nursing home performance. Catherine Hawes reported that the reform has produced change in nursing homes, including improved accuracy of information in residents' medical records and care plans, decreased use of physical restraints and indwelling catheters, and increased presence of advance directives and incontinence supports.[16] Even though OBRA '87 made provisions for improving quality of life, the primary improvements have been in quality of care. In 2001, Rosalie Kane suggested that quality of life was not being equally addressed:

> Even if there were no quality-of-care problems in nursing homes, conventional nursing homes arguably fail the quality test because of the severe strictures on life in these settings. Put simply, the total disenfranchisement associated with living in a nursing home is too high a price to pay for even high quality technical care.[17]

In reaction to this, a small grassroots movement began in the late 1980s that later became known as the culture change movement in long-term care. Leaders of this movement founded the Pioneer Network in 1997, which increased the voice of the movement.[18] The movement has endeavored to deinstitutionalize traditional models of care and replace them with person-centered, holistic models.

III. Culture Change in Long-Term Care
A. Definition

The culture change movement in long term care targets the improvement of quality of life for residents living in nursing homes; however, a uniform definition of what it is and how it works in practice does not exist.[19] Though there is no straightforward definition, there are multiple conceptualizations and examples of the practices espoused by the movement. For instance, a variety of models are widely accepted as examples of culture change in action, including the Eden Alternative, the Green House model, the Live Oak Regenerative Community, the Wellspring program, Planetree, and the household/ neighborhood model.[20] The term "culture change" as it pertains to long-term care can refer to individual components of care as well as comprehensive, organization-wide change.[21] However, there seems to be consensus that culture change was meant to be expansive in nature rather than limited to individual components or practices.[22]

Even though various models differ, Mary Jane Koren identifies some unifying features within models that comprehensively integrate culture change, including 1) individualizing care; 2) creating homelike environments; 3) promoting close relationships among staff, residents, families, and communities; 4) empowering staff to respond to resident needs and work collaboratively with management to make decisions about care; and 5) improving quality continuously.[23] She also describes how these five critical features translate into practice.[24]

Traditional nursing home care thwarts resident autonomy and decision-making. Conversely, individualized care supports elders as they make decisions every day about their lives and care. Residents direct all care and services offered by the home as much as possible.[25] Nursing home systems and practices concerning food delivery, medication administration, bathing, sleep, incontinence management, and so forth are transformed to be more flexible to accommodate choice and an individualized experience.[26]

Culture change in long-term care seeks to transform institutionalized settings from hospital like environments to homelike environments.[27] Some nursing homes have moved to smaller living environments, called "households" or "neighborhoods," where a small number of residents live. These spaces contain smaller living rooms and kitchens, where institutional markers such as overhead paging and medical carts are eliminated.[28] These smaller settings lend themselves well to the next key feature of culture change in long-term care, the development of close relationships. This practice is often called "consistent assignment," where nurse aids consistently work with the same residents to foster familiarity and caring.[29]

To truly support resident decision-making, care staff such as nurse aides must have the ability to respond to residents without running decisions through the chain of command. Therefore, culture change aims to flatten the nursing home hierarchy and encourage high levels of engagement throughout all levels of the organization.[30] Through this process, nurse aides are empowered with decision making authority, thus allowing them to respond at the bedside to resident needs.[31]

Quality excellence is highly valued within culture change in long-term care; thus, continuous quality improvement processes are essential to the adoption of culture change practices. Strong quality improvement processes, which incorporate tracking and measurement of outcomes, are essential in capturing the impact of culture change on organizations adopting it.[32]

Deep organizational change is necessary for realizing culture change in long-term care and requires extensive reconceptualization of the structure, roles, and processes of care to transform nursing homes from health care institutions to person-centered homes.[33] Person-centered (or person-directed) care is a bedrock principle of the culture change movement, and the term is often used interchangeably with the term "culture change." According to the Pioneer Network, person-directed values include patient/resident choice, dignity, respect, self-determination, and purposeful living.[34]

To achieve deep organizational change in nursing homes, the culture must change, hence the term "culture change." Edgar Schein studies culture in a context broader than long-term care and contends that there are three levels of culture: 1) artifacts, 2) espoused beliefs and values, and 3) basic underlying assumptions.[35] Artifacts are the most superficial level of culture, representing visible and felt structures and processes and observed behavior.[36] These might include objects, structures, programs, materials, and advertising. Often the artifacts are what homes concentrate on changing first because they are tangible; however, homes that do not go past this level of culture do not experience deep organizational culture change. Organizations must go into the other two levels of culture: espoused beliefs and values, which are a person's sense of "what ought to be, as distinct from what is,"[37] and basic underlying assumptions, which are things within an organization that "become so taken for granted that [one finds] little variation within a social unit."[38] A home that has comprehensively adopted culture change has addressed all three levels of culture.

B. National Implementation

Although culture change has become widely accepted as a best practice and is even supported by national policies such as OBRA '87 and other new legislation such as the Affordable

Care Act of 2010,[39] implementation has been slow. A 2007 Commonwealth Fund study surveyed nursing directors in 1,435 nursing homes. The directors were asked whether their homes had adopted 1) practices that make care more resident-directed, 2) a work environment with decentralized decision-making, and 3) a physical environment that is more homelike.[40] Only 5 percent of nursing directors indicated that their homes comprehensively met the description of a culture changed home.[41] Approximately one-third reported adoption of some culture change practices and another third indicated that they were planning to begin adopting such practices, leaving approximately one-third of nursing directors indicating no current or future adoption of culture change practices.[42] Susan Miller and colleagues conducted a similar study, finding a slight increase in culture change adoption, with 13 percent of directors of nursing in 2009 and 2010 reporting that culture change had "completely changed the way they care for residents" in all areas of the home[43] compared with 5 percent in the 2007 Commonwealth Fund study.[44]

Though implementation of person-centered care is not yet widespread, recent policy continues to push for implementation. The Affordable Care Act calls for transformation of both institutional and community-based long-term care services and supports into a more patient-centered system.[45] In July 2015 the U.S. Department of Health and Human Services (HHS), Centers for Medicare & Medicaid Services (CMS), released proposed regulation changes for nursing homes. The proposed regulation changes include multiple person-centered directives and comprehensive person-centered care planning.[46]

Despite the significant need for culture change in nursing homes, why has its adoption been underwhelming? A literature review reveals several reasons, including the lack of evidence-based outcomes of culture change, the increasing health complexity of elders now living in nursing homes, high turnover rates and staffing shortages, the regulatory environment, and the reality that organizational change is difficult.

A 2014 study by Shier and colleagues underscores the lack of empirical evidence that culture change efforts produce positive outcomes.[47] A recent comprehensive literature review concluded that studying culture change is challenging for two important reasons: 1) culture change has remained amorphous in its definition and currently lacks a solid framework for understanding and 2) multiple methodological dilemmas exist in setting up studies in nursing homes related to culture change implementation.[48] A knowledge base and outcomes are critical in pushing homes to adopt culture change. As Shier and colleagues point out:

> Nursing homes considering change need evidence-based guidance in how to invest scarce resources and operationalize culture change; residents and families need

guidance for selection decisions; and fiduciaries need evidence-based metrics for recognizing and promoting best practices through policy, public reporting, and reimbursement.[49]

Shier and colleagues also call for more studies employing quasi-experimental design that follow nursing homes over time and include a strong analytical framework for conceptualizing culture change in practice.[50]

Numerous studies have noted that nursing home residents have become more acutely impaired over the past 30 years.[51] Hospitals are increasingly pressured to move people out quickly, and nursing homes are now serving elders with these acute needs.[52] The increasing complexity of the care needed by residents, which results in increased demands on staff time and skills, and the decreased ability of increasingly impaired residents to actively direct their care contributes to slow integration of culture change. This evolution in the field means that organizations must equip their staffs differently to deal with these demands and that budgets are constrained further as nursing homes provide more services without reimbursement.

Staff turnover in nursing homes also has been an issue for years, with nurse aide turnover especially high.[53] One study found that the average yearly turnover rate for nurse aides was more than 100 percent in many nursing homes.[54] High turnover compromises relationship development, which is critical to the delivery of individualized care, and thus undermines an organization's ability to implement culture change. In addition, training is paramount to a staff's ability to deliver person-centered care, and the continuous training of new workers necessitated by high turnover is expensive and difficult to maintain. Another concern is the scarcity of specialized staff in the health care field in general, such as licensed practical nurses and registered nurses, which poses further challenges to the culture change movement. [55] To enable organizations to deliver person-centered care, specialized staff, especially nurses, is essential. Lacking such staff, organizations are ill-equipped to implement culture change. There is promise that turnover rates in nursing homes that have implemented culture change will decrease.[56]

Although federal regulations and policies demonstrate support for person-centered care, an underlying gap exists between these regulations and policies and putting person-centered care into practice. The primary problem, nationally, lies in the different and sometimes conflicting regulatory requirements nursing homes must navigate. One source of regulations, CMS, is responsible for producing and maintaining federal regulations for all nursing homes certified to accept Medicare and Medicaid residents.[57] CMS regional offices hold state agencies accountable for enforcement of the federal regulations. In addition, each state has its own nursing home licensing requirements that must parallel, yet are allowed to exceed, federal requirements. Further complicating matters, states have different approaches to licensing, the survey and inspection process, the investigation of complaints, and the identification and enforcement of deficiencies.[58] Consequently, navigating regulations while implementing culture change is extremely complicated. This hybrid regulatory scheme leaves less time and energy to devote to care and to the implementation of culture change. Though challenges exist, various stakeholders vested in culture change have met with federal regulators to work through the barriers.[59]

A final reason culture change has not been widely adopted is the reality that deep, meaningful organizational change is hard work and takes time.[60] W. Warner Burke contends that one of the major hurdles to large-scale organizational change is limited knowledge on how to plan and implement the change.[61] Continued research focused on the process nursing homes undertake to implement person-centered care[62] could yield a body of much needed knowledge, including best practices and implementation strategies that are effective in helping nursing homes implement culture change and avoid costly mistakes. Instead of leaving them to determine how to implement culture change on their own, nursing homes could also benefit from receiving additional support and tools.

C. Incentives for Implementation

Because nursing home quality has historically been lacking, some states use pay-for-performance (P4P) or value-based purchasing models to incent nursing homes to improve their quality. Rather than paying nursing homes for the quantity of services delivered, P4P or value-based purchasing models reimburse nursing homes based on the quality of care they deliver.[63] To evaluate quality and performance, states implementing P4P or value-based purchasing must evaluate homes against specified metrics.[64] In the initial six states that implemented P4P or value-based purchasing, evaluation of quality included measures related to staffing, nursing home inspection outcomes, clinical quality indicators, resident quality of life, and customer satisfaction.[65] Medicaid is a primary payer of all bed days in nursing homes (51 percent);[66] therefore, incentive payments through the Medicaid reimbursement program may be a promising way to encourage nursing homes to improve quality, including the quality of life for residents.

By 2010, 14 states had implemented or planned to implement P4P models.[67] The incentive payments in these states are based on a wide variety of measures, including "staffing, regulatory deficiencies, resident satisfaction, and clinical quality" as well as less standard measures such as "occupancy, efficiency, Medicaid use, and culture change."[68] At the time of the study, only two states, Colorado and Oklahoma, had P4P incentives specifically for culture change.[69] In March 2015, 65 state policymakers, long-term care researchers, and other stakeholders met to share information on state initiatives related to P4P or value-based purchasing. The conference, sponsored by the Minnesota Department of Human Services, Purdue University School of Nursing, and University of Minnesota School of Nursing, was supported by a grant from the HHS Agency for Healthcare Research and Quality. At this conference, representatives from Kansas, Utah, and Ohio reported including culture change components in their P4P models. These three states joined Colorado and Oklahoma in incenting culture change. Minnesota's Performance-Based Incentive Payment Program does not specifically target culture change efforts; however, facility proposals may include actions conducive to culture change implementation.[70]

Susan Miller and colleagues found that states with P4P reimbursement models that incent culture change seemed to have higher levels of culture change adoption than states without these incentives.[71] The authors also found that nursing homes in states with P4Ps that incent culture change scored higher across all practice domains investigated, including the physical environment, staff empowerment, and resident choice and decision-making, which are indicators of person-centered care.[72] This demonstrates the potential for P4P policies to promote the positive qualities of culture change regardless of nursing homes' motivation to adopt the practices associated with culture change.

Although several states are moving to P4P models and some states incent culture change specifically, states vary significantly in how this done. Some states incent quality by tying reimbursement dollars to the inputs of producing high-quality care while others pay homes once outcomes are produced.[73] This means that some states increase payments when a home engages in the process of implementing change while others increase payments once changes are in place and outcomes are demonstrated. The resulting question, then, is: Which approach is more effective in producing quality outcomes?

The measurement of quality resulting from various qualifying implementations (each state has different specifications about what qualifies for payment) under different state P4P programs has not been studied. More studies are needed to understand how process and outcome incentives impact quality improvement in nursing homes. Studies such as these will be complicated by the absence of well-established culture change outcomes, which are outlined earlier in this article. Thus, it is important to move forward with establishing valid culture change outcomes before wide adoption of outcome-based P4P

models takes place. Establishing uniform, valid culture change outcomes for nursing homes will help ensure that actual culture change is being encouraged through incentives.

IV. Conclusions and Future Directions

Culture change has been shown to be a positive approach to improving the quality of life of elders living in nursing homes. Much anecdotal evidence supports this conclusion, such as stories from providers, residents, and families; however, there is little empirical evidence that culture change produces better clinical outcomes than other models of care. Lack of empirical evidence may be related to the methodological challenges of studying a concept as complex as culture change and organizations as complex as nursing homes. Methodological challenges are likely to lessen as more nursing homes implement culture change and more efforts are made to operationalize culture change.

In addition, P4P reimbursement models show promise for incenting adoption of culture change in the states that have pursued this approach. As more states consider this approach for encouraging homes to adopt culture change, some fundamental questions must be answered by research, such as the following: a) Do extrinsic motivations such as financial reimbursement motivate the deep organizational change necessary to cause a nursing facility to adopt, implement, and maintain culture change? b) Are P4P models truly incenting higher quality? It is important to address these questions and those noted earlier in this article as more states become interested in implementing P4P programs.

The historically poor quality of care in nursing homes is improving, but improvements in quality of life have fallen behind.[74] Our population is growing at the fastest rate in history; therefore, as Bill Thomas believes, it is time to abolish the traditional nursing home and innovate new models of care.[75] Culture change holds much promise for improving the quality of life for elders in nursing homes. There is no time like the present to advocate for more provider and consumer interest in culture change as well as further research to add to the empirical evidence for culture change.

1. *Nancy Hooyman et al., Aging Matters: An Introduction to Social Gerontology 11 (Pearson 2015).*

2. Gary S. Winzelberg, *The Quest for Nursing Home Quality: Learning History's Lessons*, 163(21) Archives Internal Med. 2552, 2552 (2003).

3. Thomas J. Mattimore et al., *Surrogate and Physician Understanding of Patients' Preferences for Living Permanently in a Nursing Home*, 45(7) J. Am. Geriatrics Socy. 818, 820 (1997).

4. U.S. Dept. of Health & Human Servs., *Long-Term Care Providers and Services Users in the United States: Data*

From the National Study of Long-Term Care Providers 105, Table 4 (2016).

5. Susan M. Hillier & Georgia M. Barrow, *Aging, the Individual, and Society* 291 (10th ed., Wadsworth Cengage Learning 2015).

6. Erving Goffman, *Asylums* xiii (Aldine Publg Co. 1961).

7. *See generally* Bill Thomas, Changing Aging With Dr. Bill Thomas, *The Culture Change Movement Is Over*, http://changingaging.org/blog/the-culture-change-movement-is-over (Jan. 27, 2015) and *The Way of the Tiger*, http://changingaging.org/blog/the-way-of-the-tiger (Feb. 2, 2015).

8. *Homes on the Range: The New Pioneers*, PBS documentary (Dale Bell 2014).

9. *See generally* Victoria Shier et al., *What Does the Evidence Really Say About Culture Change in Nursing Homes?* 54(Supp. 1) Gerontologist S6 (2014).

10. Michael B. Katz, *Poorhouses and the Origins of the Public Old Age Home,* 62(1) Milbank Meml. Fund Q.: Health & Socy. 110, 132 (1984).

11. Winzelberg, *supra* n. 2, at 2552–2553.

12. *Id.* at 2553.

13. Catherine Hawes et al., *The OBRA-87 Nursing Home Regulations and Implementation of the Resident Assessment Instrument: Effects on Process Quality,* 45(8) J. Am. Geriatrics Socy. 977, 978 (1997).

14. *See generally* Omnibus Budget Reconciliation Act of 1987, Pub. L. No. 100-203, 101 Stat. 1330, Subtitle C: Nursing Home Reform (1987).

15. Sara Hunt, *Residents' Rights: Curriculum Resource Material for Local Long-Term Care Ombudsmen* 9–10 (National Long-Term Care Ombudsman Resource Center 2005).

16. Hawes, *supra* n. 13, at 981–983.

17. Rosalie A. Kane, *Long-Term Care and a Good Quality of Life: Bringing Them Closer Together,* 41(3) Gerontologist 293, 296 (2001).

18. David C. Grabowski et al., *Who Are the Innovators? Nursing Homes Implementing Culture Change,* 54(Supp. 1) Gerontologist S65, S65 (2014).

19. Christine E. Bishop & Robyn Stone, *Implications for Policy: The Nursing Home as Least Restrictive Setting,* 54(Supp. 1) Gerontologist S98, S100–S101 (2014).

20. Audrey S. Weiner & Judah L. Ronch, *Models and Pathways for Person-Centered Elder Care* 15–16 (Health Professionals Press 2014).

21. Nikki L. Hill et al., *Culture Change Models and Resident Health Outcomes in Long-Term Care,* 43(1) J. Nursing Scholarship 30, 30–31 (2011).

22. Sheryl Zimmerman et al., *Transforming Nursing Home Culture: Evidence for Practice and Policy,* 54 (Supp. 1) Gerontologist S1, S3 (2014).

23. Mary Jane Koren, *Person-Centered Care for Nursing Home Residents: The Culture-Change Movement,* 29(2) Health Affairs 312, 313-314 (2010).

24. *Id.*

25. *Id.* at 313.

26. *See generally* Kan. Dept. for Aging & Disability Servs. & Kan. St. U. *PEAK 2.0 Criteria 2015–2016,* http://www.he.k-state.edu/aging/outreach/peak20/2015-16/peak-criteria.pdf (accessed Apr. 2016).

27. Margaret P. Calkins, *Creating Home in a Nursing Home: Fantasy or Reality?* 1, https://www.pioneernetwork.net/Data/Documents/Calkins-Fantasy-or-Reality-Paper.pdf, (accessed Apr. 2016).

28. Koren, *supra* n. 23, at 313.

29. *Id.*

30. *Id.*

31. *Id.*

32. *Id.* at 314.

33. David C. Grabowski et al., *Culture Change and Nursing Home Quality of Care,* 54 (Supp.1) Gerontologist S35, S35 (2014).

34. Pioneer Network, *Introduction,* http://www.pioneernetwork.net/Consumers (accessed Apr.2016).

35. Edgar H. Schein, *Organizational Culture and Leadership* 26 (3rd ed., John Wiley & Sons 2004).

36. *Id.* at 25–26.

37. *Id.* at 25.

38. *Id.* at 28.

39. Patient Protection and Affordable Care Act, Pub. L. No. 111-148, 124 Stat. 119 (2010).

40. Michelle M. Doty et al., *Culture Change in Nursing Homes: How Far Have We Come? Findings From The Commonwealth Fund 2007 National Survey of Nursing Homes* vi, The Commonwealth Fund, Pub. No. 1131, http://www.commonwealthfund.org/usr_doc/Doty_culturechangenursinghomes_1131.pdf (May 2008).

41. *Id.* at viii.

42. *Id.*

43. Susan C. Miller et al., *Culture Change Practice in U.S. Nursing Homes: Prevalence and Variation by State Medicaid Reimbursement Policies,* 54(3) Gerontologist 434, 439 (2014).

44. Doty et al., *supra* n. 40, at viii.

45. 124 Stat. 119.

46. *Medicare and Medicaid Programs; Reform of Requirements for Long-Term Care Facilities, 2. Summary of the Major Provisions,* Federal Register, https://www.federalregister.gov/articles/2015/07/16/2015-17207/medicare-and-medicaid-programs-reform-of-requirements-for-long-term-care-facilities#h-13 (July 16, 2015)

47. Shier et al., *supra* n. 9, at S7.

48. Zimmerman et al., *supra* n. 22.

49. Shier et al., *supra* n. 9, at S7.

50. *Id.* at S14–S15.

51. David C. Grabowski, *The Economic Implications of Case-Mix Medicaid Reimbursement for Nursing Home Care,* 39(3) Inquiry 258, 259 (2002).

52. Vincent Mor et al., *Changes in the Quality of Nursing Homes in the US: A Review and Data Update,* http://citeseerx.ist.psu.edu/viewdoc/download?doi=10.1.1.516.5718&rep=rep1& type=pdf (Aug. 15, 2009).

53. Nicholas G. Castle et al., *Nursing Home Staff Turnover: Impact on Nursing Home Compare Quality Measures,* 47(5) Gerontologist 650, 650 (2007)

54. *Id.*

55. Peter McMenamin, American Association of Nurses, *RN Retirements—Tsuanami Warning!,* http://www.ananursespace.org/browse/blogs/blogviewer?BlogKey=398c2049-1b0d-405e-b065-0b0cea4eec59&ssopc=1 (Mar. 14, 2014.

56. Pioneer Network, *Positive Outcomes of Culture Change: Staffing,* http://www.pioneernetwork.net/Providers/Case/Staffing (accessed Apr. 2016).

57. Kieran Walshe, *Regulating U.S. Nursing Homes: Are We Learning From Experience?* 20(6) Health Affairs 128, 130 (2001).

58. *Id.* at 131.

59. Pioneer Network, *Federal Policy and Regulation,* http://www.pioneernetwork.net/Policy/Federal (accessed Apr. 2016).

60. W. Warner Burke, *Organizational Change: Theory and Practice* 9–10 (4th ed., Sage Publications 2014).

61. *Id.*

62. Shier et al., *supra* n. 9, at S15.

63. Rachel M. Werner et al., *State Adoption of Nursing Home Pay-for-Performance,* 67(3) Med. Care Research & Rev. 364, 364 (2010).

64. Greg Arling et al., *Medicaid Nursing Home Pay for Performance: Where Do We Stand?* 49(5) Gerontologist 587, 589 (2009).

65. *Id.* The initial states that implemented payfor-performance or value-based purchasing are Georgia, Iowa, Kansas, Minnesota, Ohio, and Oklahoma.

66. Erica Reaves & MaryBeth Musumeci, *Medicaid and Long-Term Care Services and Supports* 4 (Kaiser Fam. Found. 2007).

67. Werner et al., *supra* n. 63, at 367. States with pay-for-performance programs were Colorado, Georgia, Iowa, Kansas, Minnesota, Ohio, Oklahoma, Utah, and Vermont. States with planned pay-for-performance programs were Arizona, Indiana, Maryland, Texas, and Virginia.

68. *Id.*

69. *Id.*

70. *See generally* Valerie Cooke et al., *Minnesota's Nursing Facility Performance-Based Incentive Payment Program: An Innovative Model for Promoting Care Quality,* 50(4) Gerontologist 556 (2010).

71. Miller et al., *supra* n. 43, at 440.

72. *Id.*

73. Werner et al., *supra* n. 63, at 373.

74. *See generally* Katz, *supra* n. 10.

75. *See generally* Thomas, *supra* n. 7.

Critical Thinking

1. How does the culture-change movement increase the quality of life of residents?

2. Do you think there are other reasons that nursing home directors have not adopted culture change?

Internet References

The Commonwealth Fund
   https://www.commonwealthfund.org/

The National Long-Term Care Ombudsman Resource Center
   http://ltcombudsman.org/

Laci Cornelison is a Licensed Baccalaureate Social Worker (LBSW) and a Licensed Adult Care Home Administrator (LACHA). She holds a master's degree in gerontology.

Unit 8

UNIT

Prepared by: Elaina Osterbur, *Saint Louis University*

Social Policies, Programs, and Services for Older Americans

It is a political reality that older Americans will be able to obtain needed assistance from governmental programs only if they are perceived as politically powerful. Political involvement can range from holding and expressing political opinions, voting in elections, participating in voluntary associations to help elect a candidate or party, and holding political office.

Research indicates that older people are just as likely as any other age group to hold political opinions, are more likely than younger people to vote in an election, are about equally divided between Democrats and Republicans, and are more likely than young people to hold political office. Older people, however, have shown little inclination to vote as a bloc on issues affecting their welfare despite encouragement to do so by senior activists, such as Maggie Kuhn and the leaders of the Gray Panthers. Gerontologists have observed that a major factor contributing to the increased push for government services for elderly individuals has been the publicity about their plight generated by such groups as the National Council of Senior Citizens and the American Association of Retired Persons. The desire of adult children to shift the financial burden of aged parents from themselves onto the government has further contributed to the demand for services for people who are elderly. The resulting widespread support for such programs has almost guaranteed their passage in Congress.

Now, for the first time, groups that oppose increases in spending for services for older Americans are emerging. Requesting generational equity, some politically active groups argue that the federal government is spending so much on older Americans that it is depriving younger age groups of needed services. The articles in this section offer solutions that put a twist on traditional services that can also save funding and increase quality-of-life among older adults. Further articles focus on end-of-life care policies and advance directives.

Article   Prepared by: Elaina Osterbur, *Saint Louis University*

iHubs: A Community Solution to Aging in Place

A new collaborative spurs a creative intergenerational strategy to address the unique needs of Colorado Springs' growing elder community.

BETH ROALSTAD

Learning Outcomes

After reading this article, you will be able to:

- Identify the concept of iHub.
- Discuss the benefits of iHubs.

Russ wants someone to pay attention to his complaint of an earache that has been going on for two years. Whenever he goes to the doctor, he says, they concentrate solely on his arrhythmia and cardiac health. Delores wants a cooking and nutrition class to help her cope with her newly diagnosed diabetes. Mary wants a place to go to converse with neighbors after having her Golden Circle subsidized meal.

All of these requests and others could be more easily met when the Innovations in Aging Collaborative is able to train its local community centers to create intergenerational hubs, or iHubs, that would be situated just blocks from older adults' homes, to better serve the needs of people like Russ, Delores, and Mary.

The iHub concept involves an intergenerational social gathering place focused on older adults living in a particular area of the community, but also attracting people of all ages. iHubs could be established in existing community centers or other facilities and cultural centers that also support the needs of elders.

A Young Nonprofit Tackles Aging

The Innovations in Aging Collaborative, a new nonprofit organization in Colorado Springs, Colorado, about an hour south of Denver, started out in 2008 as a volunteer effort to identify challenges and opportunities arising with Colorado Springs' rapidly growing aging population. Incorporated in December 2012, Innovations hired its first staff member and embarked upon goals set forth by community stakeholders. Our board of directors comes from multiple sectors: business leaders, the public library system, higher education, healthcare, gerontology, neighborhood leaders, and senior service organizations. Innovations' mission is to convene the community to promote creative approaches to address the challenges and opportunities of aging.

Stakeholders as well as older adults who have participated in conversations with Innovations over the past five years stressed a preference for collaboration rather than launching a new infrastructure, and they asked us to organize resources through private partnerships, public policy, and citizen efforts. They also recognized that leveraging existing resources was going to be important to the success of iHub: creating a new program requiring large investments from funders was not going to work in a community with more than 2,000 registered public charities (Summit Economics, 2013).

Aging in Colorado Springs

Colorado Springs lies at the foot of Pikes Peak, at 6,010 feet above sea level. A beautiful city that blends an urban atmosphere with quick access to mountain recreation, Colorado Springs now is facing a "silver tsunami" as is the rest of the nation, but has unique challenges. Colorado long has been a state with a young population, but between 2000 and 2010, its ages 55 to 64 group increased by an annual average of 6.1 percent, compared to a total population increase of 1.7 percent.

According to the 2010 census, Colorado Springs' El Paso County had an older-than-age-65 population of approximately 62,000. By 2020, this will double; and by 2030, the older adult population will nearly triple to 172,394, with the general population at 981,394 (Adams, 2011).

The Colorado Springs community is geographically large, making access to and delivery of services difficult. Transportation for those with mobility barriers is a huge problem—both for people who do not own (or who cannot afford) a car and for elders dependent upon public or specialized transportation. The 2013 and 2011 *Quality of Life Indicators* reports pointed out that 42 percent of our community elders experienced a transportation barrier when engaging in activities such as buying groceries and filling prescriptions, going to medical appointments, and participating in social activities (Pikes Peak United Way, 2011, 2013). Another challenge for Colorado Springs (and Colorado in general) is the low numbers of physicians, specialists, and psychiatrists for a population the size of our community (Adams, 2011).

iHubs Get Rolling

Innovations in Aging believes that a successful community integrates and involves all of its residents. To that end, we are promoting the concept of iHubs inside existing community centers and natural gathering places to support aging in place. We have hosted two significant community events, bringing together a cross section of human service professionals, nonprofit leaders, government officials, business leaders, artists, and retirees to create an open dialog to address the issues, but also to identify potential solutions to support older adults' ability to age in place. Innovations hopes to create an intimate neighborhood model to cope with challenges such as transportation, and to have easy access to wellness, fitness, arts, culture, and education programs close to home for elders aging in place.

We currently are working, with the help of our volunteer teams, through community centers to reach out to several hundred neighborhood residents to gather input and co-create programs in their community centers that meet their needs and evolve to meet the changing needs of their neighbors. For example, hosting a semi-regular veterinarian services clinic for elders' pets; launching new community-based classes from the local community college; and bringing the experience of an art gallery to the community centers through classes taught by local artists. Innovations identified certain Colorado Springs community centers as the first potential partners for collaborating to design a neighborhood-based iHub; we considered four centers, an alternative facility in a neighborhood lacking a senior center, and a virtual hub. In the end, we selected the Westside Community Center to partner with because of its internal capacity and enthusiastic leadership.

Innovations began the program at Westside with surveys, interviews, and focus groups. The goal is to gather data for two months; evaluate current programs; identify potential gaps and opportunities; invite new collaborators; implement programs; and evaluate progress at ninety days and six months. We are working with the community center to invite elders in the neighborhood to participate in surveys and focus groups. This will help the community center in its short-term and long-term planning.

The Westside Community Center is evaluating its existing programs. So far, the feedback has been very informative. We have talked about the need for transportation and medical care, but also basic concerns around home safety and maintenance. The needs are great, and our challenge will be to connect older adults to existing service providers and trustworthy enterprises to meet them all.

Russ, Delores, and Mary participated in one of our focus groups as a part of Innovations' community outreach. Many participants want to remain in their homes as long as possible and to be connected to neighbors of all ages. The group is outspoken, well-connected, and fiercely independent; 75 percent drove themselves to lunch the day of the interview, and the average age in the room was seventy eight. Innovations looks forward to engaging with more elders like these and continuing to solicit their input to shape a community action plan.

An Involved Community Can Realize the iHub Vision

We envision our city and county having several iHubs in formal community centers, but also in libraries, fitness centers, and perhaps in residential housing complexes. We need continued involvement from all levels of our community to achieve this goal—from the mayor to the children who will participate in cooking classes with people like Delores. The greater involvement and engagement of people of all ages will create a community that will be able to care for all of its citizens. This goal is lofty, but seems achievable, given the level of interest in iHubs.

References

Adams, T. H. 2011. *Aging in El Paso County.* A report compiled for Innovations in Aging Collaborative. www.innovationsinaging.org/Resources/2011+Innovations+in+Aging+Collaboration+Report-26.html. Retrieved October 4, 2013.

Pikes Peak United Way.org. 2011. *Quality of Life Indicators Report.* www.ppunitedway.org/ourimpact/qli. Retrieved October 4, 2013.

Pikes Peak United Way.org. 2013. *Quality of Life Indicators Report.* www.ppunitedway.org/ourimpact/qli. Retrieved October 4, 2013.

Summit Economics. 2013. *Nonprofits Matter: An Economic Force for Vibrant Community.* A report compiled for the Center for Nonprofit Excellence. www.cnecoloradosprings.org. Retrieved October 4, 2013.

Critical Thinking

1. What makes iHubs different from many of the programs that senior centers and agencies offer?

2. What are the benefits of offering in iHubs in libraries, fitness centers, and communties centers?

3. Describe other ventures or iHub opportunities that could benefit your community.

Internet References

American Society on Aging
http://www.asaging.org
Innovations in Aging Collaborative
http://www.innovationsinaging.org/index.php/outreach

BETH ROALSTAD, MSW, is the executive director of the Innovations in Aging Collaborative in Colorado Springs, Colorado.

Article Prepared by: Elaina Osterbur, *Saint Louis University*

How to Save Social Security While Reducing the Deficit

Alexander Chaconas

Learning Outcomes

After reading this article, you will be able to:

- Explain the strategies to save social security.
- Identify strategies to reduce the deficit.

Last week, Rep. Mark Walker (R-NC), Chair of the House Republican Study Committee, warned that if lawmakers do not deal with the depletion of Social Security trust funds, "the program will not exist in 12 years." Despite such warnings, plus a large impending budget deficit due to the recent tax cuts and a newly proposed $4.4 trillion budget, Republicans have been proposing ineffective entitlement reforms that fail to address the Social Security crisis.

Last month, Paul Ryan proposed charging wealthier seniors higher Medicare premiums and dissolving the Independent Payment Advisory Board (IPAB), a bloated Medicare cost-cutting organization that has failed in its mission. While both measures could slightly offset burgeoning expenditures, a far more effective measure would be to remove the maximum annual taxable amount for retirement and disability insurance. If it were removed, and benefit calculations remained the same, Social Security trust funds would remain solvent for over 60 years. This would drastically reduce the deficit as well.

Medicare accounts for 3.6 percent of GDP, as of 2016. The main part, Part A, which provides uniform hospital coverage for anyone 65 or older, regardless of income, is funded through a payroll tax of 2.9 percent, half paid by the employer and half by the employee. The smaller parts of Medicare, Parts B (medical coverage) and D (prescription drug coverage), derive around 75 percent of their funding from property and business taxes;

the rest comes mostly from premiums based on beneficiaries' incomes.

Ryan's plan to increase the Part B premiums for wealthier households would barely make a dent in the deficit, since premiums only cover 23 percent of Part B revenue and 13 percent of Part D. Some economists are recommending an increase in the general Medicare payroll tax. But any effectual increase would render the most recent income tax cuts for the middle-class pointless. The focus needs to be placed on retirement insurance benefits.

Retirement insurance benefits, formally known as Old Age and Survivors Insurance (OASI), are the biggest drain on entitlement spending. They account for 4.3 percent of GDP, as of 2017. OASI is funded through a 6.2 percent payroll tax on both employees and employers. But, in contrast to Medicare, there is a taxable income limit. Anyone at least 62 years old can receive pensions, regardless of income, as long as he or she has earned a minimum of 40 Social Security credits, equating to 10 years of earned income. Earned income is income generated through wages or salaries. It does not include investment income, which is generated through passive business activities, such as interest, dividends, and stocks.

The benefits a person receives at retirement are based on average indexed monthly earnings (AIME): The earned annual incomes of up to 35 of the person's highest earning years are averaged, adjusted for inflation, and divided by 12, in order to calculate a monthly earnings average. Then, AIME is incorporated into a formula that determines monthly benefits for retirement. The higher the AIME, the more benefits received. In order to qualify for the max monthly benefit of $2,687, individuals retiring at 65 must have earned an annual income at or above the maximum taxable amount for every single year of their career, up to 35 years. This number is $128,400 in 2018. (A list of historical maximums can be found here.)

Most households in the highest quintile income bracket, which in 2015 included those making $202,366 or more, qualify for the maximum amount of $2,687 in monthly retirement benefits. Historically, enough of their AIME amount has come from earned income. Not only are higher earners, including millionaires and billionaires, only taxed on the yearly income-based limit, but they also needlessly receive these benefits after retirement.

It is vitally important to remove this yearly income-based tax limit. Imposing a 6.2 percent payroll tax on the full income of those that earn above the limit might seem unjust, given that they won't see increased benefits. But it would help balance the budget and guarantee the continued existence of Social Security for the low- and middle-income households that actually need it.

Critical Thinking

1. What are your thoughts regarding taxes and entitlement?
2. The author speaks of justice as it relates to increasing payroll tax on high earners to balance the budget and support Social Security, do you agree with the author?

Internet References

AARP

https://www.AARP.org/

Real Clear Policy

https://www.realclearpolicy.com/

ALEXANDER CHACONAS is an advocate for Young Voices and a journalist residing in Arlington, Virginia. He writes about criminal justice reform, entitlement reform, and culture.

Article   Prepared by: Elaina Osterbur, *Saint Louis University*

What Should Lawyers Know about Advance Directives for Health Care?

A Geriatrician Speaks Out

DANIEL J. BRAUNER

Learning Outcomes

After reading this article, you will be able to:

- Define advance directive terminology.
- Discuss the importance of a durable power of attorney for healthcare.
- Discuss the role of a lawyer in the preparation of advance directives.

A common response from many physicians to the question of what should lawyers know about advance directives for health care would be something along the lines of, "tell your clients to talk with their doctors about it," because creating an advance directive is a medical, not a legal, endeavor. The argument goes, who better to talk with patients about their future treatments than the physicians charged with caring for them during those difficult times? But, despite the move to make creating advance directives an increasingly medical practice, evidenced by the as-yet unsuccessful campaign to make it a billable medical procedure, I hope to show that lawyers still have an important role to play. In my (admittedly minority) opinion, this role involves helping clients understand that choosing a good person to be one's power of attorney for health care should take precedence over signing forms indicating which medical procedures to have or not have in the event of incapacity. The reason is that these forms often do not produce their intended results. Instead, patients can end up being given either too much futile medical intervention or too little beneficial care.

Obtaining an advance directive, which often includes a code status, i.e., a "Do Not Resuscitate" (DNR) versus "Full Code" designation, is becoming a routine part of being admitted to most hospitals, especially for older and gravely ill patients, and especially now that patients are increasingly cared for by hospitalists who have not previously known the patients. This trend is encouraged by the Patient Self-Determination Act, which requires that patients be asked about advance directives upon admission to a hospital. The presence of an advance directive has become an indicator for quality of care by accrediting institutions such as The Joint Commission (formerly known as the Joint Commission on Accreditation of Healthcare Organizations) and has spurred the increase in use of advance directives.

For physicians, obtaining a patient's advance directive is largely motivated by a desire to spare the patient from the often futile application of so-called "life-saving" procedures. For many patients, advance directives are seen as a means of liberation from the "tyranny of futile technology" at the end of their lives. Because many patients admitted to hospitals are not in a good position to make decisions, and because they are often taken care of by strangers, there is increasing pressure to obtain advance directives earlier in the course of patients' disease trajectory. In an effort to ensure more patients have advance directives ahead of time, many are now advocating that sooner is better. This belief has entered the realm of popular consciousness, and many older people are anxious to create their advance directives as a means of ensuring optimal care for themselves in the future.

But, despite all of this apparently positive movement toward the increased use of advance directives, the reality is that, despite their directives, many patients continue to receive futile care at the end of their lives that merely prolongs their suffering and dying. Less well-appreciated is the alternative scenario, also not uncommon, in which old and gravely ill patients who have advance directives are not given care that might actually help them. Advance directives may be ambiguous in certain medical situations. DNR orders, for example, may have meanings that go beyond simply not applying CPR. Several studies have shown that "DNR patients" tend to receive less aggressive care in general, sometimes appropriately, but also when they might have benefited from this care and might have wanted to be able to make the choice.

Why should lawyers be interested in advance directives? Given the current situation, you are uniquely situated to act as a positive force to improve the care of gravely ill and dying patients. You are consulted by clients about advance directives and, given that the original advance directives were crafted with legal experts and that their very existence is predicated on legal precedent, it is important for you to understand how and why advance directives currently function—or fail to function—and what you can do to help your clients navigate the difficult terrain of planning for end-of-life care.

The reasons that DNR patients may receive less aggressive care and that advance directives may fail to ensure desired and appropriate care can be better appreciated by taking a brief foray into the history and evolution of resuscitation and the advent of DNR and advance directives. This exploration will also suggest ways of ensuring your clients' intentions are honored when they become patients.

The beginnings of the practice of applying resuscitation to everyone whose heart stops in the hospital can be traced back to the 1950s when the therapy involved open resuscitation, i.e., cracking open the chest and massaging the heart directly. CPR was, at that time, mostly limited to cases of cardiac arrest associated with anesthesia and surgery. However, with the development of the technique of external massage in the 1950s and a 70 percent success rate reported in the first published study in 1960, CPR began to be increasingly practiced outside of the operating room. It was only a few years after the 1960 report that resuscitation in the form of CPR became increasingly widespread in hospitals.

Advance Care Planning Glossary

Advance planning terms are not well-defined. They can vary by state, by hospitals within a state, by form, and by doctor, patient, and lawyer. Clients can look to the National Institute of Aging, www.nia.nih.gov/health/publication/advance-care-planning, for some basic definitions, but they should be forewarned that

these definitions are not always applied consistently. The following offers some guidance.

- **Advance directive:** A legal document expressing your medical care wishes that goes into effect only if you are incapacitated and unable to express them yourself. An advance directive generally contains a "living will" and appoints a person to act as durable power of attorney for health care. "Advance directive" can be understood as the umbrella term for any advance care planning document.
- **Living will:** A type of advance directive addressing medical care preferences during terminal illness. It does not deal with property and is not a will at all.
- **DNR:** A code for a patient's medical chart indicating "do not resuscitate"—do not do anything to restart the heart or lungs once they have ceased. DNR orders are often the main feature of advance directives.
- **No code:** An alternative way of indicating "DNR."
- **Full code:** Do everything possible to revive. The default code that applies when DNR is not specified.
- **Durable power of attorney for health care (DPA):** A legal document naming someone to make medical decisions for you if you are unable to do so. Often contained within an advance directive. Also called a healthcare "proxy," "surrogate," or "agent." Not a power of attorney for anything other than healthcare decisions.

However, with this dramatic change in practice, it became evident that the initial success rates were not reproducible. The vast majority of patients whose hearts stopped could not be brought back with CPR. Reviewing the papers from that era, it becomes clear that the reason for the high success rates in the early studies lay in the very select population of patients receiving CPR. They had mostly suffered from iatrogenic (doctor caused) cardiac arrest from anesthesia and surgery and other procedures such as cardiac catheterization. Despite the extremely poor outcomes of CPR as it became more widespread, especially in patients who were at the end of terminal diseases, a number of forces led to the practice of performing CPR on all patients who developed stoppage of the circulation or cardiac arrest, regardless of whether CPR would help the patient.

It was not until 1974 that the first standardized order for withholding CPR was proposed by the American Heart Association and published in the *Journal of the American Medical Association*. This "Order Not to Resuscitate," which quickly became known as DNR, was first proposed as a doctor-initiated process; there was no mention of discussing it with patients or their families. It was to be used on patients in the final phases of terminal diseases, patients who would clearly not benefit from CPR.

This would change dramatically just two years later and was no doubt influenced by the case of Karen Ann Quinlan, a young woman in a chronic, vegetative state; the New Jersey Supreme Court had ruled that doctors were required to comply with the requests of her parents to withdraw life support, then provided her in the form of mechanical ventilation. This case was precedent-setting because it was the first legally sanctioned removal of life support. It also established the importance of patient preferences, voiced in this case by the patient's surrogates, in determining the application and withdrawal of therapy. It was also responsible for opening public discourse about the treatment of dying patients. Shortly after the case was decided, a series of papers in the *New England Journal of Medicine on* care of dying patients was published along with an editorial titled "Terminating Life Support: Out of the Closet!" In one of the papers, a physician, along with two lawyers, wrote that patients should make the decision about CPR and, if they were unable, family members should make the decision. The President's Commission on Bioethics also supported this idea, and so the first advance directive was established.

Ironically, by forcing patients to opt out in advance, the DNR order sealed the default status of resuscitation by opting everyone else in. It was not long before other life-prolonging procedures, such as artificial nutrition and dialysis, began to be added to advance directive forms. These procedures, too, began to be provided by default. By default, then, a patient without an advance directive was to be evaluated based on very limited sets of considerations without regard for his or her overall condition and prognosis.

The default status of these therapies places pressure on physicians to have their older and sicker patients make choices ahead of time. But this may have unintended consequences.

When I admit one of my older patients to the hospital, one of the first questions the covering medical resident asks me is, "what is their code status?" Given the present state of affairs, this is an excellent question. It signals that the resident is asking whether I have had the "advance directive conversation" and whether the patient wants "aggressive" care or not. That this is all intuited from whether patients are "DNR" or "Full Code" is understandable given the DNR's history as the first advance directive and its use as an identifier of patients who would not benefit from CPR because they are in the final phase of terminal illness. Of course, the residents also want to spare my patients from futile CPR at the end of their lives, and this is a goal that I share. But I am more concerned that patients get the consideration and therapies that might actually help them in the present moment. And so I reply, "that's not the question at hand," and I tell them about the patient and his or her latest problems.

The advance directive has also evolved into another process your clients should understand: the "goals-of-care conversation," which has become an increasingly common one for doctors to have with gravely ill and dying patients and their families. In this conversation, doctors will disclose the gravity of the situation and pose the question, "what are the patient's goals?" This can be a very useful conversation because patients can become fully informed of their prognoses and be given a voice in their care. However, the reality of the conversation is that it often signals a lack of viable medical options besides those to palliate symptoms. Patients are then given the illusion of a choice between aggressive therapy, though none may exist that will help them, or palliative care. If they choose aggressive care, the physicians will attempt to "educate" the patient and family about the problems with that choice. This usually results in patients choosing the palliative approach. If the patient or family insists on the "aggressive" approach, several possible results may ensue. The patient may receive the requested futile therapy. Or, an ethics consult may be requested to help work out an agreeable solution, and/or the doctors will make unilateral decisions based on the futility of the requested aggressive therapy.

In many ways, the goals-of-care conversation and the advance directive from which it evolved can be seen as analogous to buying protection from the mob. Physicians are offering to protect patients from the default, mostly futile, therapies at the end of their lives if they choose to "be DNR" or select nonaggressive care. Although it is good to protect patients from these types of treatments, the price they pay for this protection in many circumstances is to forfeit consideration of potential diagnostic evaluations and therapeutic interventions that may actually help them. This is fine for patients who do not want any more medical interventions, but, in my experience, the vast majority of patients will consider therapies that have a good chance of helping them.

There is always some degree of uncertainty about the outcome of any medical therapy, but thoughtful physicians are able to give some idea of the likelihood of success, which ranges from almost none for CPR from noniatrogenic causes at the end of a terminal disease, to a high likelihood of improvement from, for example, a pacemaker for complete heart blockage. Of course patients always have the right to forego therapy, even if it would help them.

In my opinion, the resuscitation choice should essentially be the last one made after all other therapeutic options and choices are exhausted, so that premature DNR orders and all that these entail can be avoided.

How can lawyers help their clients create optimal advance directives? Clients should be educated about the perils of premature DNR. Even if they think they would not want CPR (a reasonable choice), clients who would want to be considered for the full complement of potential medical therapies should be advised to wait before including a DNR order in an advance directive. The first step in creating an advance directive should be the appointment of a suitable person as a durable power of attorney for health care (DPA). Clients should be encouraged to choose a DPA who will advocate on their behalf when they are unable to do so and who can consult effectively with physicians. Appointing an effective DPA could then obviate the need for an advance DNR order entirely.

The key to choosing an effective DPA is to select someone who is able to engage in decision-making conversations with physicians. The DPA must also be able to understand the degree of impairment the patient is willing to tolerate and the degree, therefore, to which the patient is willing to continue to receive aggressive therapy. Moreover, a client should be encouraged to seek physicians who are able and willing to engage in decision-making conversations and who can be trusted to honestly disclose the chances of therapies really helping all along the course of the client's life.

In sum, I recommend that lawyers advise clients to:

- remain "Full Code," since that status will require doctors to think more about possible diagnostic and treatment options;
- concentrate on choosing a good DPA;
- insist that the DPA be educated about the perils of premature DNR and the necessity of exploring treatment options with physicians;
- discuss with the DPA the conditions under which aggressive care might be stopped and how the resuscitation choice should be the last decision after all other therapeutic options and choices are exhausted.

Lawyers may also wish to reduce their reliance on certain pre-packaged forms and concentrate instead on those that create a durable power of attorney.

A number of the ideas I have discussed here are not mainstream, since most physicians tend to believe in the inherent ethical good of an advance directive and of emphasizing code status. Many will discount the idea that the DNR order adversely affects other care. However, one can hear in the everyday discourse among doctors and read in the empirical outcome studies that the reality is otherwise. Yet many physicians feel that continued education and goals-ofcare conversations will limit the meaning of a DNR order to, "do not perform CPR at the end of life." They believe that the practice of obtaining early DNRs should, therefore, continue.

And so the ideas presented here are not officially sanctioned by any organizations, though I have presented them in papers and symposia of the American Geriatrics Society and the Center for Medical Ethics in Kansas City, as well as in various forums at the University of Chicago, including those of its MacLean Center for Clinical Medical Ethics, of which I am assistant director. Perhaps addressing attorneys and other audiences outside the medical profession will result in wider acceptance of these unorthodox views. In any event, it is important to remember that my goals and those of physicians with more standard views are the same: we all seek to provide effective end-of-life care that both honors the wishes of our patients and recognizes the limits of our therapies.

Critical Thinking

1. What are some of the ethical issues that might arise when preparing advance directives?

2. Discuss state laws that address advance directives.

3. What sort of repercussions might occur in the event the DNR is not honored?

Internet References

American Geriatrics Society
　http://www.americangeriatrics.org/
National Council on Aging
　https://www.ncoa.org/
National Institute on Aging
　https://www.nia.nih.gov/

DANIEL J. BRAUNER, MD, is a geriatrician who develops interdisciplinary approaches to medical and ethical issues affecting the elderly. He also investigates ways of improving communication with persons with dementia and he additionally studies how dementia affects care of nondementia illnesses. He is an associate professor of medicine at the University of Chicago Pritzker School of Medicine, an assistant director of the University of Chicago's MacLean Center for Clinical Medical Ethics, and a medical director of Montgomery Place Health Care Pavilion, a retirement housing and health services facility serving older people on Chicago's South Side.

Article   Prepared by: Elaina Osterbur, *Saint Louis University*

The Aging Network and Long-Term Services and Supports: Synergy or Subordination?

A national aging network is critical to providing consumers access to affordable long-term-care options

ROBERT B. HUDSON

Learning Outcomes

After reading this article, you will be able to:

- Identify long-term services and supports (LTSS).
- Discuss the challenges faced by the Aging Network and LTSS.
- Discuss how the role of the Older Americans Act (OAA) pressures the Aging Network to become involved in LTSS.

The last quarter century or so has seen a remarkable transformation in the world of policy and services regarding aging. Demographically, the older population is itself growing older; economically, much of the older population is at risk for devastating costs associated with chronic illness and disability; and politically, programs supporting long-term services and supports (LTSS) are facing unprecedented budgetary challenges at the federal and state levels. Very much caught up in this convergence is the aging network, born of the Older Americans Act and long closely tied to its objectives, guidelines, and funding. More recent developments, however, have loosened those ties, finding many network agencies—by choice or circumstance—lodged in the large, growing, and more pressured policy world of LTSS.

Network agencies face several dilemmas in this new environment. First, the world of LTSS has long been the most troubled terrain in aging-related policy. Virtually by definition, it addresses the most vulnerable members of the older population; its place in the world of health and social services has never been settled; and few actors have made it their central policy concern. Second, the aging network has always had, and continues to have, responsibilities and identities quite removed from LTSS, identities that have defined its existence and provided much of the basis for its political and budgetary support. Third, and perhaps most fundamental, there continues to be no societal consensus as to which social institutions—the family, government, the private sector—should assume principal responsibility for addressing the nation's LTSS needs.

The more recent political and administrative joining of aging and disability services and supports has further complicated these questions. Together, these elements combine to find today's network—widely redubbed an aging and disability services network—faced with an uncertain mandate to address varied populations and problems without sufficient capacity or authority to meet multiple needs and preferences.

Long-Term Care Services and Supports: A Residual Policy Arena

Until quite recently, the populations of adults needing and using LTSS have had only marginal social visibility and even less political standing. Old age was once considered an illness—and an especially problematic one because little could be done about it (Benjamin, 1993). Moreover, when mental illness was present, "public officials saw no obvious solution to the dilemmas presented by aged senile persons; some proposed that counties or family assume fiscal responsibility . . . and others insisted that sons and daughters be forced by law to meet their responsibilities toward parents" (Grob, 1986).

Persons with disabilities were often viewed yet more critically. Unlike the old, whose birthdate or widowhood could be easily ascertained, "disability has always been more problematic, both because no single condition of 'disability' is universally recognized and because physical disability and mental incapacity are conditions that can be feigned for secondary gain" (Stone, 1984). Erkulwalter [Erkulwater] (2006) expands this understanding, noting that "people in wheelchairs are regarded as the deserving disabled by most Americans, but mental disabilities . . . and chronic pain are poorly understood impairments that elicit as much skepticism as they do empathy."

In the world of LTSS, the long-standing marginal status of the affected individuals has been compounded by the world of public policy often having little interest or understanding of their vulnerabilities. Put differently, locating responsibility for providing LTSS among groups and types of providers has never been definitively resolved. Making those determinations was not nearly as straightforward as providing income through cash or in-kind benefits, or providing acute medical care services through hospitals and allied institutions. Chronic illness involved myriad vulnerabilities, and avoiding responsibility for meeting those needs was long the common practice of a variety of health and social service providers.

In the case of people with disabilities, great emphasis was placed on the establishment of disability, where historically the individual had to assume "the sick role" to which one might be confined for a lifetime and for whom care might be demeaning or intermittent. There was little movement away from this paradigm and toward social reform until the early 1970s, when people with disabilities began pressing for social inclusion. This lack of policy ownership across both populations has long meant "the long-term care individual was *marginal* to the service providers upon which she/he depends" (Callahan, 1981).

More recently, the separate streams of older people demanding community-based LTSS alternatives and people with disabilities demanding independence and choice have helped these populations move toward the center of the health and social policy stage. Both cases involved a two-stage transition wherein long-term care needs moved from being seen as an unfortunate individual condition to being viewed as a social problem in need of community recognition, and, second, from that socially recognized need to being elevated onto the public policy agenda.

LTSS: In Search of a Policy Home

Given the vagaries of population and problem definition, it is not surprising that LTSS policy long found itself lodged almost entirely in the worlds of private charity and public assistance. Much private charity was housed in community hospitals, and early public support was centered in various forms of "indoor relief" (Rothman, 1971). By the time of the New Deal, efforts were being made to move LTSS populations out of institutional settings and somehow ease them into the community. Most notable was Social Security's Old Age Assistance program, a cash benefit that "forbade payments to any inmate of a public institution."

Yet, unsurprisingly, cash proved not enough for many individuals suffering from chronic illness or disability. "Pensions, it turned out, were not a substitute for indoor relief, at least not for the elderly who were infirm as well as poor" (Vladeck, 1980). This led to the first foray of the so-called private sector to enter what is today called LTSS, through the advent of early "mom and pop" nursing homes in which proprietors took in boarders and their Old Age Assistance checks. Some decades later these homes reemerged as the modern nursing home industry.

The continued unwillingness of the public sector to own the LTSS problem was highlighted three decades later by the simultaneous enactment of Medicare and Medicaid. After failures to launch any kind of national health insurance in the Roosevelt and Truman administrations, reformers in the 1960s were determined to see acute hospital and medical care benefits finally become law through the enactment of Medicare. Central to their strategy was to omit all provisions that could detract from this core objective, anything related to LTSS being high on that list (Marmor, 1970).

Medicaid was conceived as a residual healthcare program to address the needs of a classic list of marginal populations—the poor, the chronically ill, and people with disabilities—because attention to these groups could stand in the way of Medicare's focus on a mainstream problem (acute healthcare) and a highly legitimate population ("the elderly"). Speaking of the principal LTSS benefit at the time, Vladeck (1980) pointedly noted that "the nursing home issue was not confronted directly; Medicaid, hastily created and enacted, was only a sideshow in the health insurance circus."

The last major LTSS policy episode occurred through the birth and expansion of the Supplemental Security Income (SSI) program, which federalized public assistance programs for poor elders, blind people, and people with disabilities. Over time, the program has become of special importance to the latter population. Expanding definitions of disability and political advocacy among those populations rendered SSI a major support for the community-based disability community However, as with the earlier Old Age Assistance and Aid to the Permanently and Totally Disabled, SSI involved only cash, not care.

The marginal standing of LTSS is seen most starkly in its long-standing home having been the world of public assistance: Old Age Assistance, Aid to the Permanently and Totally Disabled, Medicaid, and SSI. In these terms, the principal contribution of the stillborn Community Living Assistance Services and Supports Act (CLASS) was to at least momentarily move LTSS into the world of social insurance where it would have joined—albeit on a truncated basis—Old Age, Survivors, Disability Insurance, and Medicare.

The Aging Services Network's Entry into LTSS

The aging network today finds itself in this world where the chronically ill and people with disabilities have been existing in the shadows of social awareness and public policy. The convergence of this problem and this network represents an uneasy fit. The network developed under the auspice of the Older Americans Act (OAA), a piece of legislation marked by broad statements of purpose and miniscule levels of funding. Passed in the wake of Medicare and Medicaid's enactment, the Act was intended to acknowledge the standing and contributions of elders in American life and to provide a variety of supports to the broader older adult population engaged in community living. The legislation also provided grant and contract support to social service providers who had promoted the healthcare laws' enactment, but who wished as well to avail themselves of federal expenditures being directed to America's elders through Lyndon Johnson's Great Society.

Appropriations under the Act increased nearly twentyfold during the 1970s, reaching roughly $1 billion by the end of the decade. The Act's lofty but ambiguous goals in conjunction with these significant revenues brought great attention to how the Administration on Aging and the state and area agencies should prioritize their activities. Should "well elders" be served in the community through senior centers and congregate meal sites? Should efforts concentrate on those with "social and economic needs"? Should special efforts be made on behalf of elders of color? Should the network serve as a watchdog against elder abuse and neglect through establishment of legal services programs? These were among the dominant questions dating to sometime in the mid-1980s.

Important for purposes here, these early arguments were not centrally about elders with chronic illnesses or those who were otherwise frail. Though never explicit, regulatory language tied to the Act continued to emphasize social and economic need, ethnicity, and region—to the considerable

exclusion of questions of health and functional well-being. The first major OAA provision tied centrally to functional impairment was establishment of the in-home nutrition program under the Act's Title III in 1978. As noncontroversial as delivering meals to homebound elders might seem, there was major controversy between the ongoing congregate nutrition sites and the in-home meals program. Two issues were in play: the more elevated and goal-oriented of the two revolved around what was the larger purpose of the Act; the more political one centered on what groups of providers were going to receive services contracts. The passage of time has favored the home-delivered meals option. Grants to the state and area agencies in support of the federal government's nursing home ombudsman program in 1978 also served to extend the network's role into LTSS.

Beyond the confines of the Act, the major initiative opening the LTSS door to the aging network in the 1980s involved waivers to the Medicaid program, which encouraged maintaining chronically ill elders in home and community settings. Up to that point, nearly all functionally and cognitively impaired elders were supported only in nursing homes, publicly financed almost entirely through Medicaid. Subsequent policy developments, both internal and external to the network, have brought it increasingly into the LTSS world. Legislatively, the Americans with Disabilities Act (1990) and the 1999 Supreme Court decision, *Olmstead v. L.C.*, put legal weight behind the community-based preference. In 2005, the Deficit Reduction Act furthered the development and consolidation of home- and community-based services by allowing states to make such services part of their Medicaid plans rather than having to continue working through the cumbersome waiver process.

Within the OAA, inclusion of a Family Support Act gave policy recognition to the role of informal supports in the LTSS world. However, not until Amendments enacted in 2006 did "Congress recognize the role that the aging services network can play in promoting use of home- and community-based long-term care services for people who are at risk for institutional care" (O'Shaughnessy, 2008). A survey of area agencies on aging (AAA), conducted in 2007, found that nearly two-thirds of AAAs responded in the affirmative to the statement: "Our state limits, either through rules or legislation, what our role should be in a long-term care system" (Kunkel and Lackmeyer, 2008).

Today, the widespread place of LTSS in the aging network world is beyond dispute. Partial findings from a follow-up survey of AAAs, conducted by the Scripps Gerontology Center at Miami University of Ohio, makes this role clear: AAAs now receive more than one-fourth of their budgets from Medicaid; more than 70 percent provide, on an optional basis, health services, case management, and care-planning assessment services; 72 percent operate as Aging and Disability Resource Centers, up from only 19 percent in 2008; 70 percent are delivering diversion-from-institution services; and, with 28 State Units on Aging and Disability enrolled in Medicaid managed care systems, 32 percent of AAAs are involved in the planning and implementation of those systems (Kunkel, Reece, and Straker, 2014).

Perhaps the best indicator of the burgeoning LTSS role is the redubbing of the aging network as an aging and disability services network: 73 percent of AAAs now serve consumers younger than age 60 who qualify because of disability, impairment, or chronic illness, with more than one-half of those agencies providing LTSS eligibility assessment, case management, and care-planning assessment.

LTSS, the Aging Network, and the Role of Other Sectors

The rise of LTSS issues in the aging network's world continues unabated. Beyond the immediate developments traced above, the larger policy context is rapidly evolving. The number of likely consumers is continuing to rise—modestly among older adults until the baby boomers attain more advanced ages—but more quickly among people with disabilities. The latter development is a result of the advocacy community's demanding a range of rights and opportunities that the policy community must recognize. At the same time, state budgets are under continuous pressure, with Medicaid now constituting 23 percent of state expenditures and LTSS constituting 30 percent of those outlays. In the face of these pressures, budget officials at both the federal and state levels are demanding new LTSS delivery efficiencies. Incentives—both positive and negative—are contained in the Affordable Care Act, but demands for greater integration, coordination, and management of LTSS have been evolving at the state level for sometime.

A major consequence of these public sector pressures is the creation of new demands on and opportunities for participation of two other societal sectors relevant to LTSS: families and the private sector. The primary role of family care in LTSS has been long known, frequently estimated in the 75 percent to 80 percent range of all care provided. Given the size of the LTSS "market," it has long been anticipated that the private sector would assume a greater role, but the low take-up rate of private LTSS insurance and low Medicaid reimbursement rates have until recently limited that sector's expansion. Yet, newer opportunities, such as the push for efficient and integrated care extending along the healthcare continuum, from acute care through long-term maintenance, provides opportunities for well-resourced private entities to enter or expand in the field.

Family Care and the Aging Network

One of the core concerns of LTSS policy advocates dating back to the 1960s has been to relieve the long-term-care burden on families of long-term-care service provision. Respite care and adult daycare have been two modest efforts in that direction, and the prospect of the CLASS Act, involving insurance protections, was by far the biggest step in that direction. Yet the rise of consumer control and directed care has once again placed family members of frail elders and people with disabilities in the spotlight. The values of autonomy and choice lie behind these efforts, and they are powerful ones. Under emerging arrangements, consumers, rather than formal agencies, can devise care plans and identify providers, who can be family members and who often can be reimbursed for their time and effort with public dollars. Despite concerns among various professional groups and other observers that heightened levels of inappropriate care and outright fraud might soon follow, studies suggest that such a scenario has not emerged as a major issue (Simon-Rusinowitz et al., 2010a; Simon-Rusinowitz, et al., 2010b).

Yet there is a larger concern surrounding this new family role and involvement. The provision of cash, vouchers, technology, and the availability of a range of informal and formal providers make a variety of care choices available to consumers and family members; however, it also saddles them with additional responsibilities. Assuming that the contracted resource levels are sufficient and the underlying diagnoses are accurate, there is much to commend this approach at the delivery level. But front-end assessment and back-end accountability may well be needed to assure appropriate care, and these are initiatives where the availability of the skills and knowledge to be found in the aging network may be under-recognized. Many of these agencies have been very successful at streamlining access and coordinating services, and this is a role they can very usefully continue to play in a consumer-oriented LTSS world.

At the policy level, the question of responsibility is more profound. Provision of a fixed amount of cash or in-kind support to consumers or informal care providers is a form of defined contribution, which, unlike insurance mechanisms—including traditional Medicaid—does not assure a defined benefit. The distinction is important in that in the former model, once a contribution is made, the funder's responsibility ends; in the latter model, cash or care must be provided whatever the cost is, as stipulated by the insurance language. Under such a system in the case of LTSS, financial risk would be shifted from government (largely through open-ended Medicaid funding) to consumers (through vouchers or other capped mechanisms). The concern to be kept in mind is that the consumer choice that families may wish to have should not be confused with the financial risk, which they might well wish to avoid. In short, family choice and responsibility could well emerge as two very different sides of the same policy coin.

The Private Sector and the Aging Network

The historical relationship between the aging network and the private sector has been uneven. On the one hand, legislative language and organizational maintenance concerns have long made the network wary of private sector incursions. OAA strictures and prevailing network values calling for attention to the most vulnerable elders have long left the network little able to prevent private homecare and allied agencies from "cherry-picking" middle- and upper-class elders who could afford to pay privately for care, but the income from whom would have been of great value to the network. Equally galling was these network agencies "losing" clients they had once served as the private sector discovered "gold in gray" (Minkler, 1989).

On the other hand, some network agencies thought they could parlay their efforts with private entities to their mutual advantage. (An attempt by the National Association of Area Agencies on Aging in the 1980s to package a "care management system" to be marketed to the private sector encountered the wrath of the then commissioner on Aging in Washington [Hudson, 1994].) The network's appraisal of major developments in managed and integrated care across the healthcare continuum will be varied. Larger AAAs in states where community-oriented Medicaid waiver programs have long been in place are well-suited to working with private companies that are broadening their scope to include LTSS in the community. They have developed a template for the role, and now need only adjust—not necessarily easily—to a far larger scale of operation. Small AAAs in states with bare bones Medicaid community-based programming will continue to operate on a lesser scale, presumably hoping that providing life-enhancing services for quasi-well elders will allow them to keep their place and standing in the community. Among this population, there are both opportunities and threats as the age-friendly Village Movement and other aging in place initiatives beckon proprietary, as well as public, players.

The private sector's heaviest involvement in the rapidly evolving LTSS world will be around care integration, centered largely on Medicaid programs' increasing demand for client enrollment in managed care programs. The case for private management of these programs lies in some combination of their presumed ability to implement programs more efficiently, their willingness to quite openly be conscious of the bottom line, and reimbursement incentives that may be built into contracts incentivizing them to stay within budgets.

However, missing from how Medicaid managed care will operate in most settings is competition—the ingredient presumed central to the effective functioning of markets and the private sector. On this score, as Nightingale and Pindus (1997) note, the issue is not really public versus private, but rather monopoly versus competition. While the first is most usually associated with the public sector and the second with the private sector, that need not be so in either case. Meaningful competition may well be absent in Medicaid private sector managed care contracts in many parts of the country. As junior partners in these plans as they develop, the network must be on guard that it be neither marginalized nor, more worrisome yet, be scapegoated if referral and screening functions become associated with excessive care on the one hand or insufficient care on the other (Galewitz, 2011).

Conclusion

A final thought ties these developments and dilemmas to the long-standing residual status of LTSS and most of those involved in it. For better or worse, both the emerging aging and now disability network and the private sector's involvement serve to bring LTSS out of the shadows of public assistance. Many network agencies have teamed, at least in small scale, with private companies toward broadening their reach. The OAA and the aging network have assiduously avoided being tied to "welfare" or public assistance, with no mandatory means testing permitted under their auspice. This does not make the OAA a social insurance program akin to Social Security and Medicare, but the Act has spoken of and to elders as a normative community with a set of near-universal needs and abilities. This underlying premise of universality in the context of very limited resources available through the Act has led to some thirty years of struggles around the extent to which OAA benefits should be targeted or delivered on a more inclusive basis. The clear pull of the network toward LTSS is a move in the targeting direction; a development that elicits varied reactions from different participants.

However, finding larger and meaningful roles for the legislation and the network with their inclusive and middle-class associations—and now potentially augmented by private sector involvement—may provide a new legitimacy to those who receive and who provide long-term-care services. In the words of Browdie and Castora (2008), "A national network is crucial in giving Americans the confidence in 'the system' to provide access to affordable and attractive long-term care options even if their family is not at hand to be their advocate." The absence of any meaningful delivery system associated with Medicaid has long been a drawback to its workings, and the network has the potential to redress that long-standing shortcoming. The CLASS Act, had it survived, might have played this role, but with its passing, a robust aging and disability network may be able to bring new acceptance to the world of chronic illness and disability

References

Benjamin, A. E. 1993. "An Historical Perspective on Home Care Policy." *Milbank Quarterly* 71: 129–66.

Browdie, R., and Castora, M. 2008. "The Aging Network: State of the States." *Public Policy & Aging Report* 18(3): 26–9.

Callahan, J. J. 1981. "Delivery of Services to Persons with Long-term-care Needs." In Meltzer, J., Farrow, F., and Richman, H., eds., *Policy Options in Long-term Care.* Chicago, IL: University of Chicago Press.

Erkulwater, J. L. 2006. *Disability Rights and the American Social Safety Net.* Ithaca, NY: Cornell University Press.

Galewitz, P. 2011. *States Pushing Managed Long-term Care for Elderly and Disabled Medicaid Patients.* New York: Kaiser Health Network. http://goo.gl/yVEYoK. Retrieved May 10, 2014.

Grob, G. N. 1986. "Explaining Old Age History: The Need for Empiricism." In Van Tassel, D., and Stearns, P. N., eds., *Old Age in a Bureaucratic Society.* Westport, CT: Greenwood Press.

Hudson, R. B. 1994. "The Older Americans Act and the Defederalization of Community-based Care." In Kim, P., ed., *Services to the Aged and Aging.* New York: Garland.

Kunkel, S. R., and Lackmeyer, A. 2008. "Evolution of the Aging Network: Modernization and Long-term Care Initiatives." *Public Policy & Aging Report* 18(3): 19–25.

Kunkel, S. R., Reece H., and Straker, J. 2014. *The National Aging Network Survey.* Oxford, OH: Scripps Gerontology Center, Miami University.

Marmor, T. R. 1970. *The Politics of Medicare* (2nd ed.). Chicago, IL: Aldine.

Minkler, M. 1989. "Gold in Gray: Reflections on the Business Discovery of the Elderly Market." *The Gerontologist* 29: 24–31.

Nightingale, D. S., and Pindus, N. M. 1997. *Privatization of Social Services.* Washington, DC: The Urban Institute.

O'Shaughnessy, C. V. 2008. "The Aging Services Network: Broad Mandate and Increasing Responsibilities." *Public Policy & Aging Report* 18(3): 1–18.

Rothman, D. 1971. *The Discovery of the Asylum.* Boston, MA: Little, Brown and Company.

Simon-Rusinowitz, L., et al. 2010a. "The Benefits of Consumer-directed Services for Elders and Their Caregivers in the Cash and Counseling Demonstration and Evaluation." *Public Policy & Aging Report* 20(1): 27–31.

Simon-Rusinowitz, L., et al. 2010b. "What Does Research Tell Us About a Policy Option to Hire Relatives as Caregivers?" *Public Policy & Aging Report* 20(1): 32–7.

Stone, D.A. 1984. *The Disabled State.* Philadelphia, PA: Temple University Press.

Vladeck, B. 1980. *Unloving Care: The Nursing Home Tragedy.* New York: Basic Books.

Critical Thinking

1. With a growing aging population, how will long-term services and supports evolve?
2. Discuss the attitudes of agencies to "welfare" and "public assistance" and how it affects older adults.

Internet References

Administration on Aging
http://www.aoa.gov/AoAprograms/OAA
American Society on Aging
https://www.asaging.org
Medicaid.gov
https://www.medicaid.gov

ROBERT B. HUDSON is a professor of social policy at Boston University, Boston, Massachusetts. He also serves as the editor of Public Policy and Aging Report, the quarterly publication of the Gerontological Society of America's National Academy on an Aging Society.

2018 Medicare Costs

Centers for Medicare & Medicaid Services

Learning Outcomes

After reading this article, you will be able to:

- Identify the basic premium payments for the variety of Medicare health insurance options.
- Discuss eligibility for the each of the Medicare health insurance options.

Medicare Part A (Hospital Insurance) Costs
Part A Monthly Premium

Most people don't pay a Part A premium because they paid Medicare taxes while working. If you don't get premium-free Part A, you pay up to $422 each month.

Hospital Stay

In 2018, you pay

- $1,340 deductible per benefit period
- $0 for the first 60 days of each benefit period
- $335 per day for days 61–90 of each benefit period
- $670 per "lifetime reserve day" after day 90 of each benefit period (up to a maximum of 60 days over your lifetime)

Skilled Nursing Facility Stay

In 2018, you pay

- $0 for the first 20 days of each benefit period
- $167.50 per day for days 21–100 of each benefit period
- All costs for each day after day 100 of the benefit period

Medicare Part B (Medical Insurance) Costs
Part B Monthly Premium

The standard Part B premium amount in 2018 is $134 or higher depending on your income. However, most people who get Social Security benefits pay less than this amount ($130 on average). Social Security will tell you the exact amount you'll pay for Part B in 2018.

You pay the standard premium amount (or higher) if:

- You enroll in Part B for the first time in 2018.
- You don't get Social Security benefits.
- You're directly billed for your Part B premiums.
- You have Medicare and Medicaid, and Medicaid pays your premiums. (Your state will pay the standard premium amount of $134 in 2018.)
- Your modified adjusted gross income as reported on your IRS tax return from 2 years ago is above a certain amount.

If you're in 1 of these 5 groups, here's what you'll pay:

If your yearly income in 2016 was			You pay (in 2018)
File individual tax return	File joint tax return	File married & separate tax return	
$85,000 or less	$170,000 or less	$85,000 or less	$134
above $85,000 up to $107,000	above $170,000 up to $214,000	not applicable	$187.50
above $107,000 up to $133,500	above $214,000 up to $267,000	not applicable	$267.90

| above $133,500 up to $160,000 | above $267,000 up to $320,000 | not applicable | $348.30 |
| above $160,000 | above $320,000 | above $85,000 | $428.60 |

If you have questions about your Part B premium, call Social Security at 18007721213. TTY users can call 1-800-325-0778. If you pay a late enrollment penalty, these amounts may be higher.

Part B Deductible—$183 per year

Medicare Advantage Plans (Part C) and Medicare Prescription Drug Plans (Part D) Premiums

Visit Medicare.gov/find-a-plan to get plan premiums. You can also call 1800MEDICARE (1-800-633-4227). TTY users can call 18774862048. You can also call the plan or your State Health Insurance Assistance Program (SHIP). To get the most up-to-date SHIP phone numbers, visit shiptacenter.org or call 1-800-MEDICARE.

Part D Monthly Premium

The chart below shows your estimated prescription drug plan monthly premium based on your income. If your income is above a certain limit, you will pay an income-related monthly adjustment amount in addition to your plan premium.

If your yearly income in 2016 was			You pay (in 2018)
File individual tax return	**File joint tax return**	**File married & separate tax return**	
$85,000 or less	$170,000 or less	$85,000 or less	Your plan premium
above $85,000 up to $107,000	above $170,000 up to $214,000	not applicable	$13.00 + your plan premium
above $107,000 up to $133,500	above $214,000 up to $267,000	not applicable	$33.60 + your plan premium
above $133,500 up to $160,000	above $267,000 up to $320,000	not applicable	$54.20 + your plan premium
above $160,000	above $320,000	above $85,000	$74.80 + your plan premium

2018 Part D National Base Beneficiary Premium — $35.02

This figure is used to estimate the Part D late enrollment penalty and the income-related monthly adjustment amounts listed in the table above. The national base beneficiary premium amount can change each year. See your Medicare & You handbook or visit Medicare.gov for more information.

For more information about Medicare costs, visit Medicare.gov.

Critical Thinking

1. Can you identify benefits that should be covered under one of these Medicare "parts" that is not currently covered?

2. Discuss the community programs that provide discounted benefits for prevention services and pharmaceuticals.

Internet References

AARP
https://www.aarp.org

Administration on Aging
http://www.aoa.gov/AoAprograms/OAA

Centers for Medicare & Medicaid Services
https://www.cms.gov

Centers for Medicare & Medicaid Services. "2018 Medicare Costs", *Centers for Medicare & Medicaid Services*, 2017.